The Clinical Management of Nicotine Dependence

James A. Cocores
Editor

The Clinical Management of Nicotine Dependence

With 12 Illustrations

Springer-Verlag
New York Berlin Heidelberg London
Paris Tokyo Hong Kong Barcelona

James A. Cocores, M.D.
Medical Director
The Outpatient Recovery Centers
Fair Oaks Hospital
Summit, NJ 07901
USA

Library of Congress Cataloging-in-Publication Data
The clinical management of nicotine dependence / James A. Cocores,
    editor.
        p.   cm.
    Includes bibliographical references and index.
    ISBN 0-387-97464-4 (alk. paper). — ISBN 3-540-97464-4 (alk. paper)
    1. Tobacco habit—Treatment.   2. Nicotine—Physiological effect.
    [DNLM: 1. Nicotine—adverse effects.   2. Tobacco Use Disorder—
therapy.   WM 176 C641]
    RC567.C58   1991
    616.86'506—dc20
    DNLM/DLC
    for Library of Congress   91-4596

Printed on acid-free paper.

Typeset by Best-set Typesetter Ltd., Chai Wan, Hong Kong.
Printed and bound by Edwards Brothers, Ann Arbor, Michigan.
Printed in the United States of America.

9 8 7 6 5 4 3 2 1

ISBN 0-387-97464-4 Springer-Verlag New York Berlin Heidelberg
ISBN 3-540-97464-4 Springer-Verlag Berlin Heidelberg New York

This textbook is dedicated to the memory of the billions of people who have fallen victim to nicotine dependence. Especially to:

My grandfather James Genakos
"Old man look at my life. I'm a lot like you were."[1]

My dear friend and teacher Karen Daino
"May your song always be sung . . .
May you stay forever young."[2]

My dear friend and teacher Kothanda Gurunathan
"He likes his fags the best."[3]

---

[1] From "Old Man." Words and Music by Neil Young. © 1971 Broken Fiddle. Used by Permission. All rights reserved.

[2] From "Forever Young." Author: Bob Dylan, copyright © 1974 by Ram's Horn Music. All rights reserved. International copyright secured. Reprinted by permission.

[3] From "A Well Respected Man" performed by Ray Davies. Used by permission. Golden Rule Administrators. Copyright 1965, Jaboy Music. All rights reserved.

Preface

The 1980s have seen a remarkable degree of public and professional acceptance of cigarette smoking as the most widespread and devastating form of drug dependence. More medical schools now give required courses about drug dependence. Prestigious journals publish reports of investigations on the subject of nicotine dependence, and more conferences and workshops are held each year on various aspects of nicotine dependence. All this is in sharp contrast to the earlier prevailing atmosphere of disinterest, ignorance, or professional disdain.

These changes created an obvious place for a textbook oriented primarily toward the needs of clinicians working with patients who have nicotine dependence. Thus, in preparation of this book, most aspects of the management of nicotine dependence are incorporated, in order to address concerns of physicians in training and other health care professionals across the world. The final product, which I believe to be comprehensive and clinically relevant throughout, is a text that I hope will be of equal use to psychologists, social workers, nurses, counselors, and physicians in all specialties. An encyclopedic treatise was deliberately avoided because that approach can be cumbersome in size, readability, and cost, and for that reason, readers will find little mention of data involving animal research, nicotine-related politics, nicotine product advertising, medical consequences of smoking, psychotherapeutic techniques, and the extent of the problem. On the other hand, the well-referenced and well-balanced chapters of this text provide the reader with an opportunity to acquire a familiarity with the most common methods used to manage nicotine dependence. I hope that clinicians and educators will integrate the material presented here into their own practices.

The Clinical Management of Nicotine Dependence was not written for physicians alone. Many kinds of health care professionals have asked for information to assist them in working with patients with a wide variety of medical or psychiatric problems. The detailed discussion of a wide range of practical clinical topics are presented in a fashion that I hope will foster better cooperation and interaction among all members of the health care team.

I was taught that "if you know syphilis, you know medicine." This pageant approach has been effective in reducing syphilis to its current low level. I recommend that syphilis turn its crown over to nicotine dependence.

James A. Cocores, M.D.

Contents

Contributors

Richard A. Brown, Ph.D., Clinical Assistant Professor of Psychiatry and Human Behavior, Brown University Program in Medicine, and Project Director, Division of Behavioral Medicine, The Miriam Hospital, Providence, RI 02906

Edward B. Bunker, National Institute on Drug Abuse, Addiction Research Center, Baltimore, MD 21224

Robert P. Climko, M.D., Clinical Assistant Professor, University of Medicine and Dentistry, Robert Wood Johnson Medical School, and Clinical Director, Princeton Psychiatric Recovery Network, Princeton, NJ 08540

John P. Docherty, M.D., Medical Director, Brookside Hospital, Nashua, NH 03063

Karen M. Emmons, Ph.D., Coordinator, Behavioral-Pulmonary Research Program, Division of Behavioral Medicine, Miriam Hospital, Providence, RI 02906

Michael Fey, Ph.D., New Life Health Products Corporation, Morris Plains, NJ 07950

Patricia R. Flynn, Manager, Quality Assurance, Johnson & Johnson, Health Management Inc., New Brunswick, NJ 08901

Harold P. Freeman, M.D., Director, Department of Surgery, Harlem Hospital Center, New York, NY 10037

Christine S. Glidden, M.A., C.D.C., Manager, Employee Assistance Program, Ethicon Incorporated, Somerville, NJ 08876-0151

Mark S. Gold, M.D., Director of Research, Fair Oaks Hospital, Delray Beach Florida and Summit, NJ 07901

R. Jeffrey Goldsmith, M.D., Medical Director, Alcoholism Clinic, Division of Central Psychiatric Clinic, Department of Psychiatry, College of Medicine, Cincinnati, OH 45267-0539

Michael G. Goldstein, M.D., Assistant Psychiatrist-in-Chief, The Miriam Hospital, and Assistant Professor of Psychiatry and Human Behavior, Brown University Program in Medicine, Providence, RI 02906

Jack E. Henningfield, Ph.D., National Institute on Drug Abuse, Addiction Research Center, Baltimore, MD 21224

Mark Hollander, Ph.D., Department of Psychiatry, University of Medicine and Dentistry of New Jersey, New Jersey Medical School, Newark, NJ 07103

Norman Hymowitz, Ph.D., Department of Psychiatry, University of Medicine and Dentistry of New Jersey, New Jersey Medical School, Newark, NJ 07103

Geoffrey P. Kane, M.D., M.P.H., Medical Director, Adult Chemical Dependency Services, Brookside Hospital, Nashua, NH 03063

Aryeh L. Klahr, M.D., Medical Director, Adult Substance Abuse Treatment Unit, Fair Oaks Hospital, Summit, NJ 07901

Stuart Kutchins, O.M.D., San Anselmo, CA 94960

George Lutz, M.D., Medical Director, Employee Health, Ethicon, Incorporated, Somerville, NJ 08876-0151

Norman S. Miller, M.D., Cornell University Medical College, The New York Hospital-Cornell Medical Center, White Plains, NY 10605

Raymond Niaura, Ph.D., Director of Research, Division of Behavioral Medicine, The Miriam Hospital, and Assistant Professor of Psychiatry and Human Behavior, Brown University Program in Medicine, Providence, RI 02906

Peggy O'Hara, Ph.D., Associate Professor, Department Epidemiology & Public Health, University of Miami School of Medicine, Miami, FL 33101

Mario A. Orlandi, Ph.D., M.P.H., Chief, Division of Health Promotion Research, American Health Foundation, New York, NY 10017

Wallace B. Pickworth, Ph.D., National Institute on Drug Abuse, Addiction Research Center, Baltimore, MD 21224

A. Carter Pottash, M.D., Executive Medical Director, Fair Oaks Hospital, Delray Beach, Florida and Summit, NJ 07901

Jed E. Rose, Ph.D., Associate Medical Research Professor, Department of Psychiatry, Duke University, and Chief, Nicotine Research Lab, Veterans Administration Medical Center, Durham, NC 27705

John A. Rosecrans, Ph.D., Professor of Pharmacology and Toxicology, Medical College of Virginia, Virginia Commenwealth University, Richmond, VA 23298-0001

Terry A. Rustin, M.D., Assistant Professor, Department of Psychiatry and Behavioral Sciences, University of Texas Medical School at Houston, Houston, TX 77225

Karen Lea Sees, D.O., Clinical Instructor, Department of Psychiatry, University of California, San Francisco, California, and Assistant Chief, Substance Abuse Treatment Clinic, Veterans Affairs Medical Center, San Francisco, CA 94121

Andrew Edmund Slaby, M.D., Ph.D., M.P.H., Medical Director, Fair Oaks Hospital, Summit, NJ 07901

James W. Smith, M.D., Chief Medical Officer, Schick Shadel Hospital, Seattle, WA 98146

Wanda Taylor, M.D., Medical Director, Partial Hospitalization Program, Fair Oaks Hospital, Summit, NJ 07901

Louis Jolyon West, M.D., Professor of Psychiatry, School of Medicine, University of California, Los Angeles, CA 90024

Part I Etiology

1
Acayatl's Curse

ANDREW EDMUND SLABY

Santayana admonished that those who do not know history are doomed to repeat it. Unfortunately, knowledge alone does not mitigate change. Psychological, social, political, and economic forces converge to direct even some of the most psychologically sophisticated of us to pursue a self-destructive course.

The spread of tobacco use from Central America to Europe and Asia is a natural experiment that provides a number of insights into comparable trends in use of opiates and cocaine.[1] Patterns of use and health effects of these drugs are well documented. The challenge is not the need for more data but the need for programs that reduce the cost in terms of human life and health resources that produce effective impact on the reality of human experience.

Pre-Columbian Tobacco Use

Recreational use of tobacco is fabled to have originated with the evil and powerful sorcerer Acayatl, who is said to have convinced Native Americans to chew, to roll and smoke, and to dry and sniff tobacco leaves 5000 years before Christ.[2] Some Central American Indians actually are said to have abandoned nomadic lifestyles to allow time in one place to grow a crop of tobacco sufficient to satisfy their addiction.[2] Tobacco seeds have been found dating to 3500 B.C. in permanent settlements in both Mexico and Peru, where it is posited that tobacco may have been used to assuage hunger pangs from lack of food.[3]

Smoking in pre-Christian Europe was limited to inhalation of burning hemp. The eminent Greek historian Herodotus wrote in 450 B.C. of the practice occurring among the Scythians living in what is today Bulgaria.[4] Five hundred years later, Pliny the Elder recommended inhalation of smoke through a reed for medicinal purposes.[4]

Use of narcotic smoke for religious purposes is noted on stone records of the Mayan civilization, dating to A.D. 600–900.[3] Lack of reeds in Mexico dictated the use of bone, clay, and wood pipes to smoke, as well as the rolling of leaves to produce a crude cigar referred to as "Acayatl," after the ancient priest.[2,4]

Columbus's Discovery

Smoking did not begin in Europe until Christopher Columbus returned from his first voyage to the New World. Columbus recorded in his diary the reception of gifts of fruit, wooden spears, and aromatic dried leaves upon landing in San Salvador. The new arrivals ate the fruit, kept the spears, and jettisoned the leaves into the ocean.[5,6] In the years that followed, smoking was encountered wherever Spaniards went. Friar Ramon Pane, a Franciscan with Columbus, reported in 1493 that the Carib Indians, a cannabalistic tribe living in the Lesser Antilles, used snuff. Tobacco was hailed as the "Indian Weed."[7]

Other early explorers[3] recorded that tobacco was smoked in pipes as a symbol of goodwill ("peace pipes") and for ceremonial purposes.[8] Brazilian Indians were observed using pestles in rosewood cups to grind up tobacco and give it an aroma and to place it in decorated bone cups to use.[8,9,10]

Tobacco and ways to use it were reported with each return of explorers. Samuel de Champlain, founder of Quebec, noted the use of plug tobacco in Santa Domingo. South American natives were observed wrapping rolls of tobacco in palm leaves and smoking it to induce a stuporous state in religious ceremonies.[11] North American Indians (e.g., the Cherokees) were reported to use wild tobacco (*Nicotina rustica*) to bond warriors on the warpath, to guarantee solemn oaths, to suppress hunger, to seek omens, to facilitate councils of war and peace, to ratify peace treaties, to confirm sales and other engagements, to convene ceremonies and rituals, and to drive away witches.[12] Smoking was used in nearly every important aspect of Cherokee life. Sir Francis Drake described in 1579 that people in what is today the San Francisco Bay came daily with feathers and small bags filled with tobacco.[5] The Spaniards themselves were growing tobacco in the West Indies in 1531. In 1575, the Portugese also began to do so.[7,10]

The word *tobacco* itself derives from the San Serif Cap "Y"-shaped *tobaga* pipes from which the Central American Indians sniffed tobacco's incense.[7] These pipes were composed of baked clay, wood, or soft colored rocks with a fork to be inserted into each nostril to smoke.[8]

Tobacco "Arrives"

When tobacco first arrived in Europe, it was sought after more for its medicinal use than as a recreational diversion. Philip II of Spain's private physician Francisco de Toledo grew the plant for its aesthetic values at the same time (viz. 1559), Jean Nicot, the French ambassador to Portugese King Sebastian, used poultices derived from the leaves to heal both a venous ulcer on a servant and a laceration to his cook's hand.[4] Nicot sent some seeds to Catherine de Medici, Queen of France, who was so enthusiastic over receipt of the gift that she christened it "Nicotiana" in her benefactor's honor.[4] The name was subsequently Latinized to *Nicotania tabacum.*[13]

Sale of tobacco early in the 16th century was limited to apothecary shops for medicinal purposes, save for purchases by sailors who adopted the Native American habit.[14] The fact that native Americans regarded tobacco as a medicinal agent probably contributed to its sale by apothecaries in England.[15] In Haiti, medicine men used snuff as both analgesia and a means to clear nasal passages. Mexicans were reported in 1519 by Ocaranza to use tobacco to heal burns and wounds and by Nernera in 1525 to induce sleep.[3,10] Sir Francis Drake's plundering of Dominica in 1586 resulted in the delivery to England of a sufficient store of tobacco seeds to ensure that nearly every English gardener grew it in the 17th century.[15] In 1629, William Barclay advertised it as a panacea.[15,16]

On the European continent, there was a similar flurry of interest. Jean Nicot's successful treatment of Catherine de Medici's stomach ailment led to use by many other prominent physicians.[11] Damin de Goes, a Portugese man of letters, used seeds from Brazil to grow tobacco in Lisbon in the 1540s and used its juice as an antiseptic for sores, fistulas, and abscesses.[17] Nicot himself used this same derivative to treat *noli me tangere*, a basal cell cancer.[17] In 1556, Nicoles Monardes, the Spanish physician, penned a lengthy treatise[15,16] on the results of tobacco treatment of over 16 disorders.

Recreational smoking did not at first ignite enthusiasm. In fact, in some instances, it did the exact opposite. The first man to smoke in Europe is said to have been Roderigo de Jerez, who so frightened people by smoke coming from his nose and mouth that the Inquisition imprisoned him for demonic possession.[7] Smoking in England was given considerable impetus when, in 1586, Thomas Harot, a mathematician who spent some time in Virginia, schooled his close friend, Sir Walter Raleigh, in the art of smoking.[4,18,19,20] By legend, when Raleigh lit up, his servant poured a pitcher of water on the ignited tobacco, falsely assuming his master was aflame![7] Raleigh persuaded Good Queen Bess to try a silver pipe full herself. Wealthy Elizabethan gallants soon toted elaborated smoking paraphernalia—pipe tools and boxes and carved pipes—and courses were taught at taverns in the art of smoking.[14] Yard-long "churchwarden" pipes allowed pious clergy to smoke with a modicum of dignity. The poor used walnut shells perforated by straws.[14] Soon the first and finest of English society developed more elaborate smoking rituals than the Indians of San Francisco Bay reported by Drake in the American West.

Although the Indians had smoked reeds filled with tobacco and had made crude cigarettes from corn wrappers, it was the Spanish who developed cigars and cigarettes.[8] Their *papeletes*—paper-wrapped cigarettes—

spread to Portugal, Russia, Turkey, and Asia.[7] At first, London men seen smoking cigarettes were ridiculed, but because it was such an easy way to smoke, it flourished. The powdered form of tobacco was christened "snuff" by the Dutch, who used it widely by 1560.[3,10] In 1620, the Royal Snuff Factory was founded in Seville which became a center for manufacturing the product.[3,10] Snuff was prepared by rubbing tobacco to become a powder, at first through a grater or later through a mill with revolving stones, by human power or horsepower. It was kept in animal bladders and dried and tanned like parchment.[7] In the 1650s, snuff arrived in Japan, and during the Ching Dynasty in China. Artisans created carved and painted snuff boxes that were garnished with silver spoons. Etiquette dictated snuff to be placed on the left thumb nail and inhaled through the nose. The Chinese believed snuff to alleviate throat ailments, constipation, cold symptoms, and pains in the eyes and teeth.[3,7,10]

Tobacco use spread rapidly around the world in the early 16th century despite prohibitions in most of continental Europe,[17] arriving in Turkey in 1605, Russia in 1634, and Arabia in 1663. The Spaniards brought it to the Philippines, from whence it was introduced in to China.[3,10]

Origins of the Antitobacco Movement

As with most things of great profit or great pleasure, tobacco had both strong supporters and detractors. James I of England published a condemnation of smoking on both health and social grounds. In his *Counterblast to Tobacco*, he cited reasons to discourage use: damage to the lungs, nose, and brain.[21] Ironically, like later damnation of marijuana (e.g., "Reefer Madness"), the vitriol only stimulated greater interest . . . and use.[4]

Pope urban VIII forbade use of snuff, threatening excommunication in a papal ban issued in 1642.[5,6] Innocent XII and XIII extended the ban to smoking.[4] Smoking was reasoned to be slow suicide by the Jesuit Jakub Balde and in Lima in 1588, smoking was banned with threat of eternal damnation.[4] With the passing of Innocent XIII 34 years after issuing his edict, Pietro Francesco Orsini assumed the Papal tiara under the appellation of Benedict XIII and repealed the interdiction, enjoying with others the delight of snuff taking.[22] John Wesley, founder of Methodism, forbade smoking in Ireland. Subsequently, smoking was forbidden by the Mormons, Seventh Day Adventists, Sikhs of India, and Buddist Monks in Korea.

Russia's first czar, Michael Romanoff, ordered public flogging with a *Knout* (a whip composed of knotted untanned elk hide), confiscating of property, and exile to Siberia. Snuff users had their noses slit or ripped off.[4] Smokers suffered fines or imprisonment in Germany from 1642 to 1848, when Prince Leopole III of Anhalt Dessau lifted the ban, with a concession to nonsmokers: A pipe could legally be knocked from the mouth of those who use one in public.[4] Smoking was decreed to be against the teaching of the Koran in 1603 by Sultan Ahmed I, punishable by thrusting the pipe stem through the nose of the user and parading the guilty through town.[4] Ahmed's son, Muhrad the Cruel, went further. Disguised, he would visit coffee houses, note those smoking, have them murdered, and have their bodies placed in front of the coffee house as a warning for all to see.[4] Soldiers caught smoking were beheaded, quartered, hanged, maimed, and left for the enemy.[4]

In the East, where perhaps condemnation and penalties were the greatest, use spread from men, who early dominated use until World War I, to all both genders and ages. Chinese girls of 8 and 9 ultimately wore appendages on their dresses to hold tobacco.[5,6] While Japan penalized use in 1616 with imprisonment and confiscation of property, tobacco cultivation flourished in the 17th century, extending into the Polynesian Islands, Ceylon, and Transylvania, to which it was brought by traveling gypsies.[22]

In the United States, smoking for pleasure was seen as moral weakness, much like glutton, by the Puritans.[9] Controls were comparable on liquor and smoking in the early 17th century. Laws and taxation were imposed to help keep the lower classes from destroying themselves.

Interestingly, perhaps due to the strong positive impact of tobacco sales on the English economy, in 1725, the Royal College of Physicians presented to the House of Commons the disastrous consequences of cheap gin, but it did *not* act on the question of smoking and atmosphere pollution and their relation to cancer of the lungs until 1909.

Although Elizabeth I became nauseous after her first puff, she was aware of revenue possibilities and merely imposed a heavy tax. By the time the Virgin Queen was laid to rest in 1603, tobacco had become the national habit.[14]

The Wages and Profits of Sin

The marriage of Virginian John Rolfe of Jamestown to the ravishingly beautiful American Indian princess Pocahontas created an alliance from which the tobacco industry began to flourish. Rolfe had mysteriously acquired the seeds of *Nicotiana tobacum* from a Spanish plantation, which gave rise to plants with a milder flavor than *Nicotiana rusticum*,[7,11] and in 1612, he persuaded American Indians in Jamestown to teach the colonists how to grow tobacco to allow it to be a commodity for trading with the rest of the world. This provided the economic base for England's southern colonies and remained a major cash crop for the American republic,[23] as shown subsequently in the Old Senate Rotunda in our Capitol building, where tobacco leaves and flowers adorned the supporting pillars constructed in 1818.[23]

James I of England, not being a tobacco devotee himself, increased tobacco tax 10-fold, limited Virginian tobacco production to 100 pounds per year, and disallowed its growth in England.[14,17] These measures, like

alcohol prohibition in the United States 4 centuries later, only led to proliferation of illicit traffickers. After increasing tariff 4000%[11] without impact on use, James acknowledged his efforts as futile and allowed London
and Bristol importers privileges if licensed. Out of deference to the Crown,
English gentlemen postponed smoking until after dinner.[14] James's differences with Sir Walter Raleigh on use of tobacco and other issues eventually led to Sir Walter's beheading.[11]

Tobacco was so highly valued in the Jacobean era that eager bachelors
in Virginia in 1619 offered for marital privilege 20 pounds of tobacco for
each of 90 English women. The following year, 60 more educated women
arrived for 150 pounds per helpmate.[7] Smoking thrived in the colonies.
Virginians, Puritans, and Quakers alike lit up. Racks in taverns held the
churchwardens.[7] Short clay pipes were referred to as "nose-warmers." In
1680, Lord Culpepper, Governor of Virginia, convened a group of royal-
ists who concurred with a perpetual export duty of two shillings per hogs-
head of tobacco directly accountable to the king.[22]

An immediate economic benefit of tobacco production for England was
the need for a large merchant marine to transport tobacco to Europe.
Need for naval protection of the fleet helped establish Britain's maritime
supremacy.[20] Profits of the tobacco monopolies afforded the extravagant
lifestyles of England's upper class, and excise duties contributed to the
royalty's largesse and financed England's military ventures abroad. Ironically, profits from tobacco sales were also to be a major source of funds for
the American Revolution.[23]

High taxation failed to reduce smoking because tax did not apply to
colonial imports (Virginia and Bermuda were exempt from import taxes),
and cheaper English homegrown varieties of tobacco were available.
Collection of tobacco taxes was contracted out to business syndicates over
which the Crown had little control. Actually, antitobacco policy probably
failed because it conflicted with the rising interest of the merchant class.
The course of the development of the colonies and slavery would have
been different if it were not for this fact. Tobacco merchants would not
have had the wealth and power to manipulate governments. It was the
tobacco merchants who obstructed the antislavery movement in England
and prevented the colony of Virginia from levying a tax on slavery. It is of
historical interest to note that 100 years prior to the American Revolution,
Nathaniel Bacon was charged with treason for bloodshed that was successfully suppressed by the mother country during an attempt by the colonists
to dispose of their staple as they deemed fit.[22]

Ambivalence toward the weed continued to wage throughout the world
as it has to this very day. Robert Burton, in his famous *Anatomy of Melan-
cholia* (1621), extolled tobacco as "a sovereign remedy to all diseases."[18]
As use spread, the form of use changed related to social class. Courtiers of
Charles II introduced snuff use, although the common man preferred pipe
smoking.[20]

In the 17th century, tobacco replaced the use of coins as taxes were paid and fines levied on it.[22] The amount produced by Virginia, the chief colonial source of tobacco, rose from 60,000 pounds in 1662 to 120,000 pounds exported in 1689. Two centuries later, ending in 1850, exports of tobacco from the United States reached 10 million dollars and was seen as a factor enhancing the support of slavery.[5,6]

On the European continent, as early as 1689, the medical school of Paris espoused the official view that smoking shortened life and was associated with women's moustaches, nervous paralysis, impaired vision, and deterioration of intellectual capacity.[14,24]

Supporters, on the other hand, included physicians and nobles alike. In a mid-17th century volume, *Panacea on the Universal Medicine: Being a Discovery of the Wonderful Virtues of Tobacco Taken in a Pipe, with Its Operation and Use Both in Physick and Chyurgery*, a London physician extolled the value of smoking for headache, toothache, redness of face, cough, and stomach pains.[8] Marie Antoinette, the Duke of Wellington, Lord Nelson, Disraeli, Alexander Pope, and Samuel Johnson all used snuff.[22,25] Johnson, in fact, in the 18th century wrote a defense of smoking. Snuff reached the peak of use in the reign of Queen Anne (1702–1714). Its popularity continued during the reign of George II and Queen Charlotte (1760–1820). Charlotte was referred to as "snuffy Charlotte" because she had a room for it at Windsor Castle.[3,10]

In 1760, an 18-year-old French Huguenot immigrant, Pierre Lorillard, set up a snuff mill in New York on the High Road to Boston, using tobacco from the Old Dominion (Virginia). Some of the carefully guarded ingredients and blends may have come from George Washington's own plantation.[7] Corn husks were one of the original wrappers used to encase tobacco to smoke. In 1787, Peter and George Lorillard launched the earliest known tobacco advertising campaigns. Washington exhorted those who could not afford to send money to support the revolution to send tobacco instead. At the same time, Father of American psychiatry and signatory of the Declaration of Independence Benjamin Rush condemned its use in his *Essays* penned in 1798.[3] Dolly Madison, on the other hand, tendered snuff to White House guests,[7] and a poet of the time described snuff as the final cause for the human nose.

The Cigarette

Although 19th-century English women who smoked used clay pipes much like men's,[15] smoking pipes in America went out of fashion in the 1800s, except in rural areas, although the wives of both Andrew Jackson and Zachary Taylor smoked pipes while in the White House.[14]

The French considered snuff more socially acceptable. In the immediate antebellum United States, tobacco was primarily used as snuff, as chew, as cigars, or for pipes. By the 19th century, three major forms of snuff reigned: Scotch Snuff (a very strong unflavored finely ground version), Maccaboy (moist, highly scented snuff), and Rapee (a coarsely grated snuff).[3,10] Throughout the 1800s until the mid-1930s, there was a communal snuff box in Congress.[3,10]

During the late 19th century, the mode of recreational use of tobacco changed from pipe smoking and snuff to cigar and chewing tobacco, much to many people's alarm, although between 1880 and 1930 snuff production increased from 4 million pounds to 40 million pounds.

Plug and chewing tobacco had colorful names in the 19th century, such as Horse Shoe, Climax, Harvest Long Cut, Board of Trade and Daniel Webster.[26] The advent of the cigarette allowed a cleaner and less offensive way to use tobacco and one that was more convenient[21] and compatible to the evolving standards of hygiene of the time. Spittoons, cigars, and pipes were messy in an environment that valued cleanliness next to godliness. Dickens, during his sojourn in America, complained of Americans who chewed and spat.[3,10]

Cigarettes, first used in Spain, were considered the poor man's smoke. After a battle with the Turks in 1832, the Egyptians, on discovering that cannon fire had destroyed their pipes, found that one could enjoy tobacco rolled in paper. Two decades later, in 1854–1856, when the clay pipes of the British were destroyed in the Crimean War, the Turkish and French allies showed them how to roll tobacco into a cigarette.[2,11] The Mexican War popularized smoking cigarros and cigarillos south of the Rio Grande.[5] Cigars were either imported from Cuba or manufactured here with Havana filters and became a symbol of prosperity.[7] Cigar smokers were not men alone. George Sand and Amy Lowell flaunted their preference. Most women, however, feared the residue on the drapes.[7] Queen Victoria demanded that when her guests smoked, they do so up the chimney. In 1846, smoking rail carriages were introduced. In the United States, the high price of cigarettes limited consumption until after the Civil War.

The Englishman John Walker was the first to develop a practical friction match in 1827. Johan Lundstrom developed the safety match in 1852 by including chlorate of potash over red amorphous phosphorus. Matches allowed smoking anywhere, contributing to the spread of cigarette smoking.[23]

Prior to the mid-19th century, tobacco was of a dark color, primarily used for chewing, pipe smoking, or cigars.[23] In the middle of the 19th century, light-colored Burley and flue-cured tobaccos were developed, contributing to the popularity of cigarette smoking.[23] Flue-cured tobacco was less alkaline than the traditional dark-leafed tobacco and accordingly easier to smoke. Of note is the fact that a slave named Bill in the Ahisha Slade Farm in North Carolina discovered by chance in 1839 that intense heat during the curing process created a golden leaf.[23] The Bull Durham brand emerged and grew in popularity following the Civil War. Burley tobacco was air cured but fermented to a blond color. The structure of

Burley allowed sugar flavoring, enhancing its appeal for chewing. Flue-cured and Burley were popularly used in American blend cigarettes.

War appears consistently to have been an impetus to smoking. In the Civil War, as in the Crimean and Mexican–American War, smoking of cigarettes flourished as Union soldiers discovered the pleasures of fine Southern tobacco.[13] The fame of Durham[11] tobacco spread after the Civil War, and orders for tobacco came in from across the U.S. After Washington Duke was released from a Union prison and forced to sell his land, he and his four sons flacked, bagged, and sold tobacco themselves, obtaining a hold on the growing tobacco industry. James Buchanan Duke,[11] a descendent to Washington Duke eventually commenced large-scale production of cigarettes.

Cigarette cards were developed in the post–Civil War era by the firm Alan and Ginter in Richmond, Virginia.[23] Technical advances in lithography in the 18th century allowed full-colored production of trade cards and billboard signs.[26] The advertising trade cards measuring 3 inches by 5 inches distributed by druggists, general stores, and mail or traveling sales representatives were of cloth or paper and quite expensive. Subjects ranged from a Yale pennant, a silk flag or a map of Portugal to pictures of famous actresses (such as Lillian Russell), queens, athletes, American Indian chiefs, flowers, beasts, birds, and fruit.[7] *Metamorphic trade cards*—folded, allowing evolution from a less developed to a more developed state—were especially popular, with minidrawings.[26] These were highly sought after to complete an album, enhancing sales . . . and smoking . . . from 1885 to 1899. In 1900, use of these cards fell off dramatically, then were gone by 1905.

Images of modern American Indians, carved by the same artists[7] who fashioned carousels and figure heads for ships, painted in vivid colors, offered Victorian consumers tobacco leaves or cigars as their natural forebears had once done to Columbus in San Salvador. Only those that had wheels to retire them at night survived, as those left to stand the night were often used for fuel, mowed down by handtrucks, stolen, abused by the intoxicated, or damaged by air rifles and sling shots.[7]

Earlier in the 19th century, at the 100th anniversary of the Lorillard Tobacco Company, Century tobacco included in their tobacco packages, on a chance occasion, a 100-dollar note, fifty 2-dollar notes, or other amounts in between. This approach was so successful that authorities accused the practice of being close to a lottery.[7] At that times, more than 100 different blends of tobacco, spice, and pepper were available in gay wrapping paper.[11] The expanding rail network of the late 19th century allowed widespread and relatively rapid distribution of tobacco products, further contributing to growth of its use.

Prior to 1884, cigarettes were an upper-class luxury due to their price. Russian immigrants and women, in particular, were hired as rollers, capable of producing 2500–3000 cigarettes per day.[23] The development of a machine by 20-year-old James Stepley Bonsack of Richmond in 1884, capable of producing 200 cigarettes per minute,[13] allowed production of 120,000 cigarettes per day. (Today's modern machines produce 8000– 10,000 per minute.[23]) The first automated cigarette manufacturing machine completed its first day of work on April 30, 1884. Cigarette prices declined with the automation, with a yield equal to that of 50 men or women rolling by hand.[18] Bunsock patented his machine. J.B. Duke negotiated and reduced the royalty for use of the machine and got William O'Brian, a young mechanical genius, to maintain the machine and troubleshoot. At first, more cigarettes by machine were produced by Duke and put into a sliding cardboard box than could be sold, but increased marketing led to 30,000,000 cigarettes being sold between March and December, 1883.[11] Duke argued that cigarettes were a poor man's luxury, selling 10 cigarettes for five cents in the 1880s. Pipe, chewing, and cigarette tobacco sales flourished, allowing the merger of five tobacco firms into the American Tobacco Company in 1890, using Powhatan, father of Pocahontas, as its symbol.[11] Antitrust legislation led to its demise 21 years later. Duke himself died in 1923, establishing the trust for Duke University.

Cigarette smoking grew in the Gay 90s, with wide use of the tobacco that yielded a slightly acid smoke, as opposed to the smoke of the alkaline irritating tobacco of the dried type. The development of Burley and flue-cured tobacco, the mechanization of cigarette production, the concentration of capital in a few companies, the development of the safety match, effective advertising, and efficient transportation all contributed to the spread of the popular use of cigarettes at the turn of the century.

Nineteenth-Century Antismoking Campaigns

As the tobacco industry organized during the 19th century, so too did those opposing its use. In the 1800s, as before and after, there were those who did not rejoice in the spread of tobacco use. In 1804,[27] the first major hygienic treatise by American physician Benjamin Waterhouse of Boston condemned use of tobacco because it was unnatural and caused muscular indolence, it impaired the senses, and it inclined users to consumptive afflictions. People throughout the 19th century[18] described smoking's relationship to mouth cancer, heart disease, insanity, hemorrhoids, laziness, and many other human afflictions or traits.[18] Until 1848,[20] smoking on the streets of Berlin was forbidden by a proclamation of the Chief of Police, who characterized it as indecent, dangerous, and contrary to an orderly and civilized life.

In 1836, in *The New England Almanac and Farmers' Friend*, Samuel Green wrote on the hazards of smoking,[28] querying whether "inhaling this powerful narcotic be good for man? . . . it inflames the mouth and requires a perpetual flow of saliva." Interestingly, Alfred Dunhill, the eminent English tobacconist, noted that with cigarette smoking, the rituals of smoking and savoring of aroma give way to a habit that "flunts the edge of pleasure,"[11] recognizing addiction.

The Anti-Tobacco Society was established in London in 1853, and in 1862, the Manchester and Salford Anti-Tobacco Society was formed. The largely lay faction constituting its membership cited physicians' condemnation of tobacco as detrimental to the health of the individual and society. While Anglicans and Roman Catholics left smoking to individual conscience, the Salvation Army did not allow bondsman and officers to smoke and issued a moralistic literature.

Reports came out in 1859 linking smoking with lip and mouth cancers.[14] A paper published in the *Confederate States Medical and Surgical Journal* in 1864 cautioned users that ill effects occur due to a "poison finding a ready exit from the body." The pathogenic consequences of the habit were said to include insanity, epilepsy, and apoplexy. It was deemed an unneeded luxury but compared to alcohol, it was seen as innocuous. It was seen as infinitely less harmful than sugar and no worse than tea. In certain cases, it was actually perceived as an antidote to gluttony and a remedy for evils that lie deeper than its own, and, as such a remedy, it was presumed that it would hold its own place until those evils were removed.[29]

Nineteenth-century ladies would not join men for a smoke. If they did, they were of questionable character. Lucy Page Gaston, founder of the Chicago Anti-Cigarette League, felt that smoking by women underminded family values and the moral fabric of society.[30] Young Americans were historically protected from smoking, with 26 states prohibiting sale to minors, although the law was inconsistently enforced.[31]

Smoking, Women's Liberation, and Growing Awareness of Smoking as a Health Risk Factor

The advent of the portable safety match, obviating the need to smoke around a fireplace or to use a candle, and the proliferation of the cigarette rolling machine[18] seemed to increase cigarette use around the country and, in fact, the world. Cigarette consumption increased from 54 cigarettes per person in 1900 to 4345 per person age 18 and older by 1963.[23] W. Duke and Sons commanded nearly 90% of the manufactured cigarette market in 1900,[18] but the antitrust decision of the Supreme Court in 1911 dissolved the American Tobacco Company, resulting in the competing firms of Reynolds, American, Liggett and Myers, Lorillard, and a number of small companies.[18]

Prosmoking leagues in the 20th century replaced the 19th-century groups that sought to ban all use. Smoking was seen as an individual freedom without evidence of dire health consequences. It was not until the 1950s, with growing speculation that cigarette use may be linked to illness, that the attitude of Americans began to change.[13]

The National Cigarette League, the Non-Smokers Protective League of America, and the Anti-Cigarette League, each comprising business-persons, educators, and reformists, at the turn of the century got heavy taxation on sales in 2 states and prohibition of sales in 15 states. They felt that smoking infringed on the rights of others, had negative health effects, and caused moral degeneracy.[13] In 1904, a policeman arrested a woman for smoking a cigarette on Fifth Avenue in New York City. Smoking by female school teachers was seen as a reason for dismissal. The Sullivan Ordinance of 1908 in New York made it unlawful for women to smoke in public. Not until 1919 did Lorillard use images of women in a series of advertisements for cigarettes. In World War I, as men were converted to smoking in the service, women began to smoke in public. Women working at men's jobs in the war effort began to adopt men's habits, ironically also adopting a risk factor for a disease previously rare among women—lung cancer.[30]

Many prominent physicians early in the century, including Sir William Oslor, first professor of medicine at Johns Hopkins, perceived the perils of alcohol to be greater than those of smoking.[32] Sigmund Freud, the father of psychoanalysis, related a neurotic need to smoke to that for oral grati-fication commencing with thumb sucking. Freud himself smoked 20 cigars a day. He died of mouth cancer in 1939 in London.[18]

Cigarette sales remarkably increased at the turn of the century through the use of premiums. At first, dealers were given clocks and lighter devices along with displays. Later, customers got coupons that could be exchanged for shoelaces, garters, silk stockings, lamps, and hand-cranked wrapping machines.

The germ theory of infection changed the course of tobacco chewing. Expectorating on the floor or into a brass cuspidor was seen as leading to disease.[3,10] The peak consumption of chewing tobacco was from 1910 to 1920. Subsequently, consumption declined until the 1960s when produc-tion increased and then plateaued.[3,10] Adolescents, interestingly, at this late time in history, began to take up the habit. The emphasis on cleanli-ness enhanced cigarette sales despite the fact that early cigarette manu-facturers did not think consumers would ever want machine-made cigars. By 1910, James B. Duke and his American Tobacco Company or Tobacco Trust thought that they would controlled 86% of the cigar business, 85% of the plug business, and 76% of the smoking tobacco business.

At the turn of the century,[27] people believed that cigarette smoking prevented yellow fever. Around the same time,[33] a New Hampshire Con-gressman and a distinguished Italian dental scientist claimed that cigarettes help to maintain good oral health. This is an echo[33] of the 16th-century American Indian belief that tobacco was good for a variety of dental uses.

Now, ironically, it is known as a risk factor for stomatitis, gingivitis, and epithelial malignancies.[33]

Despite the 1908 Children's Act making it an offense to sell cigarettes to juveniles under age 16 years, enabling police to seize cigarettes from boys and girls smoking in public, the tobacco industry was not seriously threatened. Most smokers dismissed the possible danger of death.

The Great War

After the tobacco trust was broken, the Reynolds Company experimented with blended tobacco, culminating in the development of Camels, which combined a Turkish tobacco for aroma and flavor, low-pH flue-cured tobacco, and seasoned Burley tobacco, producing mildness that allowed inhalation.[23] This American blend was a smashing success. Over a million Camels were sold in 1913. Two years later, it captured 12% of the cigarette market. In 1919, it held 38.7%.[23] Premiums were dropped and, until recent years, the major cigarette companies concentrated on promoting a single Camel-like blend. The American Tobacco Company had Lucky Strikes; Lorillard, Old Gold; and Liggett and Myers, Chesterfields.

New prosmoking associations emerged during this period, to counter antitobacco figures, such as Tidswell, a physicism who in 1912[14] associated smoking with stillbirths. The Allied Tobacco League of America, Smokers Against Tobacco Prohibitions, and The Tobacco Merchants Association emerged prominently at this time, arguing that there were no ill effects and that legislation against smoking infringed on personal liberty.[13]

The First World War, like previous wars and wars that were to follow, was associated with increased numbers of men and women smoking. For men, smoking was an indication of manliness, and to women, of liberation. The endorsement of General John Pershing of smoking with his successful plan to issue cigarettes as part of soldiers' daily ration further increased cigarette sales and promoted the image that smoking was American and masculine.[18] This practice continued until the 1970s.[18] Women during this same period obtained equal access to smoking, with sales pitches targeted at women's interest in greater freedom such as: "I'm a Lucky girl—Blow some my way."[34]

While the U.S. government contracted for the entire output of Bull Durham for 1918 for soldiers,[11] the Great War brought an end to chewing tobacco's prominence in the tobacco market. Cigarettes were king.

Cigarettes as Symbol

The strong moralistic attacks of the 19th century had only faint echoes as the 20th century moved toward maturity[35] A. A. Brill, the psychoanalyst who introduced Freud to the English-speaking American readership, stated that neurotics opposed smoking. Smoking became associated with being avant-garde, sophisticated, free thinking, and liberal.[35] Many role models of the (World War I) years smoked, including a number of physicians who took it as a normal part of the culture.[27] Women of prominence took up the habit,[30] including Amelia Earhart and fashion-conscious debutantes. Ads appeared in trendy fashion magazines.

Focal efforts[13,30] to increase smoking among women showed high yield. Taking up the habit provided social status, sophistication, and liberation . . . as well as weight reduction. An especially effective campaign of Lucky Strike[8] encouraged women to "reach" for a Lucky instead of a sweet. Sales of Lucky Strikes tripled in 1 year. No advertising campaign has ever been so successful.[8] In 1923, 5% of cigarettes were consumed by women. Six years later in 1929, 12%. Once seen as the prerogative of the privileged class or the diversion of women of ill repute, cigarettes became one more indicium of the double standard to be eroded.[30] The president of Bryn Mawr College shocked people by permitting smoking rooms when it was still grounds for dismissal at other schools in 1925.[30]

Antismoking laws[13] aimed at reduction of smoking and protection of the young from cigarette use gave way. Most antismoking laws were repealed by the end of World War I.[13] Economic individualism[36] played a role in increasing permissiveness in sexual behavior in the 1920s, as well as in the use of tobacco as statements of personal choice. Opium ("hop") came to be included among recreational, but not always legal, options for those who had a cultivated taste for smoking pleasures.[37]

In 1925, Camels, Chesterfields, and Luckies had over 80% of the market and maintained this competitive edge until the 1950s, when the health scare prompted changes in buying patterns. Currently, 75% of the U.S. cigarette sales and three of the four major types of cigarettes are accounted for by products that barely counted prior to the heightened awareness of long-term cigarette smoking on health: king-size straights, filtered, and mentholated filtered cigarettes.[21] Filtered cigarettes (with or without menthol) now represent one half of sales. The old standards—Camels, Chesterfields, Luckies, and the rest—account for only one fourth.

In the 1920s, what had been known as vague physiologic disease began to be recognized to have definite causes, such as vitamin deficiencies and biochemical deficits.[38] Pathological anatomy and the germ theory not only were contributing to the developmet of the therapeutic medicine but also were raising questions of preventive medicine. In 1922, John Harvey Kellogg wrote *Tobaccoism, or How Tobacco Kills*.[38] Well connected and a supporter of research, he was both a health reformer and a founder of Seventh Day Adventist health institutions.[38] Moses Barron, pathologist at the University of Minnesota, reported in 1921 an increase in lung cancer among smokers—until that time a rare disease.[18] Concurrently, experimental pathologists demonstrated that tobacco tars gave genesis to skin cancers.[27]

The Great or Not-So-Great Depression

In the 1930, cigarette smoking arrived.[38] Rudy Vallee composed "My Cigarette Lady" in 1931, and Eleanor Roosevelt smoked in public.[30] Heroines of the silver screen smoked in films. By 1935, 52.5% of men and 18.1% of women smoked,[30] with urban women under age 40 years more likely to do so. Doctors failed to forbid cigarettes because they themselves smoked and feared hurting the U.S. economy . . . and, of course, their own if it made them unpopular with patients.[38] Smoke obfuscated lantern slides at medical meetings. How could injunctions of the medical profession be taken seriously even if it did not officially sanction smoking?

Cigarette smoking increased continuously in this century until the 1960s[23] and is still on the increase in developing countries. Ads began to appear in major middle class women's magazines in the 1930s: *McCall's, Better Homes and Gardens*, and *Ladies' Home Journal*.[30] *Good Housekeeping* and *Seventeen* refused to accept cigarette ads, but *Ms. Magazine* continued their publication into the 1980s.[30] A 1938 *Fortune* survey indicated that 81% of women did not disapprove of women smoking in public.[30] Today, educated women and college-bound women are least likely to smoke, yet for many women today, smoking remains a symbol of rebellion and liberation.[30]

The New York State Journal of Medicine published its first cigarette ad in 1933 and continued to do so for 20 years, with over 600 pages of ads, suggesting a policy of complacency, if not overt support from the medical profession.[34] The Children and Young Persons Act[31] passed in 1933, forbidding sales of tobacco to those under 16 years old. Vending machine sales, however, persisted, with only 20 annual prosecutions per year from 1945 to 1952 in England.[31]

In the 1930s, Alton Ochsner, a prominent New Orleans surgeon, reported a relationship between cigarette smoking and cancer of the lung, but because of his strong antismoking stance, his observation was minimized, if not dismissed. A critic sarcastically noted that sale of nylon stockings, like sale of tobacco, paralleled the observed increased prevalence of lung cancer.[38] In 1936, a French physician, Mauric Delubel, compiled the pathogenic effects of tobacco and included leukoplakia of the mouth, acute tobacco intoxication, chronic coryza, prolapse of the rectum, and arteriosclerosis.[38]

The Journal of the American Medical Association (*JAMA*) commenced cigarette advertising in 1934[39] and continued to do so until shortly after publication of the landmark report by Wynder Graham effective January 1, 1954.[39]

World War II

Patriotism and smoking were again linked in the World War II efforts, showing hard-working women smoking at a time when nearly a third reported doing so. Filter cigarettes appeared before the war, both to avoid wasting valuable tobacco in unsmoked butts and to appeal to the growing numbers of women smokers, who disliked soggy cigarette ends.[11,20]

Early filters offered little resistance to the flow of smoke and did not have measurable impact on cigarette flavor.[11] Reduction of tar relates to wrapping paper porousness, tobacco additives, burning temperature, tightness of the pack of the tobacco, and the length of the burning column.[11] Filters that introduced air into the smoke drawn in, by providing perforations in the filter, dilute the puff and allow more air inhaled and less tar.

At the time of World War II, smoking diseases appeared to be a definite risk factor for three diseases: tobacco amblyopia (an eye disease), neoplasia of the mouth, and cardiovascular disease.[38] In the 1940s, a Mayo Clinic group met strong reaction from skeptics when they suggested a relationship of smoking to coronary heart disease.[38] Several studies in the 1940s indicated that tobacco tar applied to the skin of animals could cause cancer. The relationship between coronary heart disease and smoking was demonstrated in 1940, and in 1941, the relationship was shown between mouth cancer and chewing tobacco.[18]

Smoking Is Dangerous to Your Health

In the 1950s, American attitudes toward smoking began to change. Demonstration of the relationship of cancer of the lung to smoking is an excellent example of how chronic epidemiologic techniques may be used to disentangle a number of differing variables in a causal chain so that possible modes of prevention may be identified and tested.[38] Physicians were at first reluctant to accept statistical evidence linking cancer and smoking.[5,6]

Evidence now suggests that tobacco *is* addictive or, as stated in an early metaphor, users are being "bound in aromatic chains."[21] Sudden cessation leads to withdrawal, with anxiety, headaches, craving for nicotine, cough, poor concentration, nervousness, and difficulty sleeping.[18] Cough increases at first because a substance in cigarettes paralyzes tracheobronchial cilia. As the cilia recover, more mucus is expelled.

The relationship between lung cancer and smoking was discussed in the landmark report by Wynder and Graham in *JAMA* in 1953. It had taken the explosion of cigarette use with World War I to create a significantly large population exposed to the putative risk factor to ascertain smoking effects on cancer and coronary heart disease.[39] Wynder and Graham presented 684 cases of lung cancer in which tobacco use appeared the principal causative factor.[39] In other studies, Wynder extracted tar from cigarettes and painted the material three times a week on the skin of mice.[40] Fifty-eight percent of the 62 who survived developed cancer. Some mice have a greater tendency to develop cancer, however, and placing tar on the skin is not perfectly analagous to placing tar on the lung.[40]

A possible relationship between emphysema and smoking was shown in 1953.[38] No cigarette ads appeared in *JAMA* after January 1, 1954. In 1958, Cuyler-Hammond and Daniel Horn[41] published a follow-up study of 200,000 people, demonstrating that smoking was associated with more ills than had been previously suspected. Total mortality among cigarette smokers was increased by 68%, as observed in men smoking regularly. Pipe and cigar smokers showed a much smaller increase, 9% and 12% respectively. Rates fell when smoking ceased but never to rates of non-smokers. Finally, increased rate of coronary thrombosis were documented among smokers. The great feat was to show that tobacco caused cancer of the mouth, lip, tongue, and lung.[41]

In 1957, the British Medical Research Council condemned smoking.[38] American physician groups were slow to follow, but in 1957, the National Cancer Institute and the American Cancer Society issued a warning that public health action was warranted despite the fact that research was not conclusive.[38] Data in 1954 indicated that one third of physicians in Massachusetts did not use tobacco, although one half of that group (i.e., one sixth of the Massachusetts physicians) had previously been smokers. Another one fifth had reduced smoking. Five years later, only two fifths of the same group remained smokers.[38]

An article in *Readers' Digest* in the 1950s associating lung cancer and smoking caused a temporary reduction in smoking that again occurred after the first Surgeon General's report in 1964.[23] There was a brief recovery in sales, but subsequently, American consumption has been falling with the counteradvertising campaign mandated by the Federal Communication Commission that resulted from Attorney John Banzhaf's (Director of Action on Smoking and Health in Washington, DC) petition.[23]

Lorillard countered attacks in the 1950s through sponsorship of the Dorsey Brothers, Paul Whiteman, Bing Crosby, Frank Sinatra, and Fred Waring and his Pennsylvanians on radio and television. The famous Old Gold dancing pack[7] was as much a friend to early TV viewers as were the California raisins of the 1980s.

The increased success of filter-tip cigarettes, such as Kents with "micronite filters,"[7] was due to the fact that some, but not all, filters removed some of the harmful ingredients of cigarettes.[8] Filter cigarette sales spread from America abroad. Aggressive marketing in England converted filter-tip sales from 2.3% in 1956 to 64.5% in 1970. Each individual cigarette is safer, due to less absorption of noxious substances, but ironically, to compensate, the nicotine addicted buy more cigarettes, thereby increasing sales. Between 1956 and 1970, the total weight of cigarette tobacco consumed fell by 9.6%, but the number of cigarette sales increased by 28.5%.[31] Alternative product production soared.[31] Cigars and cigarette sales were 315 million in 1967. Six years later, they were 1135 million. Rates of cigarette smoking continued to rise until the mid-1960s, when sales began to decline.

Smoking of tobacco, like use of other drugs, has a history of moral opposition.[42] Smoking tobacco, unlike use of other recreational drugs or excessive alcohol use, does not alter consciousness or cause escape from social responsibility. The public, therefore, until recent awareness of the impact of passive inhalation, deemed smoking a matter of individual responsibility. Shortly after the Surgeon General's report, studies in 1964 and again in 1966 found little change in smokers' attitude toward smoking.[42] A U.S. Public Health Service survey revealed that smokers regarded their habit as pleasurable and relaxing while acknowledging possible health consequences.

Consumer Beware

There was no federal involvement in regulation regarding cigarette smoking until May 23, 1961, when President John F. Kennedy was asked at a White House news conference what could be done about smoking and health.[18] He promised to investigate the question and appointed a panel of eight physicians, a chemist and a statistician. After a 30-month review of literature on the subject, the first *Surgeon General's Statement on the Health Consequences of Smoking* was released by Surgeon General Luther Terry on January 11, 1964.[10,18] The transient decline in smoking observed at the time of this report did not become permanent until the 1970s, when the norm became again not to smoke. The report of the Surgeon General's Advisory Committee on Smoking and Health concluded[10] that smoking is associated with heart disease, is a cause of lung cancer, is the most important cause of bronchitis, and is associated with increased risk of premature death.

In 1966, the legislative branch of the federal government required a warning label on cigarette packages.[18] The original label was that cigarette smoking "may be hazardous" to your health. A few years later, this was altered to read "is dangerous." The Federal Communication Commission ruled a year later that the Fairness Doctrine applied to cigarette advertising and required radio and television stations accepting cigarette advertising to provide equal time for public health and American Cancer Society announcements of health hazards of smoking.[18] The announcements of the Cancer Society were so effective that the tobacco industry ceased television and radio advertising.

Although tobacco sales have become somewhat flat, tobacco's profitability and cigarette sales volume has increased steadily since 1969. Low-

and ultra-low-tar cigarettes now account for more than one half of all cigarette sales, compared to 26.6% in 1977. Over 100 new brands of cigarettes have been introduced since 1975. The number of U.S. smokers in 1962 was estimated to be 49 million, and in 1983, there were 58 million, or 33% of the total adult population.[43]

New Targets, New Sales

The impact of smoking on the American economy has significant consequences.[13] About $1\frac{1}{3}$ million people were employed on over 276,000 tobacco farms in 1977, producing the nation's sixth largest cash crop, with an estimated value of $2.5 billion in 1970.[13] Ten states list tobacco as a major crop, with Kentucky and North Carolina holding 60% of the market.[13] Many jobs and personal fortunes have been—and in the relatively near future will continue to be—tied to the fortunes of the tobacco industry.

Awareness of the interrelationships among tobacco dependence, alcohol use, and other drug abuse arose in the 1970s,[44] together with cognizance of the ironic reality that the increasing success of women at the worksite is tied with increased rates of heart disease, lung cancer, alcoholism, and suicide for those most successful. Increased smoking by women relates to increased personal stress balancing work and motherhood in the modern world, increasing sense of freedom and independence by women, women's desire to do anything men do, and the appeal in advertising to glamour, romance, social success, and independence.[8] In both the 1970s and the 1980s, women and minority groups have become increasingly targeted for smoking advertisements. When cigarette ads were banned on TV and radio, the number of ads in the press increased.[30]

There has been an evolving interest in how licit drug use precedes illicit use. For women, for example, either alcohol or cigarette use precedes marijuana use. Alcohol, cigarettes, and marijuana use precedes other illicit drugs.[44] However, of course, use of milk also precedes alcohol use, as critics note. Stress, however, leads to anxiety and depression, which in turn, in those who are predisposed, leads to cigarette smoking and other substance abuse.[44] Alcohol users have smoking rates higher than nonalcohol users. The factors combine to increase morbidity and mortality.

Smoking Today

Currently, over 40,000 research reports exist on the hazards of smoking.[45] This research has resulted in development of less hazardous cigarettes, education programs in schools, cessation of television and radio ads for cigarettes, antismoking campaigns by citizens, and most importantly, physicians now have the best record of having quit smoking and the greatest percentage of nonsmokers of any professional group.[45] They now provide a model for their patients rather than providing the double message of the early and mid-20th century. Ironically, however, nurses smoke more than any other health professional group. Recent antismoking statutes are enforced on airplanes and in hospitals but generally not to the same degree elsewhere.[46] Labeling the habit as unacceptable, undesirable, and socially deviant is enhancing effectiveness in reducing smoking in selected circles.

Today it is realized that, indeed, smoking is dangerous to health. Smoking causes up to one third of all cancers and 90% of lung cancer. It is a risk factor for cancer of the mouth, pharynx, larynx, esophagus, bladder, kidney, and pancreas.[18] The majority of smoking-related illnesses are not neoplastic. They are respiratory and cardiovascular. Fifteen percent of chronic bronchitis and emphysema are linked to smoking.[18] Also smoking is a major cause of hypertension, stroke, and myocardial infarction. Smoking-induced peripheral artery insufficiency causes skin wrinkles and organic impotence.[18] Death rates [47] are higher among men who are regular smokers and increase with the number of cigarettes smoked per day.[47] In Hammond and Horn's study[47] in 1958, which drew attention to excess mortality, coronary disease accounted for 52.1% of the excess; lung cancer, 13.5%; and cancer of other sites, 13.5%. The major finding in this early study was the high association between cigarette smoking and the total death rate. Dr. Wynder, who originally described the relationship between bronchiogenic cancer and smoking in the 1950s, was the founding editor of the *Journal of Preventive Medicine*.[45] Today, we are aware both that smoking is, indeed, quite hazardous to health, and that a smoker of 20 cigarettes is addicted and may be expected to experience withdrawal symptoms 20 to 30 minutes after cessation of use.[48]

On October 12, 1984, the Comprehensive Smoking Education Act established the Office of Smoking and Health in the federal government, requiring ingredient disclosures for cigarettes and warning labels.[18] Strong antismoker advocates have suggested that subscriptions to all magazines with cigarette ads should be cancelled.[38] As this book goes to press, there is a move in Minnesota to ban vending machine sales of cigarettes and in California to increase cigarette tax for funding of antismoking commercials.[49]

Revenues of smoking-related industries are an important component of the national economy. The market share of tobacco products remains high, accounting for $60 billion, or 2.5% of the gross national product.[13] It is the sixth largest cash crop in the United States, with 85% coming from the tobacco belt from Georgia to Kentucky and Virginia. It is the number one crop in Virginia, South Carolina, Kentucky, and North Carolina and the second in Tennessee, Maryland, Massachusetts, and Georgia. Approximately 2.5% of the nation's work force is employed in tobacco-related services. The United States sets a minimum price for tobacco and then buys tobacco that cannot be sold above this price. Annual sales of 5 trillion cigarettes a year yields $40 billion. In 1980, Americans alone purchased

630 billion cigarettes for nearly $20 billion.[48] Growth in industrial countries, however, has been limited to 1%. The combined advertising expenditures in 1983 was $1.5 billion.[13] Tax revenues for federal, state, and local excise tax were $6.2 billion in 1977. When talking about smoking today, one is talking about a critical element in the economic life of the United States and the world and a major factor in the employment rate.

Costs of smoking, on the other hand, are a factor in rising health care costs of an aging baby-boomer population. Smokers of one pack of cigarettes per day have 50% greater illness, absenteeism, and rate of hospitalization than nonsmokers. Loss of productivity because of illness and early smoking-related deaths cost Americans $24 billion a year.[13] Smoking has been linked to cancer of the bladder, kidney, pancreas, lung, mouth, pharynx, and larnyx, and to esophageal disease, coronary heart disease, emphysema, arteriosclerosis, bronchitis, peptic ulcer disease, cerebrovascular disease, decreased birth weight, and fetal disease.[13] Fifty-one thousand die of cigarette-related chronic obstructive lung disease annually, and another 170,000 of cigarette-related coronary disease, and 12,000 more of cigarette-related cancers.[13]

Tobacco is currently used more than any other drug in the world.[23] A billion cigarettes were produced in the entire United States in 1885. Today, more than that is smoked daily, with most people having histories of beginning as adolescents. Divorced or separated men and women have higher rates of use than their married equivalents, but widowed men have lower rates than married men.[50]

For women, generally speaking, the greater the income, the greater the smoking. The same is not true for men, for whom smoking is higher among both high-and low-income than for middle-income men.[50] Professional and technical workers have continued to have the lowest smoking rates, whereas laborers, craftsmen, and other blue-collar workers have the highest rates.[50] Many ethnic groups see smoking differently, and the tobacco industry has turned to marketing targeted at high user ethnic groups such as Hispanics.[51]

During the past decade, there has been a decline in the popularity of smoking. The decline among adolescent boys, however, is due to some shift toward chewing tobacco and snuff.[18] In 1980, 640 billion cigarettes were smoked; in 1984, only 600 billion.[18] Fifty percent of men and 33% of women smoked in 1965. In 1986, the numbers dropped, respectively, to 32% and 29%.[18] Comparably, cigarette smoking is falling in selected other countries such as Italy, where there has been a decrease among currently smoking adult men from 71.4% in 1949 to 45.6% in 1983. However, the number of Italian women ages 14 and over who smoke has increased 17.7% since the 1960s.[52] Cigarette sales do not accurately reflect the decreased number of people smoking, as those who are truly addicted require more of low-tar and -nicotine cigarettes to get the same high, which maintains or increases the volume of sales.

The current trend is to stigmatize smokers by banning smoking in airplanes and hospitals and making smokers sit in special sections in restaurants.[46] This makes a smoker a social deviant and an outcast. Prosmoking groups argue that individual freedom of expression is jeopardized when smoking is prohibited. Politeness, however, has yielded to the damand for clean air and at present appears to be winning out. Acquiescence to smokes due to nonsmokers' politeness was in the past interpreted as a victory for smokers' rights.[46]

Conclusion

The spread of the use of tobacco and continued consumption despite un-equivocal evidence of its detrimental effects to health is a tribute to how a drug that is used to relieve existential pain, is a symbol of status, and is highly tied into the economic fabric of a community cannot simply be controlled by bans, fines, threats of physical punishment, or even heinous punishment itself. Neither popes nor kings and queens can dissuade those eager to use. Threat of death itself is not a deterrent. Great individual fortunes were amassed by tobacco barons, and the new America grew. The great British Navy evolved around the development and trade of tobacco. The pain of wars from the Crimean to the Korean led to more and more use. The drug became interwoven into the fabric of culture as a symbol of masculinity, free thinking, patriotism, and women's liberation. Only today can a decline be seen among those least in need of such symbols, as evidence grows to confirm the wide-ranging health consequences.

Interestingly, marijuana historically was used by oppressed black dock workers and those suffering the pain of war. It has been suggested for use in assuaging the pain of advanced cancer. As a symbol of protest against the Vietnam War, its use spread. Movies such as "Reefer Madness' did not deter its use in a generation that saw "pot" (marijuana) use as being no worse than alcohol use.

As with alcohol, prohibition of marijuana helped evolve a whole in-dustry of drug traffickers. This time, it was not bootlegging that led to organized crime, but sales of the drug was usually first to young people comparable in age to those generally beginning to smoke. These young people became aware of the profits to be made from importing, packaging, and distributing substances that seemingly facilitate interpersonal rela-tionships and help the unemployed or underutilized but talented cope with evolving problems in an overpopulated world with declining resources. Use of marijuana, cocaine, and a number of designer drugs became a symbol of the Age of Aquarius. Those who use these drugs often see themselves as more liberal, free thinking, iconoclastic, and in need of something to assuage the painful existential feelings of aloneness, impo-tency, and low self-esteem in the modern world.

Until the complex economic, psychological, and existential forces that lead to drug use are fully understood, one will continue to see problems with use, whether the drug is alcohol, nicotine, marijuana, or cocaine. Efforts at control have had only small impact on alcohol and cigarette use. Awareness of the essential human needs for self-esteem, for freedom of choice, for interpersonal support, and for a more equitable distribution of economic and other essential resources is required, in order to develop ways to prevent use of drugs that are dangerous to health that have more enduring tangible effects in a community than success in the next political campaign.

References

1. Kneist W. Oder gesundheit ein kulturhis torischer ruckblick. Z ges Hyg 1981; 27: 411–480.
2. Anderson JR. Acayatl; ancient Aztec sorcerer. Alabama Medicine 1984; 53: 14, 17–18, 20.
3. The health consequences of smoking: Nicotine addiction (20th report of the Surgeon General). Washington, DC: U.S. Government Printing Office, 1988.
4. Roxburgh J, Clarke J. The war of the weed. Nursing Time 1988; 84: 48–50.
5. Johnston FR. Hippocrates never heard of it: The anatomy of a modern epidemic. Am Surgeon 1985; 51: 1–7.
6. Johnston JFW. The narcotics we indulge in. Part 1. J of Psychoactive Drugs 1985; 17: 191–199.
7. P. Lorillard Company Lorillard and tobacco 200th anniversary—Lorillard Company, 1760–1960. Author, 1960.
8. Diehl HS. Tobacco and your health: The smoking controversy. New York: McGraw-Hill, 1969.
9. Hedrick JL. Smoking, tobacco, and health. Contract No. PH86-67-176. Bethesda, MD: National Clearinghouse for Smoking and Health, 1969.
10. U.S. Public Health Service. Smoking and Health: Report of the Advisory Committee to the Surgeon General of the Public Health Service. Publication No. 1103. Washington, DC: Public Health Service, 1964.
11. McCusker K. Landmarks of tobacco use in the United States. Chest 1988; 93: 345–365.
12. Ethridge RF. Tobacco among the Cherokees. J of Cherokee Studies 1978; 3: 76–86.
13. Perlman H. The history of policy formation on cigarette use. PA Med 1986; 89: 25–28.
14. Garrett W. Smoking: Now and then. Canadian Nurse 1973; 69: 22–26.
15. Humphries SV. Smoking—Its blessings and hazards. Central African J of Med 1975; 21: 86–88.
16. Bewby TH. Smoking: The 16th and 17th century response. Intl J of Addict 1973; 8: 191–196.
17. Harrison L. Tobacco battered and the pipes shattered: A note on the fate of the first British campaign against tobacco smoking. Brit J of Addict 1986; 81: 553–558.

18. Cooper KR. From king to culprit: Tobacco. Virginia Medical 1986; 113: 458–468.
19. Micca G. Il tabacco nella storia della medicina. Minerva Medica 1968; 59: 697–700.
20. Stepney R. The Indians' revenge: A drink without drinking. Practitioner 1980; 224: 109–111.
21. Taylor P. The smoke ring: Tobacco, money and multinational politics. New York: Pantheon, 1984.
22. Tabor SJW. Historical sketch of tobacco from 1602 to 1800. The Boston Medical and Surgical J 1851; 44: 491–494.
23. Slade J. The tobacco epidemic; Lessons from history. J of Psychoactive Drugs 1989; 21: 281–291.
24. Guerra F. American Medical Bibliography 1639–1783. New York: Harper, 1962.
25. Davis ES. On smoking and Samuel Johnson. Am J of Public Health 1979; 69: 1087.
26. Christen AG, Swanson BZ. Orally used smokeless tobacco as advertised in the metamorphic trade cards of 1870–1900. Bull of the Hist of Dentistry 1983; 31: 82–86.
27. Burnham HA. Moliere and the smoking pandemic. NY State J of Med 1986; 108–109.
28. Powers JS, Wetteman M. On the hazards of smoking: Statement from 1836. Am J of Public Health 1979; 69: 389.
29. Editorial. (unsigned). A 19th century perspective on the health consequences of smoking. J of the Med Assoc of Georgia 1979; 68: 191.
30. Ernster VL. Mixed messages for women: A social history of cigarette smoking and advertising. NY State J of Med 1985; 85: 335–346.
31. Froggatt P. Determinants of policy on smoking and health. Intl J of Epidemiol 1989; 18: 1–9.
32. Robb-Smith AHT. Did Sir William Osler have carcinoma of the lung? Part 2. Chest 1975; 67: 82–86.
33. Ring ME. Oddments in dental history: Down with toothbrushes—Up with tobacco! Bull of the Hist of Dentistry 1984; 32: 31–32.
34. Blum A. When more doctors smoked Camels: Cigarette advertising in the journal. NY State J of Med 1983; 83: 1347–1352.
35. Jaffe JH. Tobacco use as a mental disorder: The rediscovery of a medical problem. NIDA Research Monograph Series No. 17. Washington, DC: U.S. Government Printing Office, 1977: 202–217.
36. Gladwin LA. Tobacco and sex: Some factors affecting non-marital sexual behavior in colonial Virginia. J of Social Hist 1978; 12: 57–75.
37. Brennan F. Smoking of opium or hop in the '20s and early '30s. Clin Toxicol 1973; 6: 611.
38. Burnbam JC. American physicians and tobacco use: Two Surgeons General, 1929 and 1964. Bull of Hist Med 1969; 63: 1–31.
39. Lundberg GD. In the AMA, policy follows science: A case history of tobacco. JAMA 1985; 253: 3001–3003.
40. Northrup E. Science looks at smoking. New York: Coward-McCann, 1957.
41. Doll R. Smoking and death rates. JAMA 1984; 251: 2854–2857.
42. Bruhn JG. Drug use as a way of life. Postgraduate Med 1973; 53: 183–188.

43. Comerford, AW, Personal communication, 1990.
44. Battjes RJ. Smoking as an issue in alcohol and drug abuse treatment. Addict Behav 1988; 13, 225–230.
45. Steinfeld JL. Smoking and lung cancer: A milestone in awareness. JAMA 1985; 253: 2995–2997.
46. Shor RE, Shor MB, Williams DC. The distinction between the antismoking and nonsmokers rights movements. J of Psychol 1980; 106: 129–146.
47. Hammond EC, Horn D. Smoking and death rates—report on forty-four months of follow-up of 187,783 men. JAMA 1984; 251: 2840–2853.
48. Brecker R, Brecker E, Herzog A, et al. The Consumers Union report on smoking and the public interest. Mount Vernon, NY: Consumers Union, 1963.
49. Schwartz J, Hurt, III H. Catching hell for smoking: Crackdown on tobacco. Newsweek April 23, 1990; 25.
50. Schuman LM. Patterns of smoking behavior. NIDA Research Monograph Series No. 17. Washington, DC: U.S. Government Printing Office, 1977: 36–66.
51. Marin G, Perez-Stable EJ Otero-Sabogal R, et al. Stereotypes of smokers held by Hispanic and white non-Hispanic smokers. Intl J of Addict 1989; 24: 203–213.
52. LaVecchia C. Smoking in Italy, 1949–1983. Prev Med 1986; 15: 274–281.

2
Psychosocial Factors and Nicotine Dependence

GEOFFREY P. KANE

Nicotine dependence, like other diseases, results from the interaction over time of multiple causal factors.[1,2] Causal factors may include molecules, social forces, and items at any level of human organization in between. These factors are often categorized as biophysical, psychological, and social.[3] The 1988 Surgeon General's report conveys this understanding in the statement: "Cigarette smoking is a multidetermined behavior shaped by both personal and environmental variables" (p. 507).[4] This chapter examines psychological and social factors that influence tobacco use and nicotine dependence.

Development of Nicotine Dependence

Social factors related to family and peers are strong determinants of whether individuals use tobacco. Tobacco use and nicotine dependence almost always begin in childhood or adolescence, with the onset of cigarette smoking greatest during junior high school.[4] Prior to initial tobacco use, a stage of preparation or anticipation has been described wherein young people develop a positive attitude toward smoking when they observe smoking by parents and older siblings.[5] Children become accustomed to the sight and smell of cigarettes and often imitate the physical actions of smoking. Candy and gum products in packages that closely resemble actual cigarette brands abet this process. One study of family modeling showed a fivefold increase in smoking among adolescent girls from households where one or both parents or an older sibling smoked.[5] When both parents smoke, the effect is greater than when only one parent smokes.[4] Peers predominate over family and other influences at the time of first tobacco use. Fifty percent of first cigarettes are smoked with a friend; nearly 75% of first cigarettes are smoked with another teenager.[5,6]

Many young people try tobacco products, but not all go on to develop nicotine dependence. Some individuals are predisposed to this progression by various social and psychological vulnerability factors.[4] For example, children whose parents have problems with alcohol and other drugs are at high risk for smoking and nicotine dependence.[7] The following groups are also thought to be at increased risk for nicotine dependence and represent potential additional social vulnerability factors: children subjected to child abuse and neglect, children and adolescents in foster care, single teenage mothers and their children, school dropouts, unemployed youth, and ethnic minority youth.[7] As these items imply, vulnerability factors may be undesirable states from which relief is sought. This echoes the themes of relief drinking and escapism in the literature on the development of alcohol dependence.[2] Other undesirable states influencing nicotine use include physiologic factors such as pain and sleep deprivation and psychiatric–psychological factors such as anxiety and depression.[4] Several studies have shown subjective stress and negative mood states to be related to the onset of regular smoking by adolescents.[4] Longitudinal research[6] has identified psychological vulnerability factors that are predictors of smoking in adolescents. Adolescents who go on to smoke overestimate the prevalence of smoking among teenagers and adults. They tend to view events in their lives as resulting from environmental forces beyond their influence (external locus of control). Compared to adolescents who do not eventually smoke, those who do have lower academic aspirations, are more tolerant of deviance, and perceive less agreement between their parents. Delinquent behavior (conduct disorder) and experimentation with liquor, beer, and marijuana are also associated with teenage smoking,[4,8] though causal relationships here are unclear.

The products and advertising of the tobacco industry and government's influence on that industry are social factors central to the development of nicotine dependence. Tobacco products must be available to adolescents before smoking and other forms of tobacco consumption can begin. Forty-three states set a minimum age for purchase of cigarettes but lack of enforcement and the widespread presence of vending machines severely compromise the effectiveness of such legislation. Tobacco products would be much less accessible to youth if existing laws were enforced, free tobacco samples were prohibited, and all tobacco sales were over the counter.[9] Teenagers and young adults are price sensitive, and increasing the excise tax on cigarettes would reduce smoking by young people.[10,11]

Initiation of smoking is generally followed by a period of *experimental smoking*, during which the person smokes less than one cigarette per week. During experimental smoking, peers often provide social reinforcement. Tobacco advertisements wield substantial influence at this stage. Cigarette ads portray themes such as independence, strength, youthful vigor, and sexual attraction that correspond to the ideals of many teenagers.[12,13] Adolescents who are smoking experimentally and whose ideal self-image resembles models in cigarette advertisements are more likely to continue to smoke.[5] Smoking serves as a means whereby adolescents express a self-image of toughness, precocity, and sociability.[6] The tobacco industry has repeatedly denied targeting youth with advertising and products, but there has been increasing criticism of this industry for what others perceive as recruitment of new tobacco users through advertising imagery, free samples and coupons, promotion of sports events, and the introduction of "starter products," such as snuff with a low nicotine content.[12-15]

The tobacco industry admittedly aims products and advertising at those segments of the adult population known to continue to have a relatively high proportion of smokers, including women, ethnic minorities, and blue-collar workers.[12,13] Though presented by the industry as intended to induce adult smokers to switch brands, the appearance and activities of models in this advertising cater to nonsmokers, as well as to smokers and frequently to youth.[13] Smoking by teenage females now exceeds smoking by teenage males, and smoking among adult females is declining much more slowly than among adult males.[4,12] These trends are explained in part by current emphasis on slimness as a standard of feminine beauty and by cigarette advertisements and brand names that reinforce that standard.[5,12,16,17] Smoking does facilitate weight control.[4,16] Desire for weight control contributes to initiation of smoking, as well as serving as one of the reinforcements that keeps some individuals, especially females, smoking.[4]

Experimental smoking may be followed by *habituation*, which is defined as smoking at least one cigarette weekly. Habituation involves development of skill in inhalation and regulation of nicotine dose, becoming accustomized to the mood-altering and other pharmacologic effects of nicotine, and development of a pattern of conditioned reinforcement from smoking.[5] With habituation, consumption may increase to a pack of cigarettes or more per day.

Continuation of Nicotine Dependence

For more than 25 years, health authorities have pointed to the dangers of tobacco consumption.[18,19] This health education has paid off; nearly half the American men and women who ever smoked regularly have quit. Yet in addition to the 50 million or so people in this country who have successfully quit smoking, there is another 50 million who continue to smoke. Their continuing tobacco use despite actual and potential adverse consequences testifies to the addictive nature of the problem. Many try to stop smoking, but their relapse rates are high. In response to questionnaires, about half of current smokers acknowledge three or more unsuccessful attempts to quit.[20] Psychological and social factors are prominent among reasons why people continue to consume tobacco products and nicotine.

Reports of smokers, plus laboratory studies of the effects of cigarette smoking or nicotine administration, have identified two major psychological reinforcements from smoking: arousal and relaxation. Smokers state that smoking helps them concentrate; studies show improvement in attention, learning, reaction time, and problem solving. Some smokers, therefore, continue to smoke because nicotine helps them to think and perform, especially when their immediate alternative to smoking is a nicotine withdrawal state, characterized by physical and emotional discomfort and confusion.[4,21] Smokers also state that smoking helps them relax, particularly in stressful situations, and it lifts their mood. They report pleasure and reduced anger, tension, depression, and stress.[21] Rituals related to carrying and using smoking materials contribute to smokers' sense of security and control.[22] Many smokers, therefore, continue to smoke because nicotine helps them to regulate mood (pp 394–414).[4]

Among adults, smoking has been shown to be associated with nervousness, emotionality, anxiety, neurotic traits, depression, anger, and rebelliousness.[4,23] Smokers smoke more in response to stress, and individuals with psychiatric/psychological problems characterized by negative affect and difficulty coping are more likely to be active smokers than individuals who are more emotionally stable. About 90% of alcoholics smoke.[4] Individuals with a history of major depression appear to be at increased risk for smoking[24–26] and in one study did not respond as well to treatment for nicotine dependence as individuals without a history of depression.[25] Stressful situations precipitate relapse to smoking among those who have quit,[4,27] and adult smokers whose chief motive for smoking is to reduce negative affect are more likely to relapse after treatment.[4]

Black Americans have a disproportionately high rate of cigarette smoking. Multivariate analysis suggests that social and psychological factors related to class and stress account for this rather than biophysical (racial) factors.[28]

As with the development of nicotine dependence, the tobacco industry and government exert strong influences on the continuation of nicotine dependence. Cigarette advertising, by its very existence, its ubiquity in print media and on billboards, and its imagery, fosters the perception that smoking is less hazardous, more prevalent, and more socially acceptable than it is.[12,29] Cigarette advertisements provide external cues to smoke that may increase the consumption of smokers and may increase relapses among former smokers.[29] Cigarette packages and advertisements have carried warning messages since 1966 and 1972, respectively, but their effectiveness is questionable.[30,31] Analysis of the editorial content of popular magazines supports the contention that publications deriving large revenues from tobacco advertising are inhibited from printing information about smoking and disease.[12,13,29] For public health reasons, some national governments are beginning to ban advertising and/or promotion of tobacco products. Norway, Finland, and Sweden have enacted comprehensive restrictions.[13] Comparable legislation is likely in France[32] and is under debate in the United States.[12,13,29,33]

Recovery from Nicotine Dependence

Like nicotine dependence itself, recovery from nicotine dependence results from the interaction over time of multiple factors. In recovery, there are important psychological (cognitive) factors and important social (environmental) factors. It is the *interaction* of these factors that is critical, because human behavior may be viewed as being both chosen by the individual and determined by the environment, with neither dominating the other.[34] This view attributes responsibility for addictive behavior and for recovery to both the individual and the community, leaving neither free to blame the other for problems or to trust the other for solutions.[2,35] To reduce the current human and dollar costs of nicotine dependence, we must help individuals to discontinue nicotine use, and we must help communities to promote treatment for nicotine dependence and not to promote nicotine use.

Change from smoking is difficult. To even consider quitting threatens the self-image and coping mechanisms of many smokers, so they do not pay attention to the matter (precontemplation[36,37]). They begin to consider quitting (contemplation[36,37]) when they realize that continued smoking is an even more serious threat. Individualized patient education from physicians,[37–41] counteradvertising,[12,33] mass media campaigns,[42,43] and smoking policies at worksites[44,45] and schools[46] are effective means of raising smokers' consciousness that quitting is important for them. The dangers their smoking creates for others[47] gets some smokers' attention, particularly when nonsmoking peers are assertive or combative[48] or when, as smoking parents, they learn of the present (respiratory infections) and future (cancer, smoking, and drug abuse) risks to their children.

Once motivated to change, smokers are more likely to take action and succeed if certain psychological and social factors are present. Belief that one's own actions can make a difference (internal locus of control[49]) and confidence in being able to not smoke in a variety of situations (self-efficacy[34,36,50]) are important psychological factors. These characteristics may be cultivated through cognitive intervention, guided imagery, relaxation training, and other methods.[34,49] To take action, many nicotine-dependent individuals need the environmental support of treatment services. There are logistic and financial barriers to the use of treatment services, which some employers have overcome by providing treatment at the worksite.[51] Professional help would become more available and accessible to smokers if treatment for nicotine dependence were covered by health insurance plans. At present, such services are categorically excluded under most plans, and the health insurance industry is reluctant to alter this.[52]

After treatment, maintaining abstinence from nicotine involves ongoing use of cognitive and behavioral techniques.[27,53] Individuals can reduce their risk of relapse by improving stress-management skills[4] and establishing a network of interpersonal support. Factors related to family are among the strongest environmental determinants of the outcome of quit attempts; family conflict correlates with relapse, family support correlates with success.[4]

Acknowledgments. The writer is indebted to Linda Barnes and Pauline Piwarunas for their assistance in the preparation of this chapter.

References

1. Susser M. Causal thinking in the health sciences. New York: Oxford University Press, 1973.
2. Kane GP. Inner-city alcoholism: An ecological analysis and cross-cultural study. New York: Human Sciences Press, 1981.
3. Lipowski ZJ. Physical illness, the patient and his environment. In: Reiser MF, ed. American handbook of psychiatry. Vol. 4. New York: Basic Books, 1975: 3–42.
4. U.S. Department of Health and Human Services. The health consequences of smoking: Nicotine addiction (a report of the Surgeon General). DHHS Publication No. (CDC) 88–8406. Washington, DC: USDHHS, Public Health Service, Office on Smoking and Health, 1988.
5. Gritz ER. Gender and the teenage smoker. In: Ray B, Braude M, eds. Women and drugs: A new era for research. NIDA Research Monograph No. 65. Washington DC: USDHHS, Public Health Service, Alcohol, Drug Abuse, and Mental Health Administration, National Institute on Drug Abuse, 1986: 70–79.
6. Chassin L, Presson CC, Sherman SJ. Stepping backward in order to step forward: An acquisition-oriented approach to primary prevention. J of Consult and Clin Psychol 1985; 53: 612–622.
7. Jones CL, Battjes RJ. The context and caveats of prevention research and abuse. In: Jones CL, Battjes RJ, eds. Etiology of drug abuse: Implications for prevention. NIDA Research Monograph No. 56. Washington, DC: USDHHS, Public Health Service, Alcohol, Drug Abuse, and Mental Health Administration, National Institute on Drug Abuse, 1985: 1–12.
8. Gritz ER. Cigarette smoking by adolescent females: Implications for health and behavior. Women and Health 1984; 9: 103–115.
9. Kellie SE. Tobacco use: Women, children and minorities. In: Blakeman EM, Engelberg AL, eds. Final report: Tobacco use in America conference. Washington, DC: American Medical Association, 1989: 3–6.
10. Kendall D. Cigarette excise tax. In: Blakeman EM, Engelberg AL, eds. Final report: Tobacco use in America conference. Washington, DC: American Medical Association, 1989: 19–23.
11. Warner KE. Tobacco taxation as health policy in the third world. Am J of Public Health 1990; 80: 529–531.
12. Davis RM. Current trends in cigarette advertising and marketing. New Engl J of Med 1987; 316: 725–732.
13. Myers ML, Hollar J. Tobacco marketing and promotion. In: Blakeman EM, Engelberg, AL, eds. Final report: Tobacco Use in America Conference. Washington, DC: American Medical Association, 1989: 29–42.

14. McCarthy MJ. Tobacco critics see a subtle sell to kids. Wall Street Journal, May 3, 1990.
15. Deveny K. With help of teens, snuff sales revive. Wall Street Journal, May 3, 1990.
16. Rigotti NA. Cigarette smoking and body weight. New Engl J of Med 1989; 320: 931–933.
17. Waldman P. Tobacco firms try soft, feminine sell. Wall Street Journal, December 19, 1989.
18. Warner KE. Smoking and health: A 25-year perspective. Am J of Public Health 1989; 79: 141–143.
19. Warner KE. Effects of the antismoking campaign: An update. Am J of Public Health 1989; 79: 144–151.
20. Schelling TC. Opening remarks. In: Smoking cessation: The organization, delivery, and financing of services, July 13–14, 1989. Cambridge, MA: Institute for the Study of Smoking Behavior and Policy, 1990: 2–6.
21. Benowitz NL. Pharmacologic aspects of cigarette smoking and nicotine addiction. New Engl J of Med 1988; 319: 1318–1330.
22. Rustin T. Treating nicotine addiction. Alcoholism & Addiction 1988; 9: 18–19.
23. Kozlowski LT. Psychosocial influences on cigarette smoking. In: Krashegor NA, ed. The behavioral aspects of smoking. DHEW (ADM) Publication No. 79–882. NIDA Research Monograph No. 26. Washington, DC: USDHEW, Public Health Service, Alcohol, Drug Abuse, and Mental Health Administration, National Institute on Drug Abuse, 1979: 97–125.
24. Hughes JR, Hatsukami DK, Mitchell JE, et al. Prevalence of smoking among psychiatric outpatients. Am J of Psychi 1986; 143: 993–997.
25. Glassman AH, Stetner F, Walsh BT, et al. Heavy smokers, smoking cessation, and clonidine: Results of a double-blind, randomized trial. JAMA 1988; 259: 2863–2866.
26. Hughes JR. Clonidine, depression, and smoking cessation. JAMA 1988; 259: 2901–2902.
27. Carmody TP. Preventing relapse in the treatment of nicotine addiction: Current issues and future directions. J of Psychoactive Drugs 1990; 22: 211–238.
28. Feigelman W, Gorman B. Toward explaining the higher incidence of cigarette smoking among black Americans. J of Psychoactive Drugs 1990; 21: 299–305.
29. Centers for Disease Control. Cigarette advertising—United States, 1988. Morbidity and Mortality Weekly Report 1990; 39: 261–265.
30. Fischer PM, Richards JW, Berman EJ, Krugman DM. Recall and eye tracking study of adolescents viewing tobacco advertisements. JAMA 1989; 261: 84–89.
31. Davis RM, Kendrick JS. The Surgeon General's warnings in outdoor cigarette advertising: Are they readable? JAMA 1989; 261: 90–94.
32. Lipman J. Advertising: French ad ban. Wall street Journal, June 7, 1990.
33. Warner KE. A ban on the promotion of tobacco products. New Engl J of Med 1987; 316: 745–747.
34. Bandura A. Social learning theory. Englewood Cliffs, NJ: Prentice-Hall, 1977.
35. Pattison EM. Rehabilitation of the chronic alcoholic. In: Kissin B, Begleiter H, eds. The biology of alcoholism. Vol 3. New York: Plenum Press, 1974: 587–657.
36. Prochaska JO, DiClemente CC. Toward a comprehensive model of change. In: Miller WR, Heather N, eds. Treating addictive behaviors. New York: Plenum Press, 1986: 3–27.

37. Ockene JK. The psychology of quitting. In: Smoking cessation: The organiza-tion, delivery, and financing of services, July 13–14, 1989. Cambridge, MA: Institute for the Study of Smoking Behavior and Policy. 1990: 26–38.
38. Orleans CT. Smoking cessation in primary care settings. NJ Med 1988; 85: 116–126.
39. Glynn TJ. Physicians and a smoke-free society. Arch of Internal Med 1988; 148: 1013–1016.
40. Kottke TE, Battista RN, DeFriese GH, et al. Attributes of successful smoking cessation interventions in medical practice: A meta-analysis of 39 controlled trials. JAMA 1988; 259: 2883–2889.
41. Wilson DM, Taylor W, Gilbert JR, et al. A randomized trial of a family phy-sician intervention for smoking cessation. JAMA 1988; 260: 1570–1574.
42. Flay BR. Mass media and smoking cessation: A critical review. Am J of Public Health 1987; 77: 153–160.
43. Pierce JP, Macaskill P, Hill D. Long-term effectiveness of mass media led antismoking campaigns in Australia. Am J of Public Health 1990; 80: 565–569.
44. Walsh DC. Corporate smoking policies: A review and an analysis. J of Occup Med 1984; 26: 17–22.
45. Borlund R, Chapman S, Owen N, et al. Effects of workplace smoking bans on cigarette consumption. Am J of Public Health 1990; 80: 178–180.
46. Pentz MA, Brannon BR, Charlin VL, et al. The power of policy: The relation-ship of smoking policy to adolescent smoking. Am J of Public Health 1989; 79: 857–861.
47. Leads from the MMWR—Passive smoking: Beliefs, attitudes, and exposures— Unites States, 1986. JAMA 1988; 259: 2821–2825.
48. Gibbs NR. All fired up over smoking. Time, April 18, 1988.
49. Segall ME, Wynd CA. Health conception, health locus of control, and power as predictors of smoking behavior change. Am J of Health Promotion 1990; 4: 338–344, 372.
50. DiClemente CC, Prochaska JO, Gibertini M. Self-efficacy and the stages of self-change of smoking. Cognitive Ther and Res 1985; 9: 181–200.
51. Fisher KJ, Glasgow RE, Terborg JR. Work site smoking cessation: A meta-analysis of long-term quit rates from controlled studies. J of Occup Med 1990; 32: 429–39.
52. Levison DN. Financing cessation services. In: Smoking cessation: The organ-ization, delivery, and financing of services, July 13–14, 1989. Cambridge, MA, Institute for the Study of Smoking Behavior and Policy. 1990: 64–74.
53. Marlatt GA. Relapse prevention: Theoretical rationale and overview of the model. In: Marlatt GA, Gordon JR, eds. Relapse prevention. New York: Guilford Press, 1985: 3–70.

3
Smoking Control Interventions for Special Populations: Beyond Cultural Sensitivity*

MARIO A. ORLANDI and HAROLD P. FREEMAN

Introduction

Overall, cigarette consumption is on the decline. Between 1964 and 1987, the prevalence of smoking among adults decreased from 40% to 29% and it has been estimated that half of all living adults who ever smoked have quit.[1] Nonetheless, smoking is currently responsible for more than one out of every six deaths in the United States and is considered the most significant preventable cause of death in society today.

Efforts to control smoking behavior have proliferated since 1964, the year in which the U.S. Surgeon General first acknowledged the health risks of smoking. These efforts have ranged from primary prevention for non-smokers to smoking cessation for active smokers.

Since the early 1980s, smoking control interventions have been intensively evaluated in both noncontrolled program evaluation settings and controlled experimental research settings. As a result, clinicians and researchers understand considerably more now than was understood in 1980 regarding the most effective ways to facilitate smoking cessation and non-smoking in the general population.

The 1989 U.S. Surgeon General's report on smoking concludes . . . concludes that the antismoking and prohealth interventions that have been initiated since 1964, when considered in the aggregate, have unquestionably had an impact on overall smoking prevalence in American society. Unfortunately, this same report acknowledges that this progress has not been experienced uniformly across the population as a whole. In fact, one of the report's five major conclusions is that the "prevalence of smoking remains higher among blacks, blue-collar workers, and less educated persons than in the overall population" (p. 11).[1] This conclusion is in accord with more recent findings that suggest that this disparity extends beyond smoking and tobacco-related mortality to a wide variety of other health disorders as well.[2]

*The development of this manuscript was supported in part by grants CA-38219 CA-41621, and CA-50956 from the National Cancer Institute.

Recognition of this disparity between the health improvements experienced by some within society and the lack of such advancements experienced by others has led to the designation of racially, ethnically, or socio-culturally defined groups as "special populations" requiring particular emphasis if the U.S. Public Health Service's health goals for the Year 2000—which include reductions in smoking prevalence among all segments of the population—are to be met.[3]

From the perspective of smoking control, this designation was a significant, though unfortunately recent, first step toward addressing this critically important public health issue, and it led to the integration of the term *cultural sensitivity* into the health promotion lexicon.[4] In this context, the term is used rather broadly to define, both qualitatively and quantitatively, the characteristic of health-promoting messages or interventions that determines whether they will be sociologically syntonic with a particular demographically defined reference group.

In pragmatic terms, this concept implies that health-promoting communications that take cultural sensitivity into account in their development are more likely to succeed. Specifically, such communications should reflect this characteristic in (1) the perceived source of the message, (2) the channel or medium used to communicate the message, (3) the format and content of the message, and (4) the nature of the change that the message advocates.[5]

Furthermore, the implication extends to the notion that such considerations are relevant for any health-promoting communication, from an hour-long video presentation on the dangers of tobacco use, to the brief smoking-cessation advice that a physician might give to a patient.

This chapter reviews the concept of cultural sensitivity as it relates to the development and implementation of smoking-control interventions. The importance of incorporating various aspects of cultural sensitivity into program planning, development, and implementation are described, recognizing both barriers and opportunities that are inherent in existing health-care delivery systems.

This perspective is used to further define a broader health-promotion framework through which cultural issues can better be understood. In addition, recommendations are made regarding actions that should be taken to improve the cultural fit between smoking-related health-promotion activities and the population groups that are currently being underserved.

Cultural Sensitivity in Intervention Program Development

Smoking-cessation researchers have long recognized that smoking is a complex behavior influenced by a variety of physiological, psychological, cognitive, and social factors. Though interventions to aid smokers in their

TABLE 3.1. Phases of intervention development research.

Phase 1:	Basic psychosocial research and hypothesis development
Phase 2:	Methods development and feasibility testing
Phase 3:	Efficacy and internal validity testing
Phase 4:	Effectiveness and external validity testing
Phase 5:	Implementation and dissemination research

attempts to quit have been available since before the turn of the century,[6] a major emphasis has been placed since the 1970s on public health relevance and on substantiating the widely ranging claims for the various approaches, in an effort to identify those approaches that should be made widely available.

The strategy that has been employed for this purpose has been a multiphase process based fundamentally upon controlled clinical trials.[7] These phases, as described in Table 3.1 flow logically from the development of basic hypotheses regarding intervention approaches that are promising, to the development of those hypotheses into testable methods, and then to their testing in successively larger-scale evaluation studies. The emphasis in these later phases of the process shifts from the earlier highly controlled efficacy studies to determine whether the intervention works under optimal conditions, to the later larger-scale effectiveness and demonstration studies to determine the degree to which the intervention is generalizable to the less-than-ideal settings found in the real world.

In this research-focused paradigm, the question of cultural sensitivity can become relevant at either of two points during the five-phase process. Either cultural sensitivity is considered an element of basic research that can be used to generate original hypotheses regarding the development and testing of culturally relevant interventions, or it is considered a secondary issue related to the generalizability of so-called proven interventions.

Generally speaking, the latter approach has been the rule and the former approach the exception. In most cases, priority has been given to showing first that interventions are effective under more or less ideal conditions before issues such as generalizability to special populations have been considered.

From an evaluation-research perspective, such ideal conditions are typically defined by the use of homogeneous study groups in settings that are easily accessible and where follow-up is either routine or, at the very least, feasible. Because the focus of such research is on (1) minimizing measurement error, (2) identifying explainable sources of variance, and (3) maximizing a researcher's ability to detect clinically meaningful intervention effects, this approach is not only justifiable, but it also represents state-of-the-art research methodology.

Policymakers, legislators, and other decision makers require at least this semblance of experimental rigor if research such as this is to be applied in any meaningful way.[8] Special-populations research, on the other hand, requires special considerations. From the identification of study samples, to the delivery of interventions, and then the recontacting of those samples for follow-up assessments, study populations that are defined according to racial, ethnic, or cultural criteria represent formidable challenges. The fact that the majority of the researchers who have contributed to this intervention development process are not themselves members of special population groups has made these challenges even more formidable.[9]

Nonetheless, explanations and rationalizations aside, the issue remains that the progress of the 1970s and 1980s in developing effective smoking control interventions, as the Surgeon General's report correctly noted, has not involved special population groups. The current challenge and the one that this chapter addresses is to identify what steps can be taken now to rectify this deficit.

Cultural Sensitivity and Its Limitations

In order to appreciate the relevance of cultural sensitivity in the development and implementation of effective smoking control interventions, it is important to first clarify a number of errors that are sometimes made in the classification of special populations. First and most significantly, the general population cannot be usefully dichotomized as minority and nonminority. As the various subgroups within society grow in numbers, this distinction is rapidly losing salience. More important, such a dichotomy fails to even address the issue of cultural specificity and sociocultural matching between intervention approaches and population subgroups in any meaningful way.

Second, it is very important to distinguish between the culture of the underclass in society[10] and ethnically, racially, or culturally defined population subgroups. The experience of poverty in society is different from the experience of being Hispanic, for example, and each of these must be further distinguished from the experience of being both poor and Hispanic.

Third, culturally relevant interventions must take into account that the broad racial and ethnic categories frequently used by demographers (e.g., Asian American, American Indian, African American, and Hispanic) mask important differences among subgroups included within these broad categories.

Keeping such distinctions in mind, the concept of cultural sensitivity can be directly addressed. Both cultural sensitivity and its significance for intervention programs are very poorly understood by most health professionals. What is understood is that health promotion efforts such as smoking-cessation interventions involve a form of communication between practitioners and clients.

Though it may be clear to them, generally speaking, that communications that are salient, relevant, and sensitive to the needs, concerns, and

TABLE 3.2. The cultural sophistication framework.

Dimensions	Culturally incompetent	Culturally sensitive	Culturally competent
Cognitive dimension	Oblivious	Aware	Knowledgeable
Affective dimension	Apathetic	Sympathetic	Committed to change
Skills dimension	Unskilled	Lacking skills	Highly skilled
Overall effect	Destructive	Neutral	Constructive

idiosyncrasies of a culturally defined population group are much more likely to achieve their intended objectives, the implications for them specifically as deliverers of such interventions are far less clear.

The distinctions made in Table 3.2 should help to clarify some of this ambiguity by introducing the concept of *cultural sophistication*, to describe the ways in which attempts to bridge the cultural communication gap can vary with respect to degree of constructiveness. According to this framework, cultural sensitivity can be viewed as a state of mind or a general orientation in which the individual is aware that there is a problem, is sympathetic to the needs of the cultural group in question, but lacks some significant skills needed to intervene effectively. At best, the overall effect of this type of individual is likely to be neutral.

This is certainly preferable to being oblivious to the problem, apathetic, and utterly lacking in the requisite skills, the overall effect of which could be destructive. Yet neither of these types would be as culturally sophisticated as someone who fully understands the issues involved, is fully committed to change, and is highly skilled in the areas needed. Individuals of this type display a type of cultural sophistication that goes beyond cultural sensitivity to what might be called "cultural competence."

Obviously, these are only stereotyped representations of specific points along a continuum ranging from the highest levels of cultural competence to the lowest. Nonetheless, it is important to note that cultural competence should be thought of as a prerequisite to the successful communication of smoking-cessation intervention messages. It is not enough to be merely culturally sensitive.

Overview of Opportunities

Though the foregoing may shed some light on the nature of the problem, the question remains as to what form the possible solutions might take. From a public-health perspective, there are three areas in which efforts are clearly needed: first, to eliminate or at least to minimize the destructive effects of cultural incompetence; second, to develop cultural competence among those who are culturally sensitive; and third, to make the most efficacious and cost-effective use of such advances to bridge the health-promotion culture gap that persists today.

Essentially, this would involve facilitating the development and movement of individuals who are in any way involved with the health-promotion process along the cultural sophistication continuum toward enhanced competence.

First, the researchers, program developers, and others actively involved in the design and evaluation of health-promoting interventions should become more culturally competent so that the cross-cultural applicability of the materials and programs available will be improved.[11] Second, those delivering interventions or health-related communications on any level, from physicians to health educators, should strive to enhance their own cultural competence and should make use of the most effective intervention materials and approaches available.[12] Third, as advances are made in the cultural competence of smoking-cessation interventions, these should be accompanied by concomitant adjustments and modifications in the ways that these advances are disseminated to the general public. Fourth, any advances made in the development, delivery, and utilization of culturally competent smoking-control interventions will be limited in terms of their public health impact by the degree to which organizations, institutions, and society as a whole accepts these advances.

Overview of Barriers

For these opportunities for increased cultural competence to be realized, many significant barriers must be overcome. At the research and program development level, incentives must be provided that will shift the efforts of more researchers and developers toward culturally competent interventions. The federal government through its National Institutes of Health (NIH) must take the lead in developing such research and development programs through comprehensive funding initiatives.

Though several important research projects dealing with the development of culturally relevant smoking-control interventions have been funded, these have lacked the direction, coordination, and funding commitment that NIH has provided many of its better-known research programs. One of the many examples of this sort of commitment is the National Cancer Institute's School-Based Smoking Prevention Research Initiative, which funded research teams nationwide to conduct 5-year collaborative studies that resulted in a consensus document that would not have been possible without this type of direction and coordination.[13] In the area of culturally competent smoking-control interventions, this level of consensus is definitely lacking and obviously needed.

For health professionals and educators who are involved in the delivery of smoking-control interventions, the key to improving cultural competence lies in enhanced training opportunities. Such opportunities should be provided both at the basic training level (i.e., in medical school, nursing school, graduate school, etc.) and through various kinds of continuing education. National organizations such as the American Medical Association (AMA) and the National League for Nursing (NLN) must take the lead in expanding their curricula to include opportunities for developing cultural competence. This type of effort would be an important step toward the elimination of cultural incompetence among health professionals.

Related continuing education opportunities have been made available through national organizations such as the American Public Health Association, the National Coalition of Hispanic Health and Human Services Organizations, and the National Center for the Advancement of Blacks in the Health Professions. The need now is to expand these activities and to make them available to as many culturally sensitive professionals as possible.

For the public-at-large, a number of factors must be taken into consideration if dissemination and promotion efforts for culturally sophisticated interventions are to proceed effectively. These include

1. Language and semantic barriers—When language, semantic structures, and symbols are used that are not understandable or are misunderstood, promotional messages may fail to have an impact.
2. Reading level and reading interest—If printed materials are used, they must take into account the reading abilities and the degree of interest that the intended target group has in reading.
3. Models and perceived sources—If prominent individuals are used as role models or as perceived sources for promotional messages who are not well known to the members of the target group, then they are unlikely to have the desired effect.
4. Communication salience—The core of the promotion, that which is being conveyed by the communication as a whole, must be appropriate and culturally syntonic to the group that the message is trying to reach.
5. Believable objectives—The promotion must convey that, contrary to past experiences, the culturally sophisticated intervention was designed with cultural subgroup participation as a primary objective rather than as an afterthought.
6. Welfare stigma—From the perspective of the underclass in society, it is important to anticipate the commonly held view that health-promotion efforts are handouts and to be avoided therefore as a matter of pride.
7. Relevance—Individuals who are members of special populations may tend to view efforts to control cigarette smoking as irrelevant and to feel that more pressing societal concerns such as poverty, crime, unemployment, and hunger should be addressed first.
8. Entropy—Given their past experiences with social change in the United States, there may be a tendency for members of special population groups to perceive themselves as powerless or helpless when confronted

with the force of prevailing socioeconomic barriers, and to adopt a nonparticipatory attitude toward self-improvement activities as a result.

However, even significant advances in cultural competence among researchers and developers, practitioners and educators, and the general public will be tempered without analogous changes at the organizational, institutional, and societal levels.[14] Organizations and institutions that employ researchers, program developers, practitioners, and educators must provide their staff with the opportunities and the reinforcement to participate in activities that will enhance cultural competence. Corporate entities such as the train, subway, and bus companies, and magazines and newspapers that choose to accept money from advertisers who promote smoking specifically among special population groups must stop this unjustifiable practice; and no matter how unlikely it may seem, the tobacco companies themselves must be persuaded to cease and desist this disservice to racially, ethnically, and culturally defined population groups.

A Framework for Change: The Expert Linkage Approach

The issues related to cultural competence, as outlined in the foregoing, represent a type of bidirectional technology transfer problem. What is called for as part of the fundamental strategy for bridging this gap is that two disparate sources of information and expertise be brought together, analyzed, and then synthesized into a new information base that can be utilized by all concerned. Havelock[15] referred to this type of problem-solving communication system as a "linkage system," and in this case, the term would appropriately describe the type of exchange among experts that is needed—an *expert linkage system*.

One body of expertise is represented by all that is currently known in the area of smoking-control intervention research. As the latest Surgeon General's report has indicated and the foregoing has underscored, clinicians and researchers have learned a great deal about smoking control in terms of what is effective and what is not effective. It is important that this knowledge and skill base be utilized to the fullest in developing culturally sophisticated smoking-control initiatives.

The other knowledge and skill base reflects all that is known regarding cultural sophistication in communicating and collaborating with particular special populations, as the foregoing has delineated. The optimal strategy for developing and delivering culturally sophisticated smoking-control interventions requires that individuals representing these different knowledge and skill bases engage in collaborative technology transfer.

The key to making this concept a reality is that each of the knowledge and skill bases that are represented within the linkage system must be viewed by all concerned as a source of expertise that must be utilized and without which the desired end result could not be achieved. The whole then truly becomes greater than the sum of the individual parts.

It is important to note in this regard that the two conceptual systems described do not necessarily make reference to two separate and discrete groups of individuals. On the contrary, there are individuals who have the ability to contribute to both sides of the collaborative exchange described and who should be encouraged to do so.

Plans for Action and Concluding Thoughts

Many of the actions that need to be taken at both the organizational and the individual levels in order to achieve improvements in the cultural sophistication have already begun. Agencies of the federal government, such as the NIH, have begun to take a greater interest in the issues related to culturally appropriate interventions.

For example, a new multi-institutional research program project that will focus on the study of smoking behavior among African Americans has been funded by the National Cancer Institute and is scheduled to commence operations in New York City in 1991.[16] As these and similar research and development activities are initiated, opportunities for the type of collaborative exchange that is now needed will improve.

Despite these and related activities that will, it is hoped, be engaged in more and more frequently and that should be encouraged at the organizational, institutional, and societal levels, there are a number of actions that individuals who are concerned about this problem can take right now to begin to address the issues themselves, both personally and as advocates to associates.

First, and most important, an individual should characterize him- or herself (or associates) as accurately as possible according to the dimensions provided in Table 3.2. This is a useful way to acknowledge that, though well-intentioned, some individuals may be quite far from any useful level of cultural competence.

Second, an analogous assessment should be carried out to determine the breadth and depth of knowledge and skills pertaining to smoking-cessation interventions.

Third, as gaps are identified, they should be addressed specifically. Individuals should try to take advantage of any organized, agency-sponsored opportunity to learn more about the knowledge and skills required both for aiding smokers in their attempts to quit and for becoming more culturally competent.

Fourth, until more organized and coordinated training activities are made available, individuals should seek out additional opportunities on their own to learn more in these areas through reading any relevant materials that can be found, and by discussing the issues with others who are interested.

In conclusion, it should be noted that simply reading a chapter such as this is neither necessary nor sufficient for the development of either cultural competence or smoking-cessation intervention skills. On the other hand, an analysis such as this can make readers more aware of the opportunities and more motivated to overcome the barriers, and if it does so, it has more than fulfilled its primary objective.

References

1. U.S. Department of Health and Human Services (USDHHS). Reducing the health consequences of smoking—25 years of progress: A report of the Surgeon General. Washington, DC: U.S. Gov Printing Office, 1989.
2. McCord C, Freeman HP. Excess mortality in Harlem. New Engl J of Med 1990; 322: 173–177.
3. U.S. Department of Health and Human Services (USDHHS). Proceedings of prospects for a healthier America: Achieving the nation's health promotion objectives. Washington, DC: U.S. Gov Printing Office, 1984.
4. Loo C, Fong KT, Iwamasa G. Ethnicity and cultural diversity: An analysis of work published in community psychology journals, 1965–1985. Amer J of Community Psychology 1988; 16: 332–349.
5. Orlandi MA. Community-based substance abuse prevention: A multicultural perspective. J of School Health 1986; 56: 394–401.
6. Dillow GL. The hundred-year war against the cigarette. Washington DC: Tobacco Institute, 1981.
7. Greenwald P, Cullen JW. The scientific approach to cancer control. CA: A Cancer Journal for Clinicians 1985; 34: 328–332.
8. Orlandi MA. Strategic planning for school-based tobacco control initiatives: An analysis of opportunities and barriers. In: The Pennsylvania planning Conference on Tobacco and Health Priorities.
9. Schinke SP, Schilling RF, Palleja J, Zayas LH. Prevention research among ethnic–racial minority group adolescents. Behav Therapist 1987; 10: 151–155.
10. Mincy RB, Sawhill IV, Wolf DA. The underclass: Definition and measurement. Science 1990; 248: 450–453.
11. Botvin GJ, Schinke SP, Orlandi MA. Psychosocial approaches to substance abuse prevention: Theoretical foundations and empirical findings. Crisis 1989; 10: 62–67.
12. Freeman HP, Bernard L, Matory W, Smith FA, Whittico JM, Bond L. Physician manpower needs of the nation. J of the Nat Med Assoc 1982; 74 (7) 617–619.
13. Glynn T. School programs to prevent smoking: The National Cancer Institute guide to strategies that succeed. USDHHS, NIH Pub No. 90–500. Washington, DC: U.S. Government Printing Office, 1990: 1–24.
14. Orlandi MA. Promoting health and preventing disease in health care settings: An analysis of barriers. Prev Med 1987; 16: 119–130.

15. Havelock RG. Planning for innovation through dissemination and utilization of knowledge. Center for Research on Utilization of Scientific Knowledge, University of Michigan, Ann Arbor, Michigan, 1973.
16. Wynder EL, Freeman HP. Personal communication; August, 1990.

4
Smokeless Tobacco

JAMES A. COCORES

Columbus brought syphilis to the Indians, and they gave him tobacco. It is doubtful
which is worse.   *Harry S. Truman*

Cigarettes are a very recent invention when compared to the long history
of smokeless tobacco. Before the advent of cigarettes, snuff ravaged entire
towns and nations. Even European aristocracy was not exempted. Cigarettes, by virtue of their convenience and relatively "clean" delivery rapidly
replaced the disgusting habits of tobacco snuff and chew.

Smokeless tobacco is making a comeback. One of the reasons that
smokeless is becoming more attractive than cigarettes to young users is the
proliferation of messages bombarding the public regarding the dangers of
cigarette smoking. Anticigarette education campaigns, such as teaching
children to "just say no" to cigarettes, no-smoking policies in the workplace or at home, and smoking restrictions in airplanes, restaurants, and
other public places are paying off with regard to educating people about
the severity of cigarette dependence. Unfortunately, the strong anti-
cigarette message may make smokeless tobacco appear less hazardous in
comparison.

The public, especially young people, must become better educated
about the dangers of smokeless tobacco because the public has been de-
ceived before into thinking that one delivery system is safer than another.
The advent of cigarette filters was the first major attempt to quiet some of
the public fears regarding the health hazards of filterless cigarettes. Advertisements such as "L&M Filters are Just What the Doctor Ordered!"[1]
began appearing. Then more "rumors" of an association between cigarette
smoking and lung cancer, pulmonary disease, and cardiovascular problems prompted a stroke of genius, which was the marketing campaign for
"light" cigarettes. Today, it is known that light smokers just smoke more
to reach the nicotine level achieved by smokers of regular-brand cigarettes.
Society should not deceive young patients and their parents by not putting
smokeless tobacco on the same plane as cigarettes.

Prevalence

The number of smokeless tobacco users in the United States is estimated at about 12 million,[2] and it is the fastest-growing form of nicotine addiction among young adults and children.[3] The average consumer of smokeless tobacco is between 18 and 24 years of age.[4] Smokeless tobacco users are primarily male, although one study reported that 1% of the adolescent females surveyed used it daily.[5] Over 80% of smokeless tobacco users first experiment with the drug before the age of 15. Most patients treated for smokeless dependence at our northern New Jersey clinics are white male athletes in high school or college and compose about 1% of nicotine-dependent patients treated.[6] However, the prevalence of smokeless tobacco use varies greatly, depending on the town or region. Thirteen percent of third-grade boys and about 22% of fifth-grade boys in Oklahoma use smokeless tobacco regularly.[7] A study of high school students in Oregon found 23% of tenth-grade males to be daily users.[8] An alarming 21% of kindergarten children in Arkansas have tried smokeless tobacco.[9]

Methods of Use

Snuff was a popular form of nicotine delivery centuries ago. Snuff use is most similar to the way in which cocaine is sniffed or snorted; the finger tips are placed in the finely ground tobacco powder then sniffed through the nostrils. The only place where snuff boxes abound today in America is at Sotheby's, where elaborate snuff boxes from the 1700s are auctioned for thousands of dollars.

There are two basic methods in which smokeless tobacco is used today: dipping and chewing. *Chewing* involves the mastication of a wad of shredded tobacco leaves in the cheek area. *Dipping* involves placing dip tobacco between two fingers and placing the drug between the lower jaw and cheek area, where it is worked like a lozenge. Manufacturers of smokeless tobacco add alkaline materials to dip and chewing tobacco because greater amounts of nicotine enter the buccal mucosa at an alkaline pH, whereas an acidic preparation is necessary for optimal pulmonary absorption of nicotine from cigarettes. Contrary to popular belief, the blood nicotine level achieved by using smokeless tobacco often reaches that achieved by smoking cigarettes.[9] Also, smokeless nicotine blood levels remain higher in comparison to the shorter spiked nicotine blood level that results from smoking a cigarette.

Etiology

The factors contributing to the development of smokeless dependence are similar to other drug addictions. Three primary areas are involved: genetic or biological factors, familial–occupational–cultural factors, and individual personality traits.

Although a small number of animal and twin studies have been conducted specifically with nicotine, research is essentially nonexistent with respect to genetic factors contributing to the development of smokeless dependence. Based on genetic research with alcoholism, it is unlikely that a specific gene or gene group alone is at the root of smokeless dependence. It is more likely that smokeless dependence is, in part, the expression of a group of genes responsible for a neurological variant, which lends itself to ongoing substance abuse and chemical dependence in general. Smokeless tobacco abuse is chosen as a function of availability.

Much more is known about environmental influences relating to the development of smokeless tobacco dependence. Parents may perceive smokeless tobacco as less of a health risk and less addicting than cigarettes. Therefore, the image of a chewer or dipper may be viewed positively in comparison to cigarette smokers. Although using or nonusing parents and relatives can influence a child's decision to try smokeless tobacco, this is not the strongest environmental influence. The most influential noncommercial advertisers for smokeless tobacco are friends and siblings who use. A nonuser is more likely to begin chewing tobacco by having more peers or close friends that chew.[10] The marked resurgence of smokeless tobacco use among young people is also a direct result of marketing by tobacco companies, which use prominent sports figures and entertainers to promote their product. This is done in movies, as is also the case with cigarettes. Sports figures, especially baseball players[11] and rodeo stars, are a few other forms of smokeless tobacco advertising that impress young viewers. The beer industry is a prime example of how a legal drug can be marketed very effectively when coupled with sporting events. Like cigarettes, smokeless tobacco is used by "cool" personalities and athletes. Children idolize and emulate such figures.

Specific personality traits preexist or develop as a direct result of drug dependence. Dependence-prone personality traits—such as lacking moderation, constantly blaming others, and difficulty with impulse control—also contribute to the etiology of smokeless tobacco dependence. There is also evidence to suggest that smokeless tobacco users have more difficulty trusting others and are more aloof, reserved, detached, tough-minded, likely to have used marijuana/alcohol, unsentimental, and more group-dependent when compared to nonusers.[8] Dippers are more group-dependent than chewers. Smokeless neophytes also choose to experiment because the behavior may be perceived as rebellious, antiestablishment or oppositional. It is most important to realize that smokeless neophytes often choose to disregard the health hazards of nicotine use and believe that they are invincible and will beat the odds of becoming dependent. Most neophytes cannot comprehend the involuntary bondage of drug dependence. Neophytes also believe that they are intelligent enough to use in moderation or to stop before any problem surfaces. Smokeless tobacco can look incredibly "cool" in the eyes of the beholder.

Medical Consequences

Smokeless tobacco is not safe. It increases the risk of oral and pharyngeal cancer.[12] Gingival blood flow is reduced by smokeless tobacco, resulting in ischemia and necrosis. Epinephrine release is augmented, which contributes to hypertension and cardiac anomalies. Other oral problems include gingival recession, soft tissue alterations, and leukoplakia.[3]

Although these and many other physical consequences of smokeless tobacco are useful educational deterrents for adults and children who have not yet experimented, conveying this information to smokeless neophytes is unlikely, in itself, to motivate the user toward abstinence and recovery. Instead, it is important to focus on the medical consequence that most often follows experimentation, which is smokeless tobacco dependence. It is most important to understand that once children or adolescents first use smokeless tobacco, they are in an extremely high risk group for

1. Progression to smokeless dependence
2. Progression and transfer to cigarettes
3. Experimentation and progression with alcohol
4. Experimentation with marijuana and other addictive drugs
5. Polydrug dependence

Therefore, the most common and devastating medical consequence of experimentation with smokeless tobacco is polydrug dependence. Users are more likely to relate to the topic of drug progression rather than a distant consequence such as oral cancer.

Prevention and Treatment

The prevention, diagnosis, and treatment of nicotine dependence is similar in all its forms: cigarette, cigar, pipe, smokeless tobacco, nicotine gum, or any combination. There are more similarities than differences between cigarette dependence and smokeless tobacco dependence. Only some of the treatment considerations specific to smokeless tobacco are discussed here.

Education is prevention, and that is the single best weapon clinicians have against smokeless dependence. One must first be aware of the regional incidence and the medical, psychological, and social risk factors involved. It is not only important to educate patients in our offices but also to present the topic at local elementary and junior high schools.

Because most of the patients treated for smokeless tobacco abuse or dependence are young, they are not as physically dependent as their older counterparts. It is also unlikely that they were treated previously. Therefore, it is important to begin treatment by involving a friend or relative and educating them both about nicotine dependence. Behavioral and cognitive approaches are also essential components of the treatment plan. For example, it is extremely important for smokeless users initially to avoid people with whom they used smokeless tobacco and stores at which they purchased smokeless tobacco.

Nicotine fading with someless tobacco can be difficult, compared to cigarette fading. Cigarettes are dispensed in more consistent measurable quantities, and therefore it can be easier to gradually taper nicotine doses using cigarettes. Smokeless tobacco also lends itself to specific settings or places because it augments salivation, while cigarettes are smoked almost anywhere, but this is changing. Hard candy or non-nicotine-containing chewing gum can be especially useful during the fading and abstinence phase. patients report that chewing gum is especially useful because of the oral gratification it provides. For a chewer, the oral gratification includes motor aspects, texture, and flavor. It is unfortunate, interesting, and ironic to note that Sigmund Freud could not get enough oral gratification from tobacco even after decades of a 20-cigar-per-day habit and 33 surgical interventions for oral cancer.[13] Chewing gum is a helpful practice during early recovery from smokeless tobacco. It is also very useful when treating nicotine polacrilex dependence.[14]

If nonpharmacologic methods are unsuccessful, or when severe physical dependence to smokeless tobacco exists, such as smokeless addicts over the age of 25 years nicotine replacement or other medicines or both may be needed. Transdermal nicotine is probably superior to nicotine gum for chew dependence. That is, the chewing behavior is replaced by using non-nicotine-containing gum, and the physical dependence is addressed by gradually reducing or fading the nicotine blood level using transdermal nicotine patches. Chewers are more likely to abuse nicotine polacrilex gum. Dippers, on the other hand, are accustomed to parking tobacco between their jaw and cheek already and therefore are much more likely to use nicotine gum properly.

When medically appropriate, transdermal clonidine can be used alone or in conjunction with nicotine replacement. Other experimental smokeless-tobacco-cessation medicines, such as low-dose imipramine, transdermal scopolamine, or bromocriptine, are being used in clinical practice to treat smokeless dependence, but there are insufficient data to substantiate claims of efficacy objectively.

The most important prerequisite to treatment planning is that the clinician does not leave the patient with the impression that smokeless recovery is focused around either a medicine or nicotine replacement. The recovery program should be well balanced to include behavioral–cognitive techniques, relapse prevention, family or friend involvement, education, nutrition, exercise, and ongoing support.

Conclusion

Smokeless tobacco use and dependence is on the rise. Clinicians should familiarize themselves with this often-overlooked form of nicotine dependence. Often, we will not find smokeless tobacco dependence unless we look for it. Therefore, smokeless tobacco should be included in the nicotine portion of the adolescent drug history.

References

1. Carrell S. When more doctors smoked Camels. Am Medical News 1989; 6(23): 36.
2. U.S. Public Health Service. The consequences of using smokeless tobacco: A report of the Advisory Committee of the Surgeon General. Department of Health, DHEW Publication No. (PHS) 86–2874. Washington, DC: U.S. Government Printing Office, 1986.
3. Glover ED, Schroeder KL, Henningfield JE, et al. An interpretive review of smokeless tobacco research in the United States. Part I. J of Drug Educ 1988; 18(4): 285.
4. Maxwell JC. Maxwell manufacturing products report: Chewing stuff is growth segment. Tobacco Rep 1980; 107: 32.
5. Severson HH, Lictensten E, Gallison C. A pinch instead of a puff? Implications of chewing tobacco for addictive process. Bull of Soc Psychi Addict Behav 1985; 4: 85.
6. Cocores JA. Nicotine addiction. In: Miller N, ed. Handbook of drug and alcohol addiction. New York: Marcel Dekker, 1990: 437.
7. Glover ED, Edwards SW. Current research in smokeless tobacco. Shangrila, OK: Annual Association for HPER, 1984.
8. Edmundson EW, Glover ED, Alston PP, et al. Personality traits of smokeless tobacco users and nonusers: A comparison. Intl J of Addict 1987; 22(7): 671.
9. Young M, Williamson D. Correlates of use and expected use of smokeless tobacco among kindergarten children. Psychia Rep 1985; 56: 63.
10. Ary DV, Lichtenstein EL, Severson HH. Smokeless tobacco use among adolescents: Patterns, correlates, predications, and the use of other drugs. Prev Med 1987; 16: 385.
11. Wisneiewski JK, Bartolucci AA. Comparative patterns of smokeless tobacco usage among major league baseball personnel. J of Oral Pathol Med 1989; 18: 322.
12. Hoffman D, Hecht SS. Nicotine-derived N-nitrosamines and tobacco related cancer. Cancer Res 1985; 45: 2285.
13. Fleiss W. Is tobacco truly addicting? South Medical J 1988; 81(9): 1084.
14. Cocores JA, Sinaikin P, Gold MS. Scopolamine as treatment for nicotine polacrilex dependence. Ann of Clin Psychi 1989; 1: 203.

5
The Biobehavioral Effects of Nicotine: Interactions with Brain Neurochemical Systems*

JOHN A. ROSECRANS

Possibly except for caffeine, nicotine is consumed (via a variety of tobacco products) by more humans than any other drug humans have thus far discovered. Its popularity greatly transcends the knowledge of its potential long-term toxic effects, suggesting that nicotine has powerful psychopharmacological effects that appear to be important to the initiation of use and the development of dependence to tobacco. As described by several authors, this drug induces a very powerful dependence in humans, which appears to surpass that induced by even heroin or alcohol. Thus, what is it about this unique chemical agent that makes it reinforcing from a biobehavioral perspective?

An examination of nicotine's chemical structure reveals few unique features (Figure 5.1) that might suggest it to be extremely active as a drug of dependence. On the other hand, few other chemicals have a pharmacological profile of action similar to this chemical,[1] which may indicate that this drug is quite specific as to how it interacts with active sites in the brain. Except for its less active optical isomer, (+)-nicotine, and a chemical relative, 3-pyrridyl-methyl-pyrrolidine (a chemical isomer), there are relatively few other compounds that appear to act like nicotine; both of the other compounds possess about one 10th the potency of nicotine in several behavioral tests.

To better understand how nicotine might be producing its rewarding effects (that is, self-administration by humans), we need to appreciate the complexity of how the brain communicates and how nicotine might interact with brain neurochemical systems that make it pleasurable to humans. We also need to look at how these neuronal interactions make it so difficult for tobacco users to reduce this drug-taking behavior. This chapter attempts to shed some light as to potential answers to these questions, at least from the perspective of how nicotine may be interacting with neurons involved

*This work was partially supported by a grant from the National Institute on Drug Abuse (DA-R01-04002-4).

53

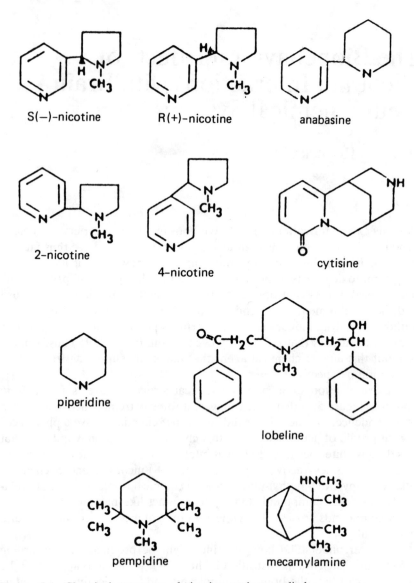

FIGURE 5.1. Chemical structures of nicotine analogs studied.

in maintaining behavior. This work will not be all-inclusive of the research reported in this area, as there are several reviews on the subject, not the least of which is the recent report of the U.S. Surgeon General.[2] Rather, this review attempts to provide an overview of how I view nicotine's interactions at cholinergic and other receptors that enable nicotine to provide a rewarding stimulus.

Effects of Nicotine on Cholinergic Neurons

Peripheral Versus Central Receptors

Students enrolled in pharmacology courses are taught that nicotine acts peripherally at specific receptors, which are cholinergic in nature—that is, nicotine mimics the neurotransmitter acetylcholine (ACh) at specific nicotinic–cholinergic receptors (n–AChRs). These receptors are located primarily within the autonomic nervous system (ANS) at preganglionic sites of both the parasympathetic (in which Ach is the major transmitter released from postganglionic neurons) and the sympathetic (in which norepinephrine is the major transmitter released from postganglionic neurons) divisions of this system. Nicotinic receptors are also the major postsynaptic receptors of neurons innervating both the neuromuscular junction and the adrenal gland. Neurons of both ANS divisions, for the most part, are arranged in a series in which the first neuron is nicotinic and the second muscarinic or noradrenergic.

Domino,[3] using neuropharmacological strategies, developed a model of the brain, which views n–AChRs and muscarinic–cholinergic receptors (m–AChRs) as being innervated by cholinergic neuronal systems independent of each other. Domino showed that nicotine-induced EEG arousal was antagonized by *mecamylamine*, a centrally (central nervous system— (NS) acting nicotinic antagonist, while *atropine*, a centrally acting muscarinic antagonist, was unable to block nicotine's effects. In contrast, the EEG-arousing effects of *arecoline*, a potent CNS-acting muscarinic agonist, was completely attenuated by atropine but not by mecamylamine. This research clearly provided a working model of central AChRs (acetylcholine receptors) in which these receptors were physiologically independent of each other. From a neuroanatomical and/or neurophysiological point of view, however, little is known about the specific pre- and postsynaptic localization of either of these receptor populations.

Furthermore, more recent findings suggest that a portion of the n–AChRs located in the brain may be located on presynaptic cholinergic and/or noncholinergic neurons, which is reminiscent of the arrangement in the ANS. Thus, these peripheral and central systems may not be as different as we have recently thought.

Nicotine-Induced n–AChR Desensitization

The preceding concept that nicotine is acting primarily as an agonist at these cholinergic receptors by mimicking the effects of ACh also needs to be revised. More recent research has provided us with a somewhat different view, especially as to what is occurring at the n–AChR. An important contribution to this work was the finding that nicotine, when administered repeatedly, induces an upregulation of n–AChRs,[4,5,6,7] which is contrary to what one would expect, considering that nicotine is acting as an agonist. Modern receptor theory assumes that agonists down regulate, while antagonists upregulate receptors, as a function of an active negative feedback mechanism resulting from the drug–receptor interaction. The logic of this suggests that nicotine may be inducing an antagonism of the n–AChR.

While difficult to reconcile with what we know about nicotine's action, this finding has assisted in understanding how nicotine may be affecting behavior. First, nicotine does not appear to be acting as an antagonist, as evidenced by the fact that mecamylamine (Figure 5.1) is extremely effective in antagonizing nicotine's effects on behavior, at least its acute effects. Furthermore, if nicotine was acting as an n–AChR antagonist, then one might expect mecamylamine to act similarly to nicotine, which has yet to be demonstrated. Second, the ability of nicotine to upregulate n–AChRs does appear to correlate with nicotine-induced tolerance[8] in studies involving schedule-controlled responding. Interestingly, mecamylamine, which has been shown to antagonize nicotine's acute effects on the same behavior, was unable to attenuate the development of tolerance to the same acute disruptive behavioral effect, suggesting that tolerance development and acute behavioral disruption may be occurring via a different mechanism. Supporting this behavioral finding, Kellar and coworkers[9] have also shown that mecamylamine was unable to antagonize the upre-

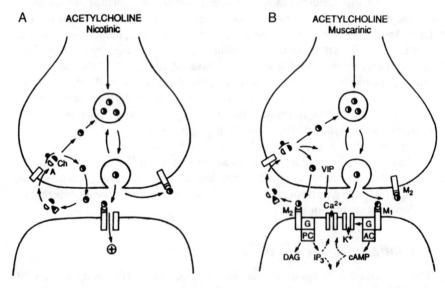

FIGURE 5.2. A schematic comparison of (A) nicotinic and (B) muscarinic cholinergic neurons. The n–AChR is viewed as linked to a cation channel, while the m–AChR appears to mediate its effects via a second messenger, IP$_3$, inositol triphosphate or c-AMP, adenosine 3',5'-cyclic monophosphate. (Redrawn from Shephard[32] with permission.)

gulation of n–AChR binding following chronic nicotine administration, showing again, a dissociation between nicotine and mecamylamine's sites of action.

The importance of these findings is twofold. First, the data suggests that nicotine and mecamylamine, even though appearing to be mutually antagonistic, may be acting at different sites of the receptor, and, as suggested by Stolerman,[10] the differences might be related to a direct effect of mecamylamine at a postsynaptic neuronal channel. Second, the finding that nicotine is capable of inducing an upregulation of the nicotinic receptor brings forth a concept that nicotine at some level may be producing these effects by desensitizing the n–AChR. This concept has been discussed by

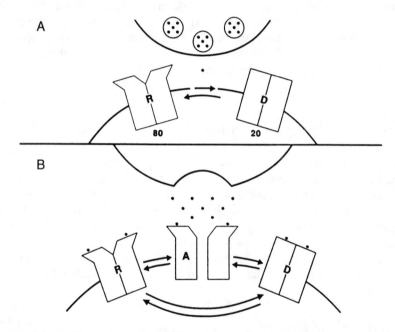

FIGURE 5.3. Mechanisms of n–AChR desensitizations. This figure represents an idealized nicotinic–cholinergic synaptic cholinergic junction containing acetylcholine (black dots), which is contained within synaptic vesicles (shown in circles) and postsynaptic membrane. (taken from Ochoa et al.[12] with permission.) A: The receptor exists in an equilibrium condition of a mixture of two forms—resting (R) and desensitized (D) states. B: An action potential facilitates the release of ACh. The result is a sudden increase in ACh concentration at the synaptic cleft and occupies one of the two receptor states, R and D. This induces a conformational change, which leads to the activated state (A), in which the channel opens, allowing cation movements essential for the development of a postsynaptic action potential. As soon as ACh occupies its sites, the affinity of the receptors toward ACh increases, and the D state is promoted, which results in the termination of the action of ACh.

many investigators, such as Susan Wonnacott,[11] who consider desensitization mechanisms as potentially important to smoking behavior.

This concept suggests that the nicotinic receptor is sensitive to ACh or substances that mimic its effects, and that agonists acting at this receptor will induce an initial opening of a neuronal postsynaptic channel, allowing the entrance of some cation as Ca^{++} (calcium), K^+ (potassium), or Na^+ (sodium) (Figures 5.2 and 5.3). The entrance of the cation serves as a second messenger or signal, which initiates a secondary postsynaptic effect, resulting in the transmission of information; an inhibitory or excitatory signal can be transmitted. Data obtained[12] by evaluating the effects of ACh at the cation channel indicate that both ACh and nicotine may act similarly, in that following an initial opening of the channel, they are also capable of inducing a transition state—receptor desensitization—which closes the receptor, to prevent further entrance (into the cell) of some cation, such as Ca^{++}. An additional correlate to this mechanism suggests that mecamylamine may be acting directly at the channel, inducing a similar transitional desensitized state, which would result in an antagonism of nicotine's effects.

Effects of Nicotine on Noncholinergic Neurons

Research conducted over the past 20 years has provided much data that nicotine, in addition to its effects at specific n–AChRs, may also interact with other amine-containing neurons, such as serotonergic (5-HT), dopaminergic (DA) and noradrenergic (NE) systems[13] (Figure 5.4). As demonstrated by many investigators, these systems make up a very important brain modulatory system, which can influence a variety of behaviors and feeling states. In addition, nicotine also appears to influence brain neuroendocrine systems, which have a lot of control over peripheral endocrine systems.

Relationships Between n–AChRs and Noncholinergic Neurons

A major question that arises from this work concerns whether nicotine produces its effects by acting directly on these amine-containing neurons or whether nicotine must first activate (or inhibit) an n–AChR adjacent to the neuron in question to elicit a response. This has been an intriguing question, and at present, the data suggest that nicotine's effects are primarily indirect. Thus, it seems that n–AChRs are present on a variety of neurons that are not cholinergic in nature, and recent data suggest that many of these receptors have a presynaptic location (Figure 5.4). Wonnacott,[11] for example, has provided data indicating that presynaptic n–AChRs can greatly influence the release of DA from specific neurons. Further-

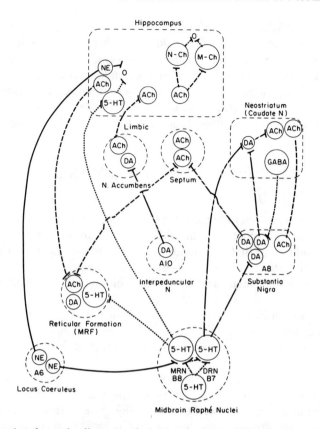

FIGURE 5.4. A schematic diagram of the interrelationships among brain amine systems. Abbreviations: N–Ch nicotinic–cholinergic; M–Ch muscarinic–cholinergic; DA dopamine; NE norepinephrine; 5-HT 5-hydroxytryptamine (serotonin); GABA gamma-amino-butyric acid; MRN medial raphe nucleus; DRN dorsal raphe nucleus. (Taken from Rosecrans et al.[33] with permission.)

more, the research of Kellar et al.[14] and Rosecrans[15] indicate that the neurotoxic destruction (6-hydroxydopamine) of DA neurons can greatly alter the concentration of n–AChRs, as well as the behavioral effects of nicotine. These data further support Wonnocott's research, indicating that many n–AChRs have a presynaptic location on noncholinergic neurons, which can greatly influence the pharmacological effects of nicotine.

Thus, what is the role of the n–AChR on these receptors, and is there a nicotinic–cholinergic neuronal pathway that will release ACh postsynaptically via presynaptic stimulation? These questions are extremely important, and we are still searching for some answers. Several investigators, for example, have conducted studies attempting to map nicotinic binding sites by using a variety of brain-imaging and receptor-binding techniques. The data suggest that nicotinic binding sites, as measured by ^{3}H-nicotine, are similar to n–ACh binding sites, as measured by ^{3}H-ACh.[16] Similar data have been obtained using 2-deoxyglucose, which has the ability to estimate increases in neuronal activity following nicotine doses. This approach has yielded a good correlation between neuronal activity and the cholinergic system[17]. Thus, there does appear to be a semblance of a nicotinic–cholinergic system, but whether it is a contiguous system, such as that of other biogenic amine-projecting systems, remains to be determined[13] (Figure 5.4).

Role of DA-Containing Neurons to Nicotine's Behavioral Effects

More recent research indicates that there appears to be a parallel relationship between nicotine binding sites and the mesolimbic dopaminergic system, indicating that DA neurons may influence how nicotine affects behavior (Figure 5.4). This is important from the point of view that several workers have suggested that this DA system might be involved in the reinforcement properties of several drugs of abuse, especially those that are stimulant in nature.[18,19] Thus, does nicotine serve as a reinforcer to behavior because of some DA interaction? This question is again quite intriguing, and we have only circumstantial information to substantiate this relationship.

Clarke[20] et al. have been cataloging information to suggest that nicotine's behavioral stimulatory effects are the result of a stimulation of the aforementioned mesolimbic DA-projecting system. In addition, DiChara and Imperato[19] provide data that nicotine is capable of releasing DA from the same mesolimbic system as has been shown for methadone, morphine, and cocaine. These workers fashion a generalization that drugs abused by humans have similar effects on DA-containing neurons. While it is an interesting proposal, much work needs to be done, especially by conducting experiments comparing these neurochemical effects in experimental animals self-administering nicotine and the other drugs in question. Too many times, in vivo and in vitro neuroscience is conducted in isolation, and because of failure to combine both approaches, erroneous conclusions result.

Relationships to Other Neurochemical Systems

In addition to its potential effect on DA neurons, nicotine has also been implicated in a variety of other neurotransmitter systems, including 5-HT and NE.[13,21,22] Neuropeptides such as the enkephalins and endorphins have also been implicated in several of nicotine's effects,[13,23] including mechanisms of physiological withdrawal, but unfortunately, our data base is still too small to take any stand as to a causal relationship between these endogenous substances and nicotine's effects on behavior. Researchers such as Hollt[24] have, more recently, been carrying out experiments involving the molecular biological aspects of nicotine's in vivo effects, which hold much promise for a better understanding of how nicotine can alter neuropeptide as well as other neurochemical systems.

Thus, the information before us is still quite speculative, but we do have a more complete picture as to how nicotine might affect a variety of different neuronal pathways important to nicotine's effects on behavior (Figure 5.3). We now suspect that in addition to a possible nicotinic–cholinergic neuronal pathway, n–AChRs may also be located presynaptically on other noncholinergic neurons, which may help us understand why nicotine is such a dependence-inducing substance. However, it seems reasonable to suggest that nicotine probably does affect many of these neurochemical and neuropeptide systems, and over time, we should be better able to relate many of nicotine's behavioral effects to some chemical interaction. Furthermore, nicotine may have an added ability to affect neurochemical function by virtue of its ability to desensitize n–AChRs. Thus, nicotine may be able to alter a specific neuronal system by exciting or inhibiting a specific neuron population via its action at some presynaptic site. In fact, it may be this quality to act as both an agonist and an antagonist at the n–AChR which is central to the ability of nicotine to elicit dependence in humans.

Role of Nicotine and n–AChRs in Alzheimer's and Parkinson's Disease

The finding that n–AChRs are significantly reduced in patients dying with Alzheimer's disease (AD)[25] has greatly increased interest and research output in the nicotine field. These findings have lead to several clinical trials with peripherally and centrally administered[26] nicotine to patients suffering with AD, but as yet there are few data to suggest that exogenous nicotine will alter the course of this cognitive disease. In addition, this research has created an interest in using brain imagery techniques (e.g., positron emission tomography—PET), which has demonstrated much concerning the localization of nicotine binding sites in control subjects and patients with AD.[26] Further support for a role of the cholinergic system in the AD syndrome comes from the work of Hodges et al.,[27] who were able to reverse the behavioral deficits of brain-lesioned rats (an AD-like syndrome) with cholinergic-rich fetal-tissue hippocampal transplants. Interestingly, cholinergic neurochemical parameters also returned to normal.

In addition to AD, recent interest in another related neurological disease, Parkinson's disease (a disease characterized by a loss of DA cell bodies from the substantia nigra), has also produced an added interest in nicotine research, especially because several investigators have presented data indicating that smokers are less likely to develop this progressive neurological disease than nonsmokers.[28] Even though the data are not as overwhelming as in AD, much interest exists for determining a role for the n–AChR in this syndrome as well.

An explanation of why smokers might be less susceptible to Parkinson's disease is very speculative at this time. However, research conducted by Fuxe and coworkers[29] suggest that nicotine could be acting by reducing dopamine neuronal activity to a level whereby they might be less susceptible to exogenously or endogenously synthesized neurotoxins such as 6-hydroxy dopamine 1-Methyl-4-phenyl-1,2,3,-tetrahydropyridine or MPTP. The theoretical model developed suggests that nicotine has the capacity to attenuate neuron function by desensitizing n–AChRs located at presynaptic DA neuron sites. Additionally, nicotine could also be expected to attenuate excess neurotoxin-facilitated Ca^{++} entrance into the cell by its closing the cation channel[11] via desensitization of the receptor; Ca^{++} in high concentrations can cause cell death. This is an attractive hypothesis and is supported by data indicating that the n–AChRs in smokers may be in a desensitized state by virtue of evidence that they have more nicotinic binding sites than do nonsmokers.[30] A strategy similar to that of Fuxe[29] was also used by Villaneuva et al.,[31] in which these workers were able to show that chronic nicotine dosing was able to reduce the cholinergic neurotoxicity of AF64A, ethylcholine mustard aziridinium ion[32] an acetylcholine–nitrogen mustard compound. Memory deficits, as well as ACh reductions, were attenuated by nicotine treatment, again suggesting that nicotine attenuated neuronal activity via n–AChR desensitization, making these neurons less susceptible to neurotoxic destruction.[33]

Summary and Conclusions

Our current view of how nicotine can alter and control behavior has changed drastically over the past 25 years. We originally viewed nicotine as a classic agonist drug, which had the capacity to mimic the physiological effects of ACh. The view at this point is more complicated and suggests that nicotine is working at its n–AChR by opening a membrane ion channel at some pre- and/or postsynaptic neuron site, allowing the entrance of some cation into the cell. This simple but complicated mechanism, the cell entrance of a cation via the channel, appears to be the signal by which nicotine can alter neuron function and consequently behavior.

A second aspect of this molecular mechanism is the finding that following initial opening of the channel, the receptor can become quickly desensitized, which attenuates further cation entrance into the cell. This cellular alteration has the in vivo effect of terminating nicotine's behavioral effects, and may also significantly attenuate the effects of a second dose of nicotine (i.e., acute tolerance or tachyphylaxis). The ability of ACh and agonists such as nicotine to desensitize the n–AChR appears to be an important mechanism by which ACh's effects can be terminated. In addition, it may be this effect, the ability to desensitize the n–AChR, which may be central to nicotine's ability to alter behavior. Because n–AChRs are so widely distributed, nicotine has the potential to affect a number of neurotransmitter and neuropeptide systems, which may explain also why it is such a popular pharmacological agent—that is, via tobacco use.

References

1. Rosecrans JA. Nicotine as a discriminative stimulus. J of Substance Abuse 1989; 1: 287–300.
2. U.S. Department of Health and Human Services. The health consequences of smoking: Nicotine dependence. DHHS (CDC) Publication No. 88-84-06. Washington, DC: U.S. Government Printing Office, 1988.
3. Domino EF. Neurophysiology of nicotine and tobacco smoking. In: Dunn WL, ed. Smoking behavior: Motives and incentives. Washington, DC: Saunders, 1973: 5–31.
4. Kisir C, Hakan RI, Kellar KJ. Chronic nicotine and activity: Influences of exposure and test dose. Psychopharmacologia 1987; 92: 25–29.
5. Collins AC, Minor LC, Marks MJ. Genetic influences on acute responses to nicotine and nicotine tolerance in the mouse. Pharmacol Biochem Behav 1988; 30: 269–278.
6. Marks MJ, Burch JB, Collins AC. Effects of chronic nicotine infusion on tolerance development and nicotinic receptors. J of Pharmacol Exper Ther 1983; 226: 817–825.
7. Nordberg A, Wahstom G, Arnelo U, Larsson C. Effect of long-term nicotine treatment on [^{3}H]nicotine binding sites in the rat brain. Drug and Alcohol Dependence 1985; 16: 9–17.
8. Rosecrans JA, Stimler CA, Hendry JS, Meltzer LT. Nicotine-induced tolerance and dependence in rats and mice: Studies involving schedule-controlled behavior. In: Nordberg A, Fuxe K, Holmstedt B. Nicotinic receptors in the CNS: Their role in synaptic transmission. Progress in Brain Res 1989; 79: 239–248.
9. Schwartz RD, Kellar KJ. Nicotinic cholinergic receptor binding sites in the brain: Regulation in vivo. Science 1983; 220: 214–216.
10. Stolerman IP. Psychopharmacology of nicotine: Stimulus effects and receptor mechanisms. In: Iverson LL, Iverson SD, Snyder SH, eds. Handbook of psychopharmacology. New York: Plenum Pub. Vol-19 1987: 421–465.
11. Wonnacott S. Brain nicotine binding sites. Human Toxicol 1987; 6: 343–353.
12. Ochoa ELM, Chattopadhyay A, McNamee MG. Desensitization of the nicotinic acetylcholine receptor: Molecular mechanisms and effect of modulators. Cell Mol Neurobiol 1989; 9: 141–177.
13. Pomerleau OF, Rosecrans JA. Neuroregulatory effects of nicotine. psychoneuroendocrinology 1989; 14: 407–423.
14. Schwartz RD, Lehman J, Kellar KJ. Presynaptic nicotinic receptors labelled by ^{3}H-acetylcholine on catecholamine and serotonin neurons in brain. J of Neurochem 1984; 42: 1495–1498.

15. Rosecrans JA. In vivo approaches to studying cholinergic receptors. In: Rand MJ, Thurau K, eds. The pharmacology of nicotine. Washington, DC: IRL Press, 1988: 207–226.

16. Clarke PBS, Schwartz RD, Paul SM, Pert CB, Pert A. Nicotine binding in rat brain: Autoradiographic comparisons of ^{3}H-acetylcholine, ^{3}H-nicotine and ^{125}I-alpha-bungaroatoxin. J of Neurosci, 1985; 5: 1307–1315.

17. London ED, Connolly RJ, Szikszay M, Wamsley JK, Dam M. Effects of on local cerebral glucose utilization in the rat. J of Neurosci 1988; 8: 3920–3928.

18. Wise RA, Bozarth MA. A psychomotor stimulant theory of addiction. Psychol Rev 1987; 94: 469–491.

19. DiChiara G, Imperato A. Drugs abused by humans preferentially increase synaptic dopamine concentrations in the mesolimbic system of freely moving rats. Proc of the Natl Acad of Sci USA 1988; 85; 5274–5278.

20. Clarke PBS, Fu DW, Jakubovic A, Fibiger NC. Evidence that mesolimbic dopaminergic activation underlies the locomotor stimulant action of nicotine in rats. J of Pharmacol Exper Ther 1988; 246: 701–708.

21. Hendry JS, Rosecrans JA. Effects of nicotine on conditioned and unconditioned behavior in experimental animals. Pharmacol Ther 1982; 17: 431–454.

22. Svensson TH. Peripheral autonomic regulation of locus coeruleus neurons in brain: Putative implications for psychiatry and psychopharmacology. Psychopharmacology 1987; 92: 1–7.

23. Rosecrans JA, Hendry JS, Hong JS. Biphasic effects of chronic nicotine treatment on hypothalamic immunoreactive beta-endorphin in the mouse. Pharmacol Biochem Behav 1985; 23: 141–143.

24. Hollt V, Horn G. Nicotine and opioid peptides. In: Nordberg A, Fuxe K, Holmstedt B, Sundwall A, eds. Nicotinic receptors in the CNS: Role in synaptic transmission. Progress Brain Res 1989; 79: 187–193.

25. Whitehouse PJ, Martino AM, Antuono PG, Lowenstein PR, Coyle RT, Price DL, Kellar KJ. Nicotinic acetylcholine binding sites in Alzheimer's disease. Brain Res 1986; 371: 146–151.

26. Adem, A, Jossan SS, d'Argy R, Brandt I, Winblad R, Nordberg A. Distribution of nicotinic receptors in human thalamus as visualized by ^{3}H-nicotine and ^{H}-acetylcholine receptor autoradiography. J of Neural Transm 1988; 73: 77–83.

27. Hodges H, Gray JA, Allen Y, Sinden J. Role of the forebrain cholinergic projection system in performance in the radial-arm maze in memory-impaired rats. Paper presented at effects of nicotine on biological systems: International symposium on nicotine, June 28–30, 1990, Hamburg, Germany.

28. Aquilonius SM. Parkinson's disease—Etiology and smoking. In: Nordberg A, Fuxe K, Holmstedt B, Sedwall A, eds. Nicotinic receptors in the CNS: Role in synaptic transmission. Progress in Brain Res 1989; 79: 329–333.

29. Janson AM, Fuxe K, Sundstrom E, Agnati LF, Goldstein M. Chronic nicotine partially protects against the 1-methyl-4-phenyl-2,3,6,-tetrahydropyrridine-induced degeneration of nigrostriatal dopamine neurons in the black mouse. Acta Physiol Scand 1988; 132: 589–594.

30. Smith G. Animal models of Alzheimer's disease: Experimental cholinergic denervation. Brain Res Rev 1988; 13: 103–118.

31. Balfour DJK. Influence of nicotine on the release of monoamines in the brain. In: Nordberg A, Fuxe K, Holmstedt B, Sedwall A, eds. Nicotinic receptors in the CNS: Role in synaptic transmission. Progress in Brain Res 1989; 79: 165–172.

32. Sheppard GM. Neurobiology. 2nd ed. New York: Oxford University Press, 1988: 155.
33. Rosecrans JA, Krynock GM, Newlon PG, Chance WT, Kallman MJ. Central mechanisms of drugs as discriminative stimuli: Involvement of serotonin pathways. In: Colpaert FC, Rosecrans JA, eds. Stimulus properties: Ten years of progress. Amsterdam: Elsevier/North Holland Press. 1978: 83–98.

6
Nicotine Addiction as a Disease

NORMAN S. MILLER

Introduction

Definitions

Before an intelligent discussion of whether a condition qualifies as a disease can take place, the basic rationale for defining a disease must be understood. A disease, according to *Webster's Ninth New Collegiate Dictionary*, is "an impairment of the normal state of the living animal or plant body that affects the performance of the vital functions, and a synonym is a sickness." An obsolete definition is "trouble."[1] *Dorland's Illustrated Medical Dictionary, Twenty-fifth Edition*, contains a definition of disease as "any deviation from or interruption of the normal structure of function of any part, organ, or system (or combination thereof) of the body that is manifested by a characteristic set of symptoms and signs, and whose etiology, pathology and prognosis may be known or unknown." Most other definitions of disease make references to terms such as *sickness* or *illness*.[2]

Victim State

Victim state implies an "*affliction*" not under the control of the victim. Although the victim state is missing in most formal definitions of disease, it is inherent in the strict concept of disease. The victim state is an unstated requirement for a medical, as well as a philosophical, definition of disease and must be met before the issue of whether a condition qualifies as a disease is completely settled. If there is an aspect of the malady that involves the power of choice, then any criteria will be insufficient for complete acceptance of a disease state.

Free Will

In a purely medical sense, in order for a condition to be a disease, it simply must be diagnosable and treatable by medical means. The "cause" of the condition must not be under the control of the victim; otherwise, it becomes a moral issue of free will. Interestingly, very few conditions ultimately withstand the rigorous application of the victim state according to these stringent criteria. In almost any condition, some exercise of free will or choice is possible, at least, to avoid exposure to the etiology of the disease, or to seek detection for early treatment. Accepted diseases such as coronary artery disease, hypertension, and cancer have an element of choice at some point in the initiation, evolution, and course of the disease—particularly in early diagnosis and treatment.[3]

Secondary Status

Physicians, psychologists, sociologists, and others have traditionally viewed alcoholism and other drug addiction as adaptive or secondary to a chosen lifestyle or caused by psychodynamic, psychiatric, or psychosocial factors that compel the individual or that leave the individual with little other alternative than to use drugs. The adaptive model states that these underlying conditions or conflicts provide a framework for the individual to identify and adopt drug addiction as an escape from intolerable stresses and to self-medicate in order to cope. In this way, addiction is an adaptive manifestation of deeper, underlying mental and social disturbances that must be corrected before the drug use can be controlled.[4]

Addiction as a Disease

The disease concept defines alcoholism and other drug addiction as primary and independent conditions that do not owe their initiation and sustentation to other conditions, illnesses, or diseases. Addiction is an identifiable and unique disease that is not a secondary adaptation. Nicotine dependence is, according to *DSM-III-R*[5] criteria, an addiction to the drug nicotine. Nicotine as a drug, therefore, qualifies as enabling a drug addiction. Alcoholism is an addiction to alcohol, and alcohol is a drug. Drug addiction such as alcoholism has always had a controversial status as a disease.[6] The background and essential reasons for the reluctance to accept addiction as a disease is explored herein.

Nicotine Addiction as a Disease

Addiction to Nicotine

Drug addiction is defined by the behaviors of addiction, which are (a) the preoccupation with the acquisition of alcohol (or other drugs), (b) the compulsive use of the drug (in spite of adverse consequences), and (c) a pattern of relapse to alcohol and other drugs in spite of their adverse consequences. Pervasive among these three criteria for addiction is a loss of control underlying the preoccupation, compulsive use, and relapse. The addictive use of nicotine inevitably leads to the development of adverse consequences because of the persistent loss of control in conjunction with the toxicity of the drug. This loss of control, once established appears to exist for a lifetime for nicotine, as it does for alcohol and other drugs. In other words, the nicotine addict will not be able to use nicotine without consistently experiencing a loss of control, at some point following a resumption of use after a period of abstinence.[7,8]

The primary foundation for considering nicotine addiction to be a disease rests on the acceptance of the loss of control over nicotine by the nicotine addict. The loss of control is the cardinal manifestation of the disease of addiction and substantiates the victim state.[9] The loss of control is the essential feature that leads to the multitude of adverse consequences, such as medical, psychiatric, and spiritual sequelae. The key point that is difficult for dissenters to the disease concept to accept is that the nicotine addict has lost this control over the use of nicotine because of a disease of the body, mind, and spirit. The dissenter contends that the addict has chosen to smoke because of an exercise of the will, albeit often to relieve some intolerance condition. The fallacy in the free will explanation of abnormal nicotine use is apparent but difficult to refute if the evidence for the loss-of-control component of addiction is not accepted.

Several studies have been performed to examine the loss of control over alcohol use in alcoholics. These studies have demonstrated that alcoholics cannot use alcohol normally or nonaddictively over their lifetimes after periods of abstinence once the diagnosis of alcoholism is made. One longitudinal study of initially abstinent alcoholics confirmed that less than 1% of the alcoholics returned to controlled drinking or drank without serious consequences, and there was significant doubt that even the 1% drank normally.

According to the first step in Nicotine Anonymous, the nicotine addict must accept his or her loss of control over nicotine, which, although not explicitly stated, extends over a lifetime. "We admitted we were powerless over nicotine—that our lives had become unmanageable." The word *powerless* is equivalent to the loss of control, and the word *unmanageable* represents the adverse consequences from the powerlessness. In order for the addict to begin recovery from the nicotine addiction, acceptance of the loss of control must be initiated. A common reason for the difficulty in achieving abstinence or relapse to cigarette smoking is an inability or unwillingness to accept this fundamental aspect of the disease. Relapse may occur after weeks, months, or years of abstinence because of the lack of acceptance of the loss of control.

A practical consequence of the disease concept is that it is much easier for the nicotine addict to comprehend the first step and to recognize the loss of control over nicotine if it is attributed to a disease rather than to a moral dilemma. Because will power over the loss of control of nicotine use is ultimately ineffective, insistence on correcting a weak character or treating an underlying psychiatric or emotional disorder will not initiate abstinence or prevent relapse to nicotine. Nicotine addicts are already filled with self-condemnation, and a further exaggeration of the guilt by making the addicts at fault for their smoking will further impede the addicts accepting responsibility for treatment of the nicotine addiction and its consequences.[10]

Alternatives to Nicotine Addiction as a Disease

Psychoanalysis

Psychodynamic theory has provided a useful conceptualization and terminology for the description of some of the intradynamic processes involved in addiction. The concepts of the conscious, the unconscious, and defense mechanisms are useful as descriptions of the addictive process, including the intrapsychic consequences of the addictive mode. Conscious and unconscious denial, minimization, rationalization and other psychodynamic processes are psychological mechanisms by which nicotine addiction is abetted intrapsychically.[11,12]

However, psychoanalytic theory neither explains the origin of addictive behavior nor provides a framework for the treatment of addiction. There is no evidence available that confirms that unconscious conflicts lead to addictive use, and subsequently that the uncovering and resolution of these unconscious conflicts lead to a cure or an arrest of the addiction. Studies do show that the continued expression of an addiction can lead to serious and significant psychodynamic conflicts that will complicate the course of the addiction.[10,13]

Although these psychodynamic explanations for self-medication may be valid for some drug use per say, it does not account for addictive use, nor is it indicative of a disease. Psychoanalytic theory can only provide a rationale for motivated use of alcohol and other drugs, but it cannot explain why alcoholics continue to use nicotine long after the benefits outweigh the adverse consequences (e.g., "I wish I could quit"). The conflicts created by addictive smoking often exceed those that may have motivated the smoking in the first place. The original distress to the ego is lost in its overwhelming disruption from diseased smoking.[12]

Biological Psychiatry

The self-medication hypothesis is also used in the biological psychiatry approach to explain addictive drug use. The assumption is that drug addiction is due to some other psychiatric illness; this assumption has not been substantiated in controlled studies. According to the self-medication hypothesis, major psychiatric illnesses such as anxiety, depression, and personality disorders are responsible for cigarette smoking and other drug addiction. The emphasis is on the apparent need to self-medicate with drugs, such as nicotine, the distress that originates and emanates from the underlying psychiatric disease.

A common example is the assumption that the use of nicotine and alcohol ameliorate the symptoms of anxiety and depression. The theory is that because anxiety produces psychological pain, the sufferer of anxiety will pursue drugs to obtain relief, as in the psychoanalytic model. Once again, this is a model that is based on the popular and old conception of motivated use of drugs. It not only fails to justify addictive or diseased use, but it also does not fit the clinical picture of the pattern of nicotine and other drug use in those who are anxious.[4,14]

Although it is generally accepted clinically that psychiatric states lead to alcohol and other drug use and addictive use, no studies have demonstrated that anxiety or depression or personality disorders lead to either nonaddictive or addictive use of nicotine, alcohol, and other drugs. There are many anecdotal reports whereby that interpretation is forwarded, but self-medication is not substantiated in controlled studies. Addiction as a manifestation of an underlying psychiatric disorder is only assumed. In fact, studies show that the use of drugs such as alcohol may decrease in anxious individuals during particularly anxious periods.[14]

Adaptive Model for Nicotine Addiction

The adaptive model states that economic, familial, individual, and social problems, stresses, and deprivations lead to addictive nicotine use. The nicotine addict, prior to the onset of nicotine addiction, has failed to achieve maturity in economic independence, self-reliance, and responsibility toward self and others. Because of these failures, the individual seeks and chooses to use nicotine and other drugs to further enhance self-identity. The important ingredients to the equation in the adaptive model is that the addiction results from a lack of adult maturity, related to environmental problems.[4]

Although this may be an appealing theory, it does not explain why some individuals choose nicotine and other drugs, while others do not who come from the same set of environmental circumstances. It also does not account for the vast numbers of individuals who do not come from deprived backgrounds yet develop nicotine addiction. The majority of smokers have jobs, families, and a reasonable integration into society. It is the minority of smokers who are disadvantaged and disengaged from society.

Causality in the Disease Model of Addiction

The interaction between alcohol (and other drugs) and the brain is responsible for the initiation of the disease of addiction. The disease model of nicotine addiction states that a vulnerability to addiction is expressed when there is exposure to nicotine. Nicotine affects neurotransmitters and receptors in key areas of the brain that may be responsible for the initiation and sustentation of addictive behavior.[15]

Nicotine has very specific actions that involve stereospecific receptors for nicotine in dopaminergic pathways that may underlie the vulnerability. These receptors can be blocked with mecamylamine but not with muscarinic cholinergic or adrenergic blocking agents. Nicotine causes the release of norepinephrine and dopamine from brain tissue and, depending on the dose, increases or inhibits the release of acetylcholine.[16-18] Nicotine causes an increase in hand tremor, an arousal electroencephalogram (EEG) (low voltage, fast activity), decreased muscle tone, and decreased deep tendon reflexes.

Although environmental stress, availability, attitudes, and morality regarding alcohol and other drugs are important factors that determine exposure to and use of alcohol and other drugs, including nicotine, there is little evidence that they cause addiction, as claimed by the adaptive model. The disease model does state that economic, familial, individual, psychological, psychiatric, physical, social, and moral consequences do ensue from addictive drug use. The important link in the disease model that is juxtaposed is that adverse consequences result from and do not cause addictive drug, such as nicotine, use.

Comparison to Other Diseases

The disease of nicotine addiction illustrates the paradoxical nature of many aspects of other diseases with both a physical component and many behavioral and mental effects. Of critical importance is that nicotine addiction compares favorably to other well-accepted medical diseases.

As with addiction, physicians are more uncertain about the diagnosis of coronary heart disease as a disease because the root etiologies are being increasingly attributable to lifestyles under the individual's control and not an invasion of some external forces rendering the individual a total victim. The diagnosis of coronary artery disease has become increasingly complex as a greater number of the etiologic factors are viewed as being under the control of the so-called victim.[3]

Interestingly, effective treatment of early coronary heart disease appears to depend much more on changing lifestyles than on receiving medical treatments. Coronary artery disease has been associated with diets high in some specific fats; obesity; type A or hard driving, stress-oriented personalities; smoking; and high blood pressure. All of these conditions are believed to be under the personal control and will of the individual, and for this reason alone, coronary artery disease may be becoming less a disease in the sense that disease is readily accepted by the public and by physicians.[3]

It may be that any condition that involves some volition on the part of the individual to initiate or sustain it will never fully qualify as a disease. A paradox is that in order to recover from an addiction, an individual must exercise some commitment of will toward abstinence from the drug consumption, according to the disease concept, just as commitment of will is involved with the prevention and treatment of coronary artery disease. However, the term *disease* explicitly means that the individual has lost the capacity to consistently control how much and how often she or he smokes and the ability to accurately predict the consequences of the smoking. From where does the control arise in the individual to offset the autonomous state of addiction, ask the objectors to the disease concept for addiction? The answers to these questions lie in the treatment of addiction and the utilization of sources of control outside the addicted individual.

Nicotine addiction is also like essential hypertension, in that neither has a known specific etiology, but both conditions cause physical disease. Moreover, hypertension is heavily affected by personal and social factors similar to those of coronary artery disease. The physical and psychological adverse complications from hypertension are as devastating and costly as those caused by nicotine addiction.

The preferred treatment of hypertension is frequently a change in diet, loss of weight, reduction in stress, and other aspects of lifestyle that are commonly recognized as under the power of the will. The treatment of nicotine addiction requires a change in lifestyle and attitudes in some ways similar to hypertension. Furthermore, adverse consequences accrue in both conditions if left untreated—generally, the greater the consequences, the longer the course of the diseases.

Cancer offers another example of the victim state. A *cancer victim* is someone who has developed a *malignancy*, which is defined as an uncontrolled growth of a tissue in the body. The tissue growth overtakes the normal functions of the organs, and eventually the ability of the body to sustain life. We do not ordinarily hold the individual responsible for the cancer. Yet do we not hold the individual responsible to seek and accept any treatment that is available? Individuals who continue to deny they either have or can have cancer will not seek early diagnosis and treatment. Are these choices not conscious decisions over which the individual has control and the freedom to exercise that control? How many victims of cancer see themselves as invincible and therefore unrealistically deny that they may develop cancer, thereby avoiding detection and treatment.

Moreover, studies are showing that individuals may have more control over the onset and development of cancer than we have previously thought. Many of the types of cancer that are readily accepted as diseases are traced to environmental conditions that initiate and sustain diseases, and where volition and responsibility may play an active role. For many types of cancer, prevention is becoming a reality (e.g., lung cancer is caused by cigarette smoking, cervical cancer is caused by certain sexual practices, stomach cancer is associated with particular types of diet, and breast cancer with taking birth control pills).

DSM-III-R Criteria for Dependence

The *DSM-III-R*[5] criteria for nicotine dependence contain six criteria for addiction and three criteria for tolerance and dependence. The criteria for addiction are reflected in the preoccupation, compulsive use, and relapse to nicotine. The dependence syndrome reflects addictive behaviors that lead to social, psychological, legal, and medical complications because of the loss of control.[7,9]

The diagnosis of nicotine addiction is straightforward and requires the application of the criteria of addiction. The preoccupation with acquiring nicotine is very dramatic, in that addicted smokers are rarely without cigarettes and will go to great lengths to obtain an adequate supply of nicotine. The compulsive use of cigarettes in spite of adverse consequences is vividly evident. Clinical studies clearly show that continued smoking is dangerous to one's health and can lead to a high rate of morbidity and mortality. Physicians can recall unfortunate accounts of chronic lung patients who turn off the oxygen on which they are dependent to survive in order to light up a cigarette. Moreover, the relapse or return to cigarette smoking after periods of abstinence is a common occurrence in nicotine addicts. Studies have confirmed a relapse rate of as high as 70% within the first 12 months.[5,19]

The daily and repetitive use of nicotine in the form of inhalation or oral absorption is striking and easy to diagnose clinically. The clinician is not met with the typical denial and rationalizations that are presented in addiction to other drugs. In fact, the nicotine addict may express a strong desire to quit smoking but also admit the inability to do so. It is the one addiction that often can be examined with the co-operation of the addict; however, the treatment of the nicotine addiction is no less difficult and challenging than with other drug (e.g., alcohol) addictions.[20,21]

The criteria for tolerance and dependence are illustrated by a diminishing effect at a particular dose and an abstinence-withdrawal syndrome on the cessation of the use of the drug. The course of nicotine tolerance and dependence is predictable and variable as with other forms of drug addiction. The intoxicating effects of nicotine are difficult to measure under laboratory conditions in humans and animals and for smokers to report. The intoxicating effects of nicotine are alertness, muscle relaxation, facilitation of memory or attention, and a decrease in both appetite and irritability. Also, nausea and vomiting are not uncommon acute effects in the nontolerant user.[19,22-24] Tolerance develops to many, but not completely to all, of the effects of nicotine stimulation. Tolerance may develop incompletely to the increase in heart rate, blood pressure, arousal, and hand tremor, and to the increase in plasma concentrations of some specific hormones. However, tolerance develops readily to the nausea and vomiting. The development of tolerance, as with other drugs of addiction, is due to pharmacodynamic changes rather than to drug disposition.[19]

The essential feature of nicotine withdrawal is that it occurs abruptly on the cessation of nicotine use. It occurs with all forms and routes of administration of nicotine. Changes in mood and performance due to withdrawal can be detected within 2 hours of the last nicotine use, peak within 24 hours, and gradually subside within a few days to several weeks.[5,25]

Physiological correlates associated with nicotine withdrawal are slow waves on the EEG, decreased catecholamine excretion, decreased metabolic rate, tremor, increased coughing, rapid-eye-movement (REM) sleep changes, gastrointestinal disturbance, headache, insomnia, and impairment of tasks requiring vigilance.[5,19]

The clinical signs and symptoms of withdrawal are a drive or strong desire to use nicotine, irritability, frustration, anger, anxiety, depression, difficulty in concentrating, restlessness, decreased heart rate, and increased appetite or weight gain. The withdrawal is suppressed by the resumption of nicotine use, as with other drugs that produce pharmacologic dependence.[19,26]

Self-administration as a Model for Addiction

Although nicotine may provide a mild-to-moderate euphoric response to acute administration, tolerance develops rapidly so that continued use of nicotine does not appear to depend on euphoria as a psychological driving force. The current theory is that the reward center in the hypothalamus, which contains dopamine neurons in the ventral tegmentum, underlies the craving or the drive to use drugs. Use of drugs that stimulate the dopamine neurons is neurochemically reinforced by the reward center.[27] Nicotine has not yet clearly been shown to affect these dopamine neurons.

A measure of the reinforcing ability of a drug is its ability to induce self-administration. *Self-administration* is when a drug is sought after for its effects and not motivated by some other reason for use. Nicotine is a self-administered drug under controlled conditions in laboratory animals. In a typical experiment, an animal is given access to a lever that delivers an intravenous injection or inhalation of nicotine. Although animals will self-administer nicotine under these conditions, the strength of self-administration is less than with other addicting drugs. However, alcohol, another drug that rivals nicotine as a clinically addicting drug, is not a particularly strongly or avidly reinforced drug under these same controlled conditions in comparison to other drugs. The more strongly self-administered drugs are stimulants and opiates. Of interest is that in humans, under controlled and uncontrolled conditions, the use of amphetamines, heroin, and alcohol increase cigarette smoking.[28]

In contrast to the intense feelings of pleasure that follow the administration of amphetamine or heroin, there are no sensations produced by injections of nicotine or smoking, which can be described as highly enjoyable similar to these other drugs. In fact, the number of smokers who claim to smoke for pleasure is rather rare, and even those state that the pleasure is coincidental with some other pleasurable activity, such as following a meal.[29]

With all these limitations, when studies are performed, nicotine is a self-administered drug that follows the patterns of reinforcement of other addicting drugs and behaviors, although less than some more potently addicting drugs. Results of studies provide direct evidence that in doses comparable to those delivered by cigarette smoking, nicotine is a reinforcing drug and is addicting. Nicotine meets the criteria for self-administration required by other drugs that are considered addicting (e.g., barbiturates, amphetamines, and morphine).[28,30-33]

Interactions with Other Drug Use

Further evidence for nicotine addiction as a drug addiction is the rate of nicotine addiction among alcoholics and other drug addicts, as well as the reverse—the rate of alcoholism and drug addiction among nicotine addicts. A high percentage—over 85% of alcoholics—are also addicted to nicotine, whereas only 29% of Americans are addicted to nicotine.[33,34] Preliminary evidence suggests that cocaine and marijuana addicts reduce their cigarette consumption during the active use of these other drugs. However, they tend to return to higher levels of nicotine use when the other drugs are not being used.[35]

Importantly, nicotine is often the first drug used by alcoholics and other drug addicts in the succession of the development of multiple drug addictions. Studies clearly show that nicotine (smoking) is present in the majority of alcoholics and other drug addicts prior to the initiation of alcohol and other drug use.[33,34]

Intervention and Treatment

There is growing evidence that traditional 12-step approaches work for nicotine addiction, as with other drugs of addiction. Nicotine Anonymous is a growing organization that has patterned itself after Alcoholics and Narcotics Anonymous. The first step, requiring abstinence, is readily applicable to nicotine addiction, as are the other 11 steps. The peer support is a powerful outside influence that assists the nicotine addict into recovery and into maintaining a sustained and continuous abstinence from nicotine.[36,37]

The disease concept is employed for Nicotine Anonymous in the treatment of nicotine addiction, as it is for alcohol and other drug addictions. This transferability in treatment of addictions confirms that the disease model applies to a broad range of drugs, including nicotine.

The use of pharmacological agents to treat the withdrawal state is also indicative of a medical condition that responds to medical treatments. Silver acetate, nicotine polacrilex, clonidine, and scopolamine are agents that can be administered to alter the signs and symptoms of nicotine dependence. As with other drug addictions (including alcoholism), there is no satisfactory pharmacological treatment for the addictive process and for the prevention of relapse to nicotine. If that occurs, nicotine addiction will probably achieve full disease status.[38]

References

1. Merriam-Webster, Inc. Webster's ninth new collegiate dictionary. Springfield, MA: Author, 1986: 362.
2. Saunders WB. Dorland's Illustrated Medical Dictionary. 27th ed. Philadelphia: Author, 1988.
3. Vaillant GE. The natural history of alcoholism: Causes, patterns and paths to recovery. Cambridge, MA: Harvard University Press, 1983.
4. Alexander BK. The disease and adapative models of addiction: A framework analysis. J of Drug Issues 1987; 20(1): 35–67.
5. American Psychiatric Association. Diagnostic and statistical manual of mental disorders. 3rd ed, rev. Washington, DC: Author, 1987.
6. Jellinek EM. The disease concept of alcoholism. New Haven, CT: College and University Press, 1960.
7. Miller NS, Gold MS. Suggestions for changes in *DSM-III-R* criteria for substance use disorders. Am J of Drug and Alcohol Abuse 1989; 15(2): 223–230.
8. Helzer JE, Robins LN, Taylor JR, et al. The extent of long-term moderate drinking among alcoholics discharged from medical and psychiatric treatment facilities. New Engl J of Med 1985; 312(26): 1478–1482.
9. Edwards G, Gross MM. Alcohol dependence provisional description of a clinical syndrome. Brit Med J 1976; 1: 1058–1061.
10. Milam JR, Ketchum K. Under the influence. Seattle, WA: Madrona Publishers, 1981.
11. Brenner C. An elementary textbook of psychoanalysis. New York: Doubleday, 1974.
12. Khantzian EJ. The self-medication hypothesis of addictive disorders: Focus on heroin and cocaine dependence. Am J of Psychi 1985; 142(11): 1259–1264.
13. Schuckit MA. Alcoholism and other psychiatric disorders. Hospital and Commun Psychi 1983; 34(11): 1022–1027.
14. Johanson CE, deWit H. The use of choice procedures for assessing the reinforcing properties of drugs in humans. In: Fischman MW, Mello NK, eds. Testing for abuse liability of drugs in humans. NIDA Research Monograph

No. 92. Rockville MD: U.S. Department of Health and Human Services, Public Health Service, Alcohol, Drug Abused Mental Health Administration National Institute of Drug Abuse, 1989: 171–210.

15. Tabakoff B, Hoffman PL. Alcohol and neurotransmitters. In: H. Rigter, Crabbe, JA eds. Alcohol tolerance and dependence. New York: Elsevier, Biomedical Press, 1980: 225.

16. Warburton DM. Brain, behavior and drugs. London: Wiley, 1975.

17. Jarvik ME, Henningfield JE. Pharmacological treatment of tobacco dependence. Pharmacol Biochem Behav 1988; 30: 279.

18. Cocores JA, Sinaikin P, Gold MS. Scopolamine as treatment for nicotine polacrilex dependence. Ann of Clin Psychi 1989; Vol. 1 1: 203–204.

19. Taylor P. Ganglionic stimulating and blocking agents. In: Gilman AG, Goodman LA, Rall TW, Murad F, eds. The pharmacological basis of therapeutics. 7th ed. New York: Macmillan, 1985: 215–221.

20. Noland MP, Kryscio RJ, Riggs RS, et al. Saliva cotinine and thiocyanate: Chemical indicators of smokeless tobacco and cigarette use in adolescents. J of Behav Med 1988; 11(5): 423.

21. Nanji AA, Lawrence AH. Skin surface sampling for nicotine: A rapid, noninvasive method for identifying smokers. Intl J of Addict 1988; 23(11): 1207.

22. Wesnes K, Warburton DM. Smoking, nicotine and human performance. Pharmacol Ther 1983; 21: 189–208.

23. Cox BM, Goldstein A, Nelson WT. Nicotine self-administration in rats. Brit J of Pharmcacol 1984; 83: 49–55.

24. Jaffe JH, Kanzler M. Smoking as a psychiatric disorder. In: Pickens RW, Heston LL, eds. Psychiatric factors in drug abuse. New York: Grune &

25. Pomerleau OF, Rosecrans J. Neuroregulatory effects of nicotine. Psychoneuroendocrinology 1989; 14(6): 407–423.

26. Shiffman SM. The tobacco withdrawal syndrome. In: Krasnegor NA, ed. Cigarette smoking as a dependence process. Washington, DC: National Institute for Drug Abuse, 1979.

27. Wise RA. Neuroleptics and operant behavior: The anhedonia hypothesis. Behav Brain Sci 1982; 5: 39–53.

28. Henningfield JE. Pharmacological basis and treatment of cigarette smoking. J of Clin Psychi 1984; 45: 24–34.

29. Warburton DW. The puzzle of nicotine use. In: Lader M, Ed. The psychopharmacology of Addiction. New York: Oxford University Press, 1988: 27–49.

30. Russell MAH. Cigarette smoking: Natural history of a dependence disorder. Brit J of Med Psychol 1971; 44: 1–16.

31. Schuster CR, Thompson T. Self-administration of and behavioral dependence on drugs. Annu Rev of Pharmacol 1969; 9: 483–502.

32. Mello NK, Mendelson JH, Sellers ML, et al. Effects of heroin self-administration on cigarette smoking. Psychopharmacology 1980; 67: 45–52.

33. U.S. Department of Health and Human Services. The health consequences of smoking: Nicotine addiction (a report of the Surgeon General). Washington, DC: U.S. Government Printing Office, 1988.

34. U.S. Public Health Service. The consequences of using smokeless tobacco (a report of the Advisory Committee of the Surgeon General). DHEW Publication No. (PHS) 86–2874. Washington, DC: U.S. Government Printing Office, 1986.

35. Miller NS, Gold MS, Belken BM, Klahr AL. Family history and diagnosis of alcohol dependence in cocaine dependence. Psychi Res 1989; 29: 113–121.
36. Alcoholics Anonymous World Services, Inc. Alcoholics Anonymous, 3rd ed. New York: Author, 1976: 58.
37. Jeanne E. The twelve steps for smokers. Center City, MN: Hazeldon Foundation, 1984: 3.
38. Cocores JA, Goias PR, Gold MS. The medical management of nicotine dependence in the work place. Ann of Clin Psychi 1989; 1: 237–240.

Part II Treatment

7
Engagement of the Nicotine-Dependent Person in Treatment*

R. JEFFREY GOLDSMITH

If smoking tobacco is the greatest preventable cause of death in the United States today,[1] then health caregivers must be trained to engage smokers in an abstinence treatment program. Millions of nicotine-dependent people (called "smokers" in this chapter) have already quit, many of them without professional assistance. In fact, the number of smokers per capita has been cut in half over the past 30 years. However, the remaining smokers may be the ones most dependent on nicotine and, therefore, most in need of professional help. Engaging these smokers in a treatment program (i.e. ensuring that they become involved with a plan or even make a pledge to participate[2]), is the key to their—and the nation's—greater health. Yet, this engagement is often difficult to effect. Like other uses of this term, *engagement* here brings with it an aura of commitment ("engaged to be married") as well as an aura of struggle ("engaged in battle"). Both senses of the word fit this situation: addicted smokers battling the urge to smoke will emerge victorious only if they are possessed of a firm commitment to do so. With so much at stake, it is important for health caregivers to understand the analysis of the engagement phase—its structure, content, and process—so that they can maximize their own talents as well as the success of their patients.

Engagement Is a Three-Party Process

It's important to appreciate that engagement involves more than two parties. Not only are the therapist and the nicotine-dependent person committed, but also the entire support system of the smoker is involved and, one would hope, committed. The support system might include the immediate family, lovers and spouses, friends, and colleagues, as well as

* The development of this manuscript was supported in part by Grants 89-35 and 90-50 from the Ohio Minority Health Commission.

health caregivers other than the designated therapist. They may all be significantly involved in the motivation of this person to get treatment for nicotine dependence. The motivation must be kept alive in the treatment. The attitudes, intervention skills, level of interest, and understanding of these three parties—smoker, therapist, and support system—can all become a significant force in the motivation for and engagement of the smoker in treatment.

Because therapists bring attitudes about smoking, tobacco, nicotine, and nicotine dependence to the treatment situation, they must address critical questions. For example, does the therapist see treatment as an event or a process? Does she or he consider smoking a bad habit or an addiction to the drug nicotine? Does he or she believe that smokers can successfully quit, or is it really a hopeless venture because so few of them ever really succeed? Does smoking really cause these diseases that are written about so frequently, or is this just a bunch of media hype? How therapists feel about these issues affects their efforts toward engagement and their definitions of treatment. If cigarette smoking is seen as a bad habit, then the therapist may be tempted to give her or his nicotine-dependent patients a stern admonishment and send them on their way. On the other hand, someone who considers smoking a dependency on the drug nicotine would be much more interested in a comprehensive program involving detoxification and relapse prevention, as well as quitting. Therapists who do not take the process seriously may see it as trivial, compared to the treatment of a so-called real problem, such as hypercholesterolemia or chronic emphysema.

The smoker brings a similar array of attitudes to the engagement process. The nicotine-dependent person frequently considers quitting to be an event and not a process. For smokers who have tried to quit and failed, those previous unsuccessful attempts may be seen as evidence that the smokers themselves are failures. This attitude not only leads to a negative self-image but also makes any subsequent commitment difficult to sustain. Denial of the addiction and the loss of control over their lives because of the addiction further complicates smokers' self-image. By denying the addiction and loss of control, dependent persons feel defective and unable to live without the drug. The image of being defective is used to explain both failed attempts to quit and drug-seeking behavior. This becomes a major obstacle. Such a conviction must be pointed out and carefully discussed before it diminishes. Even then, it may be a formidable barrier.

In this precarious situation, the support system can play a crucial role, for good or for ill. Significant others, as well as close friends and colleagues who smoke, can undermine the motivation and can sabotage the efforts to quit. While the supportive people may not know how to help smokers quit, they can be instrumental in getting people to a treatment source and encouraging them to stay involved in the treatment. Ex-smokers or colleagues and friends who are sensitive to the quitting process can be an enormous help during the time of withdrawal when craving and difficulties in concentrating disrupt the smoker's usual moods. Health caregivers who do not see this as an important health concern can inadvertently undermine the process by not respecting and appreciating the magnitude of what is about to occur. Despite the 400,000 deaths per year directly attributed to smoking and despite the powerfully addictive nature of nicotine, few members of the medical profession see nicotine withdrawal as a major metabolic event. For this reason, smokers are not yet allowed to be detoxified in the hospital. This attitude may make it difficult to legitimize the struggle that some smokers go through whenever they try to quit.

Motivation Not to Smoke

Because the smoker must embrace at least some of the reasons to give up this addiction, the issue of motivation is central to the engagement process. Health caregivers should, therefore, have at their fingertips the myriad reasons to stop smoking—physical/medical, social, and psychological reasons. The long list of tobacco-related illnesses, often leading to tobacco-related deaths, includes diseases well-known to be connected to cigarettes, such as lung cancer, as well as those not generally recognized as being tobacco related, such as osteoporosis.[3] Loss of energy and impaired breathing during vigorous activity are physical by-products of smoking recognized by much of the general public. The changes in the smoker's skin, the odor of smoke, and the general annoyance felt by nonsmokers are also becoming important motivations not to smoke. Counteradvertising on posters, radios, and television may tap into people's inner wishes to quit and be healthy. Periodically, there are public campaigns with health awareness activities, which also reinforce these messages, such as the Great American Smokeout every November and the Nondependence Day, which occurs in the summer. Health ordinances and regional laws that restrict smoking in public places are placing considerable pressure on smokers. In 1989, there was a federal law banning smoking on domestic air flights. Less recognized are the psychological motivations not to smoke (e.g., guilt and shame). These are crucial motivators to evoke during a successful treatment for nicotine dependence. Other reasons, such as "I'll live longer," may be remote and may not sustain the person during difficult times when there is a craving to use tobacco.

Guilt and shame can be generated by almost any interaction because they are psychological forces lingering in the unconscious psyche. Guilt among smokers is frequently attached to the awareness of causing physical harm to self or others. It is experienced as doing something wrong for which you will be punished. Shame is frequently connected with the loss of control over smoking and the difficulties in quitting. There is frequently denial about feeling guilty and feeling out of control. While engaging the patient in treatment, evoking or uncovering this shame about the loss of control can be very productive as a motivation to quit.

There is also a lot of guilt and shame tied up in the lying and deception that is necessary to maintain nicotine dependence. Lying and deception occur after promises to quit or after confrontations about the hazards of smoking by doctors and loved ones. Smokers are frequently aware of this deception, which they use when feeling defensive and under attack. Ultimately, the smoker deceives her- or himself to avoid the pain of guilt and humiliation. Being rid of such lying and deception brings a wonderful spiritual freedom during recovery.

Most smokers know that tobacco products are harmful to their health and want their children to learn this. When the children in turn confront them and ask why they continue to use these tobacco products, the adults are frequently at a loss about how to respond. These can be critical moments in motivating the smoker to attempt quitting. Significant others can be a tremendous influence in quitting or relapsing. One private program on the West Coast reported that the relapse rate was three times higher in smokers who quit and went home to a smoking spouse, compared to those who went home to a nonsmoker.[4]

The Process of Engagement

A review of the psychotherapy literature shows that there are common stages to psychotherapy no matter what the theoretical model for psychotherapy happens to be. There also seem to be common items that are considered to be standard for each stage of psychotherapy. Beitman suggests that each stage has six components: goals, techniques, content, resistance, transference, and countertransference.[5] Each component is considered specific for the stage. While there are some differences between psychotherapy and the treatment of nicotine dependence, there are also many similarities. Because engagement is such an important part of the treatment of nicotine dependence, a careful analysis of engagement from a psychotherapeutic point of view can be very helpful.

Goals

The goals of engagement, regardless of the type of treatment, are the establishment of trust, credibility, and the therapeutic alliance; the establishment of the ground rules of the therapy and the therapeutic contract; and the elucidation and enhancement of motivation to participate in the treatment. Many people, both doctors and lay persons, still frequently consider smoking cessation a matter of willpower and interest in correcting bad habits. The facts are that 90% of smokers would like to quit smoking, as many as 60% have made serious attempts to quit, and slightly more than

60% are concerned about their personal health.[6] Smokers are frequently *ambivalent*, meaning that they both want to quit and do not want to quit. This struggle makes them embarrassed that they cannot make up their minds and take action. As long as they cover over this confusion and uncertainty with denial, there is no need for them to be anxious or embarrassed. Engagement in the treatment of nicotine dependence must involve uncovering this confusion and the feelings that go with it. Health caregivers must demonstrate their capacity to deal with such sensitive issues before smokers will trust them with these feelings in all of their intensity. Hand in hand with trust is the establishment of credibility, the belief that the health caregiver has the skills and knowledge to treat nicotine dependence. Failure to establish trust or credibility could lead a highly motivated smoker to look elsewhere for treatment and could give the ambivalent smoker another reason to avoid taking action at that moment.

With trust and credibility established, the therapist can work on the development of a therapeutic alliance, which Beitman refers to as "the self–observer alliance."[5] Such an alliance requires some motivation on the part of the nicotine-dependent person, as well as a reasonable belief that the health caregiver can provide assistance in quitting. Without the alliance, there is no commitment or bond to carry out the treatment. A strong alliance can provide the nicotine-dependent person with the faith to carry out the treatment contract during an especially difficult time, when assailed by doubts and urges to abort the treatment process.

Enhancing the smoker's motivation becomes crucial as soon as an alliance appears, especially in the unmotivated smoker. All too often, we assume that motivation is something that one either has or does not have, like a light switch that is either on or off. Motivation enhancement may be the only way to activate the unmotivated smoker. For the ambivalent smoker, treating the low motivation may be essential to eliciting a commitment to the proposed treatment.

There are several basic principles for working with smokers who have low motivation. A careful assessment is essential, to rule out chronic illnesses, such as depression and alcoholism, which interfere with the maintenance of consistent motivation and commitment. Exploration of the symbolic meanings of smoking and smoking cessation can evoke special individual meanings to these processes. A woman may be terrified of gaining weight because she once saw someone gain 30 pounds upon quitting. Some smokers fear losing contact with colleagues, family, and friends with whom they smoke. It may be unnerving on the job to lose smoking buddies and to have no one with whom to socialize during coffee breaks.

After a careful assessment of the person's motivation, the therapist can then identify both the amount of motivation and the areas of weakness. Interventions can be devised to tackle denial, shore up low self-esteem, and avoid the bad influence of inveterate smokers. The nicotine-dependent person in denial about the loss of control due to nicotine may need to go through a period of treatment during which the awareness of nicotine and its impact on her or his life is broadened. As the awareness of the loss of control and unhealthiness increases, the growing uneasiness around continuing use of tobacco products also increases. This obviously interferes with enjoyment of the nicotine and makes it easier to let go of the addiction. Something as simple as a cigarette log or journal in which the smoker records the time and situation of each cigarette throughout the day, frequently causes the smoker to cut down the number of cigarettes smoked.[7]

The establishment of the ground rules of the treatment is also important during the engagement phase. The ground rules involve items such as cost, payment, frequency of visits, and time and place of meetings. These ground rules can be crucial during the engagement phase because economic factors regarding treatment of nicotine dependence are different than they are for other illnesses. It is ambiguous whether insurance companies will cover treatment for nicotine dependence. (Insurance companies do seem to cover certain aspects of standard treatment by individuals or by programs.) Coverage may vary according to comorbidity factors, which may or may not be related to nicotine and nicotine dependence. Attempts by the smoker to negotiate these ground rules for his or her own special reasons offer the therapist an important arena in which to establish trust and credibility, as well as an opportunity to learn something unique about this smoker.

Techniques

Empathy is one of the most important techniques in establishing and maintaining any engagement during a treatment. It is important to appreciate that empathy comprises two steps. The first step is to gain an empathic understanding. This means that the observer puts her- or himself in the position of the informant and tries to understand from an emotional point of view as well as a cognitive point of view what that experience would be like.[5] Beitman points out that "when therapists construe their patients as members of categories, empathic understanding may be also conveyed by questions that reflect knowledge of the experience of others in similar circumstances."[5] The second step involves the expression of this understanding to the informant so that the informant *feels understood.* Without this second part, the person may not believe that the listener has correctly understood.

The use of role definitions can be very important during the engagement phase. Role induction for new patients has been shown to be effective in enhancing outcome.[8] Defining the smoker's role in treatment can provide considerable support by clarifying the boundaries of the treatment. Role definition should clarify who to turn to during crises. Role definition expresses the therapist's belief that the smoker has the ability to change. The therapist's expressed belief can be extremely important for the frustrated smoker who has made unsuccessful attempts at quitting in the past.

Different therapists may define roles differently. The choice of treatment may also dictate the role definition chosen. Beitman lists different types of role preferences, which correspond to different doctor–patient relationships and different interpersonal styles.[5] One model is called the "medical model." In the medical model, for example, the therapist takes an authoritarian stand, while the smoker's role is to follow directions. In this model, the smoker is supposed to provide sufficient detail for the therapist to make a recommendation. Many people find this role comfortable because it corresponds to the interactions that they have had in the past with doctors. Some smokers prefer to engage in a collaborative relationship, which they can use to problem solve. With this relationship, the smoker reserves the final judgment and uses the therapist as an expert consultant. Still others prefer a warmer, more supportive alliance in which the therapist and smoker explore together. The exact role definition does not matter so much as the fit between the therapist and the smoker.[9] The therapist can instruct the smoker about the way she or he works, or the therapist can listen to the smoker and try to fit with the role that the smoker is seeking. One would hope that there is some capacity to negotiate both ways.

Two other techniques were mentioned by Beitman.[5] One is the expression of specialized knowledge, and the other is the use of effective suggestion. In a demonstration of specialized knowledge, the smoker may come to understand that the therapist has a special theoretical framework, which comprehends the range of problems that the smoker is experiencing. The patient develops confidence that this therapist will know how to bring relief. Making effective suggestions has the same benefit. In smoking-cessation programs, the effective suggestions often convey the specialized knowledge. It is important to appreciate that some peope want to manage quitting on their own and will reject suggestions. It may be that the smoker wants to be in charge of the treatment, and once in charge, the smoker may relax and ask for suggestions (see the aforementioned collaborative interpersonal style). Because of the need to be in control, these persons need to ask for the suggestion before they can hear it and entertain it seriously. This may apply to the setting of a quit date or to the decision whether to use medication or to go "cold turkey" (i.e., full, unmedicated abstinence on the quit date).

Management of the treatment contract is, of course, an important part of any treatment. Firm, clear guidelines can serve as a message that the therapist is in control of the situation. Willingness to be flexible and to accommodate some of the idiosyncratic needs of the smoker can also be an important communication of an empathic understanding. Negotiating the contract is an important technique in order to differentiate when it is important to be firm and in control versus when it is important to be flexible and accommodating. Smokers' failure to live up to his or her side of the contract may reflect a serious reservation in his or her commitment to the treatment. If this is addressed early, it may elucidate the need for remedial work before the commitment can be made. Failure to address such reservations can lead the therapist down a path of frustration and annoyance and smokers down a different but equally dissatisfying path, one of embarrassment and defensiveness.

Cultural Sensitivity and the Engagement of Ethnic Minorities

The research literature suggests that ethnic minority smokers frequently wish to quit smoking but are not successfully engaged and retained in traditional smoking-cessation programs.[10] There are several possibilities as to why this has occurred. It may be that the ethnic minority communities have different priorities and that smoking cessation is not a high priority within the community. It is also possible that the standard programs have some culturally insensitive attitudes that offend the minority smoker. In addition, it is possible that the different world views inherent to the different cultures cause a clash in the negotiating of an empathic connection and a suitable treatment plan. Health caregivers who work with ethnic minority populations are beginning to develop culturally specific and culturally sensitive techniques in an attempt to engage, more successfully, the ethnic minority community for health care services.

In working with African-American smokers, it is important to appreciate the differences between Afrocentric thinking and Eurocentric thinking.[11] Afrocentric cultures emphasize *spirituality*—a holistic world view in which spiritual and material are one. There is great emphasis on the interconnectedness of individuals: "I am because we are; and because we are, therefore, I am." Faith and intuitive knowledge is valued more highly than sensate knowledge. The group is considered more important than the individual, and decisions are made according to this relative importance. Disease and illness may be seen from a nonscientific world view, called "personalism," in which objects have energy or essences that pervade them. Causal factors include other possibilities than are included in the traditional medical explanation.[11]

In contrast Eurocentric thinking has a different set of values and measuring sticks. They value scientific knowledge based on the five senses. Time is experienced as a linear process; objects, produced or owned, measure importance. The individual is considered more important than the group. Ideas are frequently expressed in an either/or fashion, such as is reflected in the United States legal system, in which things are determined to be right or wrong. Disease and illness is explained scientifically, and interventions are based on these explanations.

One can see very quickly that two people, each with a different world view, could misunderstand the subtle valence expressed by the other person. A Eurocentric therapist may see a smoker's missing of an appointment as a resistance, while an Afrocentric smoker may feel that the family has made demands that were considered obligatory. Communicating scientific knowledge may not impress the ethnic minority smoker the way it would a white educated smoker. Tuning in to the spiritual conflict of the ethnic minority smoker may impress him or her much more.

The cultural identity of minorities can also be variable. Peter Bell and others have identified four interpersonal styles that reflect the different cultural identities in the African-American community.[12] These are not to be construed as pathological or rigid and immutable. They can be dynamic, and one person can shift from one style to another. They reflect ways of coping with the biracial world from an ethnic minority perspective. Each style has its own strengths and weaknesses, and the culturally aware therapist can tap into the different styles and make interventions that are consistent with the ethnic minority smoker's own self-identity. For instance, the *acculturated* smoker may be very Eurocentric in thinking and actually may be quite impressed by scientific knowledge and scientific interventions. The acculturated smoker may be offended by ideas suggesting that her or his cultural roots are African in nature. In contrast, the *culturally immersed* smoker may see the issue of cigarette smoking in terms of the struggle between the dominant white culture and the oppressed African-American culture. Tapping into this world view may lead the culturally aware therapist to capitalize on the issue of racial genocide, which is stirred up by the cigarette companies targeting the African-American community as superconsumers.[13]

OASIS is a culturally specific treatment program for Ohio's ethnic minority smokers. It is based on the principles of a standard multi-component program. OASIS provides medication when it is considered appropriate by the smoker and the collaborating physician. The program consists of five one-on-one sessions. The smokers are required to develop an extended support network, with at least one family member and one friend. The smoker and therapist work toward a quit date and practice the skills of problem-solving, coping, and relaxation techniques while discussing the cultural relevance of smoking, along with fears and relapse triggers.

The referral network of OASIS is an important part of this program. There are extensive connections in the African-American community, and people in the referral network understand that the approach is Afrocentric and that the counselors are African-Americans. The program is stationed along popular bus routes. Appointments must accommodate smokers with jobs, as well as those who are unemployed.

Like many multicomponent programs, OASIS uses written material and homework exercises. The handouts have been tailored in a culturally specific way to incorporate language and phrases common in the African-

American community. They are also somewhat simplified in the language, to accommodate the Afrocentric preference of the spoken language over written materials. Cartoon illustrations obviously depict African-American individuals and not white people.

Cultural identity is assessed early on in the program, and counseling styles are adapted to the smoker's own interpersonal style. The counselors have been trained to be culturally sensitive and have been instructed in culturally specific techniques while counseling. This training in cultural awareness does not ensure success, but it gives the counselor a greater chance at understanding the subtle meanings and implications of the smoking cessation process for this particular ethnic minority smoker. This training also helps avoid some of the cross-cultural triggers when the counselor and smoker have different interpersonal identity styles.

Summary

Engagement is an extremely crucial process in the treatment of nicotine dependence. It includes the establishment of trust, credibility, and a belief in the therapist's expertise. By combining the strength of a therapeutic alliance and an appropriate treatment plan, the therapist and smoker can tackle the vicissitudes of nicotine withdrawal and nicotine dependence. In doing so, the therapist must be alert to the smoker's resistances to the process of quitting. These resistances may involve denial, low motivation, fear, and depression. The effective therapist must develop interventions for all of these obstacles.

Ethnic minority smokers offer a unique challenge to the culturally aware therapist. African-American smokers seem to have more difficulty quitting despite wishing to quit. It may be that these smokers are inadequately engaged by the programs constructed for white Americans. Awareness of the cultural differences between the African-American community and the ethnically European white community can help the therapist understand the priorities driving the desire to enter treatment. Awareness of the different interpersonal styles within the African-American community can help the culturally sensitive therapist tailor her or his intervention. Development of culturally specific programs may increase trust, credibility, and the therapeutic alliance, thereby improving the long-term recovery rates.

References

1. U.S. Department of Health and Human Services. The health consequences of smoking: Nicotine addiction. Washington, DC: Author, 1988.
2. Morris W, ed. The American heritage dictionary of the English language. New York: American Heritage Publishing and Houghton Mifflin Company, 1973.

3. U.S. Department of Health and Human Services. Reducing the health conse-quences of smoking: 25 Years of progress. Washington, DC: Author, 1989.
4. Smith JW. Long term outcome of clients treated in a commercial stop smoking program. J of Substance Abuse Treatment 1989; 5: 33–36.
5. Beitman BD. The structured individual psychotherapy. New York: Guilford Press, 1987.
6. Huber GL. Tobacco: Its history, economics, and political influence. Sem in Respir Med 1989; 10: 278–296.
7. Ferguson T. The smoker's book of health. New York: Putman, 1987.
8. Frank JD. Expectation and therapeutic outcome—The placebo effect and the role induction interview. In: Frank JD, Hoehn-Soric R, Imber SD, Liberman BL, Stone AR, eds. Effective ingredients of successful psychotherapy. New York: Brunner/Mazel, 1978.
9. Strupp H. Psychotherapy: Clinical, research, and theoretical issues. New York: Aronson, 1973.
10. Hoffman A, Cooper R, Lacey L, Mullner R. Cigarette smoking and attitudes toward quitting among black patients. J Natl Med Assoc 1989; 81: 415–420.
11. Asante MK. Afrocentricity. Trenton, NJ: Africa World Press, 1988.
12. Bell P, Evans J. Counseling the black client. Center City, MN: Hazelden Foundation, 1981.
13. Tuckson RV. Race, sex, economics and tobacco advertising. J Natl Med Assoc 1989; 81: 1119–1124.

8
The Role of Family and Friends in the Management of Nicotine Dependence

JAMES A. COCORES

Nicotine-dependent peers and family members serve as a powerful form of advertising that significantly contributes to the experimentation and use of nicotine by young neophytes. This deadly example set by peers and family members strengthens the youthful perception of invincibility, which also contributes to the progressive addictive process from social use to nicotine dependence. Fortunately, an antinicotine posture on the part of peers and family members, which acts as a powerful form of antinicotine advertising, can also influence and prevent nicotine use and can guide nicotine addicts into recovery. Negative peer pressure triggers the process of nicotine dependence; positive peer pressure triggers the process of nicotine recovery. Though support from a friend, spouse, or parent is related to long-term abstinence from nicotine,[1-3] this social sword is double edged. That is, friends and family can serve either to enhance coping and relapse prevention skills or to help precipitate relapse.[1,4] The misinformed, uneducated family member or friend can inadvertently sabotage any progress made by the clinician or patient toward beginning treatment and recovery. Therefore, the importance of involving family members or friends from the outset in treatment planning cannot be overemphasized.

Nicotine-dependent patients with friends or family members either who have never smoked or who are ex-smokers are more likely to achieve long-term abstinence than nicotine dependents whose close social circle includes smokers.[1-4] However, what about the treatment of nicotine-dependent patients whose significant others are also nicotine dependent? This common situation can deter engagement into treatment, can foster relapse, or can strengthen denial in the identified patient. Clinicians tend to view this scenario as a frustrating obstacle instead of viewing it in a positive manner. In this and other smiliar instances, clinicians view the glass as half empty rather than half full. One patient is multiplied by two once the nicotine-dependent patient is convinced of the positive symbiotic clinical experience gained by recruiting a nicotine-dependent friend or family member into the treatment process. Where possible, this multiplication approach converts a once potential treatment saboteur into an ally. This can be accomplished once a number of facts are understood and believed: 90% of smokers would like to quit smoking, as many as 60% have made serious attempts to quit, and slightly more are concerned about their personal health.[5] Also, smokers who enter treatment with a friend or relative, establishing a "buddy system," are more likely to recover than addicts who go it alone.[6]

Giving each patient options shows flexibility. The initial discussion between the patient and the clinician revolves around possible support candidates. Addicts then select one or two treatment partner(s) from among the numerous active and nonsmoking candidates. When a fellow nicotine dependent is chosen, the pair often take pride in helping and supporting each other. A form of healthy competition usually ensues between male pairs, while female pairs more often take advantage of the verbal and social support that the buddy system fosters. When a non-smoker is selected, the smoker usually does not want to impose on the friend or relative. This stance usually is resistance and denial in disguise. Most smokers are amazed at the amount of time and support friends and relatives are gladly willing to offer.

Whether the support person chosen is a smoker or not, nicotine-dependent patients become more motivated and take treatment more seriously when a family member or friend is involved in the recovery process.[7,8]

Education

Whether the support person is nicotine dependent or not, education about the disease concept of nicotine dependence is the first step.[9] The goal of this first clinical intervention is to take the shame, blame, or fault out of nicotine addiction by convincing the addict and the supportive significant other about the disease concept, as outlined by Miller in Chapter 6. In this way, the patient and the support person understand that it is futile to try and understand the hows or whys of nicotine dependence. It is the quest for these answers that permits the denial of nicotine dependence to flourish. For this reason, I like to cut to the chase with my patients during the first meeting. I prefer to expose the addict's postponing and denial game during the first session.

When smokers' say, "I smoke more when I am stressed," I say "Smokers smoke most when they are bored!"

In response to, "I have money problems and when things get better I'll stop," I tell them about the lottery winner who began smoking three times the amount plus became addicted to cocaine *after* winning millions.

When they say, "I have too much on my mind now. When we go on our vacation later this month I'll stop," I say, "Sure, people drink and smoke even more during their vacation."

Reviewing some common rationale for continued use enlightens the significant other about a common form of denial. Reviewing some common rationale for continued use also exposes the addict's defenses as invalid excuses. At the same time, the addict feels transparent but understood. This adds to the mystique and shamanism of the clinician.

The educational path used to convey the disease concept is not as important as the common destination. The goal for patients and their significant others is to understand that the how or why of nicotine dependence really does not matter. What is important is that the disease is present and that it can be treated by any one of a host of single and combined methods. The patients are led to believe that they are powerless or not responsible for what has happened with regard to their progression to nicotine dependence, but that they are responsible for their recovery. By conveying the disease concept, it is hoped that the patient is viewed by the support person as a victim. The conversion from an interpretation of ignorance and weakness to victim status permits recovery to begin. The willpower theory fosters arguments and shouting matches and blocks recovery. There is no better way to (alienate) addicts than for a clinician or support member to become judgmental or offensive. Knowledge, empathy, love, and understanding are the best ways to enable the addict to progress with recovery. I ask support persons to imagine that the smoker already has lung cancer and that the smoker is refusing chemotherapy, surgery, and other treatments. I ask them, "How would you try to convince the cancer patient to try the treatments?" The support person rapidly realizes that they would probably not call the resistant cancer patient a "stupid idiot" for not accepting the treatment being offered. I try and show them that the way one would approach a cancer patient is the same way one would approach a nicotine addict.

Patients are also taught the second half of the First Step of Nicotine Anonymous, which is covered elsewhere (Chapter 27) by Jay L. This second half involves recognizing the consequences of nicotine dependence and how the nicotine habit has become unmanageable. The support person accompanying the addict often can uncover consequences that the addict forgot. The examples of unmanageability must be personalized, as suggested by Rustin in Chapter 10.

Recovery Is a Process

Significant others must be trained, along with addicts, in understanding that addiction is a process that gradually progresses from pleasurable experimentation to increasingly pleasurable voluntary regular use to advanced stages, which involve regular and less voluntary use, with less pleasurable results. The final stage is ridden with silent disgust, guilt, and shame, which accompanies the seemingly alien behavior characteristic of nicotine dependence. The addict and the significant other must understand the process of addiction before they can understand that recovery is the same process in reverse. It takes time to achieve a smooth blend of vintage recovery; it takes about a year.[9] Long-term abstinence and recovery may take many attempts and treatments, usually involving relapse.

Relapse is in many ways a necessary evil. In most cases, long-term recovery is impossible until a period of abstinence is ended by the harsh reality of relapse. It is important for support persons to view relapse as a part of the recovery process. Relapse is also part of the disease, but more importantly, it adds to the seriousness of the illness and can fortify motivation. The significant other should be drained of any guilt or fear that their own behavior has led or will lead to the smoker's relapse. Family members and friends can help a smoker's recovery, but they cannot make the user resume nicotine use. The support person must understand that relapse is not failure but is an opportunity to thoroughly learn a new relapse-prevention strategy.

Significant others learn about the meaning of nicotine abstinence and how this differs from the process of nicotine recovery. Abstinence is required before recovery can progress. The significant other learns that abstinence involves mourning, bereavement, and anger on the part of the addict. The addicts have surrendered the drug that they used to cope with life's problems. They also surrendered the drug that allowed them the greatest pleasures in life. The psychosocial stressor closest to smoking cessation is about equivalent to the death of a spouse. This is why nicotine-dependent persons who try to stop "cold turkey" (i.e., with full, un-medicated abstinence) make Freddy Krueger look like a boy scout. In contrast, recovery involves being abstinent from nicotine, coping with life's problems, and enjoying life. Abstinence is wild mood swings and intense craving for nicotine; recovery involves the ups and downs of daily living with an occasional memory of the good old days of cigarette smoking.

Conclusion

Support persons should be recruited into treatment whenever possible. Significant others can be trained to refrain from their occasional impulsive and sometimes aggressive interventions. They are encouraged to lovingly and empathetically support the addict's responsibility of following through with the treatment plan. After the addict has agreed to a treatment plan, then the support person helps monitor compliance without posing as a police officer. The nicotine addict should have at least one support person at home and one at work. The significant other's communications regarding the addict should be supportive, brief, and nonjudgmental. Nicotine addicts easily become angry, stubborn, incorrigible, nasty, and hostile, and most importantly, they will not listen or take direction if they detect that the significant other is preaching or being judgmental. Depending on the persons and the stage of their nicotine dependence, successful recovery may require little support for some smokers, yet other smokers may be unable to recover after completing 10 treatment programs, each involving numerous support persons. The point is that significant others need to understand that their support is likely to be needed over an extended period of time. The American Cancer Association sums it up well: family members and friends can "Adopt a Smoker." The only prerequisites required are knowledge, love, and patience. The rest is up to the nicotine addict.

References

1. Horwitz MB, Hindi-Alexander M, Wagner TJ. Psychosocial mediators of abstinence, relapse, and continued smoking: A one-year follow-up of a minimal intervention. Addict Behav 1985; 1: 29–39.
2. Mermelstein R, Cohen S, Lichtenstein E. Social support and smoking cessation and maintenance. J of Consult Clin Psychol 1986; 54: 477–453.
3. Coppotelli HC, Orleans CT: Partner support and other determinants of smoking cessation maintenance among women. J of Consult Clin Psychol 1985; 53: 455–460.
4. Ockene IS, Benfari RC, Nuttall RL. Relationship of psychosocial factors to smoking behavior change in an integrative program. Prev Med 1982; 11: 13–28.
5. Huber GL. Tobacco: Its history, economics, and political influence. Sem in Respir Med 1989; 10: 278–96.
6. McIntyre-Kingsolver K, Lichenstein E, Mermelstein RJ. Spouse training in a multicomponent smoking cessation program. Behav Ther 1986; 51: 67–74.
7. Cocores JA. New treatment for co-addiction disorder. Psychiatric Times 1988; 5: 13–15.
8. Cocores JA. Outpatient treatment of drug and alcohol addiction. In: Miller NS, ed. A handbook of drug and alcohol addiction. New York: Marcel-Dekker, 1990.
9. Cocores JA. The 800-COCAINE book of drug and alcohol recovery. New York: Villard Books, 1990.

9
Behavioral Treatment of Cigarette Dependence*

RICHARD A. BROWN and KAREN M. EMMONS

Cigarette smoking remains the largest preventable cause of death in the United States. More than 390,000 Americans die each year due to cigarette smoking, accounting for 22% of all deaths among men and 11% of deaths among women.[1] The annual costs associated with smoking are estimated to be $47.5 billion in medical care, absenteeism, decreased work productivity, and early retirement or death.[2] This figure does not include the cost of illness for exposed nonsmokers from involuntary or passive smoking, which has now been established as a cause of disease, including lung cancer.[1] These facts provide compelling reasons for the development and delivery of effective and economical smoking-cessation programs.

There have been impressive gains in the public's knowledge and beliefs about the health risks of smoking, which have translated to accelerated quit rates.[1] From 1965 to 1987, smoking prevalence among adults in the United States has decreased from 40% to 29%.[3] As the prevalence of cigarette smoking declines, the population of smokers is changing. The percentage of heavy smokers may be increasing,[4] which suggests that they will experience more withdrawal symptoms, stronger urges, and greater difficulty quitting.[5,6] Sociocultural changes are also evident, as smoking prevalence is higher among less educated individuals, among blue-collar workers compared to white-collar workers, and among blacks, Hispanics, and other ethnic minority groups.[7]

As the population of cigarette smokers changes, so do the characteristics of those individuals who use smoking-cessation programs. Between 80 and 95% of ex-smokers have quit without the benefit of formal treatment programs, and smokers who attempt to quit on their own are twice as likely to succeed as those who seek help in quitting. Thus, smokers who seek assistance in quitting are heavier smokers who have made more quit-

* This chapter was supported in part by the National Cancer Institute Grant No. CA50108 and Biomedical Research Support Grant funds to Karen M. Emmons.

smoking attempts than those who quit without assistance. Smokers who are middle-aged, better-educated, and white are also most likely to participate in smoking-cessation programs.[3]

All of these changes will have a significant impact on smoking-cessation treatment in the 1990s and beyond. Treatments must be tailored to individual needs and must be culturally sensitive. Traditional clinic treatment approaches may be relevant for an even smaller number of smokers. Consequently, many investigators have adopted a public health orientation to smoking cessation, using minimal professional involvement and focusing on public clinics, worksites, community, mass-media, and physician-delivered strategies. There is a related surge of interest in developing and evaluating self-help and minimal-contact intervention approaches.

However, it is likely that, as time goes on, more of the smoking population will become *less successful* with minimal treatment approaches. Thus, in parallel with the need for public health interventions, there is an equally strong need for more basic research. Powerful and intensive programs are needed, including pharmacological adjuncts to detoxify and treat heavily dependent smokers. Yet, an interesting dilemma presents itself: What we know currently about smoking and cessation, based on the past 10–20 years of research, may be less relevant in the next 10 or 20 years, given the changing demographics of the smoking population.

Fortunately, along with this challenge has come an increasing sophistication about the multidimensional and complex determinants of the nicotine-dependence syndrome. The earliest behavioral work viewed cigarette smoking as a discrete, observable, and easily measurable behavior, which was guided by the principles of learning–both respondent and operant conditioning. This simplified view has gradually given way to a more complex, biopsychosocial model, which recognizes interactions among the multiple physiological and psychosocial factors that come into play across the several stages of a smoker's career: initiation, acquisition, maintenance, cessation, and relapse.

The focus of this chapter is on behavioral treatment approaches to smoking cessation that have been developed and evaluated in the clinic setting. Our review will be selective, rather than exhaustive, and we will offer recommendations for clinical practice wherever possible. While we consider the movement toward a public health orientation to be extremely relevant and meaningful, a discussion of self-help, worksite, mass-media, community, and physician interventions is beyond the scope of this review. Suffice it to say that these approaches have traditionally drawn heavily from the behavioral treatment technology developed through clinic trials and will likely continue to do so. Likewise, we view recent advances in the use of pharmacological adjuncts to treatment to be quite promising, yet we discuss them only briefly because they are covered in greater detail elsewhere in this volume.

The Social Learning Approach

In discussing behavioral treatments, we believe that the social learning approach is the most applicable and provides the best framework for recommendations on implementing smoking-cessation programs. Social learning theory can be viewed as a broadening of behavior modification to include modeling and other cognitive processes.[8] While the social learning approach focuses on observable antecedents and consequences of smoking, the model also acknowledges biological and physiological factors as predisposing conditions that moderate learning and behavior. Covert events—thoughts, feelings, mood states—are readily incorporated within this framework, providing they can be reliably self-monitored by the smoker.

Thus, smoking can be viewed as a short-term method of coping with a variety of life problems, including stress, anger, boredom, low self-image, and social situations, as well as a method of modulating physiological functions, such as arousal or fatigue. Setting can automatically trigger smoking, often long after an individual has quit. The general rationale for treatment is that with practice and alternative skills training, the smoking behavior can be unlearned and replaced with more adaptive patterns.

Readiness-for-Change Model

An important theoretical contribution of more recent origin is the work of Prochaska, DiClemente, and colleagues. Their "readiness-for-change" model holds that quitting smoking is a dynamic process, repeated over time and taking up to 7 years from first thoughts about quitting to continuous abstinence. The different stages of change (precontemplative, contemplative, action, maintenance, and relapse) reflect different degrees of motivation that exist as individuals approach a behavior change. Individuals use different cognitive and behavioral processes within the different stages. Cognitive processes are more likely to be used by individuals who are in earlier stages of readiness to change (e.g., contemplative), whereas behavioral strategies are more typically used in the action stage.[9]

The findings of Prochaska and colleagues emphasize the importance of viewing smoking cessation as a process and suggest that tailoring behavioral and cognitive strategies to the stage of readiness of the individual smoker may accelerate the quitting process and improve overall outcomes. These investigators have studied the natural course of smoking and quitting and have developed several psychometrically sound measures of stages of motivational readiness to quit, pros and cons of decision-making about quitting, and of processes that individuals use during the various stages of change.[9,10]

Tenacity of the Smoking Habit

United States data indicate that the majority of smokers wish they could quit and that 70% have made at least one unsuccessful attempt to do so.[1] Every year, less than 10% of smokers who try to quit are successful.[3] Most formal smoking cessation programs have 1-year success rates of between 20 and 40%.[2]

The concept of cigarette smoking as a dependence on or addiction to nicotine has gained widespread acceptance.[11,12] Smoking delivers nicotine to the brain within about 7 seconds, and maximum nicotine concentrations in the brain are reached within 1 minute.[12] Nicotine is a powerful primary reinforcer that is strengthened by the sheer number of learning trials associated with every puff of the 7300 cigarettes smoked each year by the pack-a-day smoker.

Inextricably linked with this powerful pharmacological reinforcement are the multiple and ubiquitous psychosocial factors that play a role in the conditioning process of cigarette smoking. While modeling and peer influence are important in the initiation of the habit, other learning influences serve to maintain it.

Smoking occurs in a wide variety of settings, some of which become discriminative cues that act as learned reinforcers for smoking. An urge is subjectively experienced when these cues are encountered. Smoking is reinforced by the enjoyment of the oral, manual, and respiratory manipulations involved in the process of lighting, puffing, and handling cigarettes; by the pleasure and relaxation associated with using alcohol, finishing a good meal, or having a cup of coffee; and by the perceived diminution of the unpleasant affective states of anxiety, tension, boredom, or fatigue. Smoking is further reinforced by the reduction of withdrawal or anticipated withdrawal reactions during short-term abstinence.

In sum, cigarette smoking is a highly practiced, overlearned behavior reinforced by both physiological events and a wide variety of psychosocial events. No other substance can provide so many kinds of reinforcement, is so readily available, and can be used in so many settings and situations. While there are numerous immediate positive consequences, the negative consequences are delayed and probabilistic. It is little wonder that many polysubstance abusers report more difficulty giving up tobacco than alcohol or other drugs.[13]

Multicomponent Treatment Programs

While the earliest behavioral treatments tended to focus on the application of a singular approach or technique, multicomponent programs have proliferated in recent years. Greater success has been achieved through combining various techniques in a multicomponent package, most probably because they can address the multiple factors maintaining smoking, as well as the considerable individual differences among smokers.[2,14]

The most effective multicomponent approaches have achieved long-term abstinence rates on the order of 50% or better.[2,12] A decade ago, these programs invariably employed some form of aversive smoking as one component,[14] but recently, several programs incorporating both pharmacological and behavioral treatment approaches have achieved comparable success.[15,16] Treatments involving nicotine fading, when used in a multicomponent program, have achieved cessation rates in the 40% range,[2] representing a promising nonaversive and nonpharmacological alternative.

The research literature, as well as our own clinical experience, lead us to recommend the multicomponent approach. It is useful to think of multicomponent cessation programs as comprising three interrelated phases: preparation, quitting, and maintenance. They are interrelated in the sense that they overlap in time, and some principles and methods are useful in more than one phase. The discussion of each phase includes a brief summary of the research literature on various strategies and methods, as well as our own recommendations for clinical applications.

Preparation

Some programs urge participants to quit immediately. We recommend, however, that there be a preparation period prior to quitting, the length of which can vary according to program needs. There are three key objectives for the preparation period. First, the participants' motivation to quit and commitment to the program should be reviewed and strengthened. Second, there should be a clearly established target quit date that allows participants the time to mentally prepare and to develop the coping strategies needed to quit smoking. Third, participants should self-monitor their daily smoking in order to establish baseline levels and to begin to learn about smoking signals and consequences.

MOTIVATION–COMMITMENT TRAINING

Most smokers are likely to be ambivalent about the prospect of quitting smoking. While acknowledging rational reasons for quitting, they may dread the prospect, lack confidence, feel hopelessly addicted, and secretly question whether the health risks could ever really have impact on them (i.e., most smokers have a healthy, 75-year-old Uncle Fred or Aunt Mabel who has smoked two packs a day for 55 years!). Motivation is a critical factor, which determines whether a person will be successful in the effort to quit smoking, and the preparation stage offers the opportunity to help smokers resolve their ambivalence and strengthen their commitment to quitting successfully.

The development of new approaches to help smokers increase their motivation or readiness to quit smoking is a major challenge for smoking researchers. Brown and Niles (unpublished data) designed a motivational intervention for *contemplators* (persons contemplating quitting), involving cognitive and behavioral treatment strategies, with the express goal of allowing smokers to learn about and experience changes in their smoking behavior and thoughts. Self-efficacy was increased and smoking rates were decreased during the program, but they returned to baseline at 6-month follow-up. None of the participants chose to attempt cessation. Further attention to issues of perceived self-efficacy, outcome expectancies, personalized health beliefs, and decision making[17,18] is warranted.

Health Information

While scare tactics are likely to be nonproductive, concern about the health risks of smoking motivates many people to attempt cessation.[19] Eighty-five percent (85%) of current smokers believe that cigarette smoking causes lung cancer, yet only 18% are "very concerned" about the effects of smoking on *their* health, and 24% are "not at all concerned."[1] The challenge is obviously to move smokers from general acceptance ("Cigarette smoking is dangerous to health") to personalized acceptance ("Cigarette smoking is dangerous to *my* health").[18]

We recommend providing personalized health risk information to smokers whenever possible. Physicians are particularly well positioned to do so, given their knowledge of their patients' health status. However health-risk information should be coupled with specific directives as to what the person can do to eliminate her or his smoking behavior. It may also be useful to provide health-related information to participants during the maintenance phase of treatment, when this information will serve as positive reinforcement for their having quit successfully. Finally, a concurrent focus on the health *benefits* of quitting may be more important to the prospective quitter than the fear of negative health consequences from continued smoking.[19]

Reasons for Quitting and for Smoking

Another approach to enhance motivation involves having participants write down their specific reasons for wanting to stop smoking and for wanting to continue smoking, as well as the short-term and long-term consequences of each. Identifying reasons to continue smoking may seem contradictory, but this makes it possible to identify the likely barriers to quitting so that they may be addressed.

The Decisional Balance Scale, which has been shown to differentiate among five readiness-for-change stages and to predict changes in smoking status, is a valuable clinical tool for use with individual smokers and for evaluating the effects of preparation-stage interventions.[20]

Contingency Contracting

Increased commitment to abstinence may be achieved by establishing an agreement in which monetary consequences are provided for smoking or not smoking. Contingency contracts have generally been effective in producing short-term abstinence, but relapse is common once the contract is withdrawn.[12] Contracting for short-term abstinence may provide a useful addition to a multicomponent program with a strong maintenance component, due to the obvious need for participants to first achieve success at initial cessation.

TARGET QUIT DATE

We strongly recommend the establishment of a target quit date at the very beginning of a program. This gives participants a specific date to work toward and should allow sufficient time for the acquisition of coping skills needed to maintain cessation and to prevent relapse. The time prior to the quit date may also be used to reduce nicotine consumption by changing brands and/or by reducing the number of cigarettes prior to quitting "cold turkey" (i.e., full abstinence, without pharmacological aids). However, reductions below 50% of baseline rate, or about 12 cigarettes a day (whichever is lower), are likely to increase the reinforcing value of the remaining cigarettes, and thus to be counterproductive.[21]

SELF-MONITORING

Keeping a written record of the number of cigarettes smoked is a standard behavioral procedure. This serves to establish baseline data, to increase knowledge about the factors cuing and maintaining one's smoking habit, and to track progress throughout the program. Self-monitoring is likely to be a reactive procedure, resulting in a self-recorded rate at least several cigarettes per day less than the real baseline.

A preprinted card or sheet, which can be attached to the cigarette pack, will facilitate self-monitoring. Participants are typically instructed to self-record each cigarette *prior* to smoking it, and to record the time of day, and the situation in which the cigarette was smoked (e.g, "with coffee," "talking with friends who smoked"). Assessment of mood at the time of each cigarette (e.g., tense, relaxed) is also useful. The situational notations allow for a functional analysis of smoking episodes, revealing the enviornmental influences that trigger smoking. These events or triggers that are associated with smoking need to be delineated, as they may become future high-risk situations for relapse,[22] requiring effective coping responses.

Quitting

An exhaustive review of smoking-intervention methods derived from social learning theory is beyond the scope of this chapter. The interested reader should consult two recent comprehensive reviews of the treatment literature.[2,12] We devote our attention to the three major types of social learning-based approaches that are typically included in multicomponent programs: self-management, aversion, and nicotine fading.

SELF-MANAGEMENT

Self-management (sometimes termed "self-control" or "stimulus control") refers to those strategies intended to rearrange environmental cues that trigger smoking or alter the consequences of smoking. The assumption is that as a learned behavior, smoking is strengthened through its association with environmental events, as well as by the immediate positive consequences of smoking. Smokers intervene actively in their natural environment to break up the smoking behavior chain (situation—urge—smoke) by using one of two general strategies: (1) alter or totally avoid the controlling signals whenever possible; and (2) substitute an alternative behavior to replace smoking cigarettes in those cue situations that cannot be altered or avoided.

Several specific stimulus-control techniques may be useful in disrupting the associations between smoking and the particular situations that prompt the smoking response. Increasing the time interval between cigarettes is a strategy that allows smoking only at particular times, which may be signaled by a cuing device or an automatic timer.[21] Smoking is thus gradually reduced and eventually eliminated, while previous associations between cue situations and the act of smoking are effectively severed. In hierarchical reduction, smokers reduce or eliminate smoking in progressive fashion from the easiest to the hardest situations. Finally, by smoking only in "deprived situations" (e.g., in the basement, or the garage), smokers narrow the range of discriminative stimuli for smoking while breaking up the pleasurable associations between situations and smoking.

In considering alternative behaviors, relaxation techniques are a logical choice for self-management because smokers frequently report that they smoke to cope with stress and because relapses frequently occur in negative-affect situations.[22,23] These techniques may be particularly useful for those who are extremely anxious about the prospect of quitting.[24] However, while relaxation training has been incorporated into some successful multicomponent programs, its use has failed to demonstrate incremental treatment effects when combined with other procedures.[19]

Stimulus-control procedures can help participants to gain increased awareness of their smoking patterns and to achieve initial reduction leading up to a quit date attempt via cold-turkey. Because smoking cues often precipitate relapse,[7,22] it will be important for participants to anticipate these high-risk situations and to develop effective coping strategies.[25,26] We recommend that stimulus-control procedures be incorporated into smoking-cessation programs in conjunction with aversion, nicotine fading, and/or pharmacological approaches.

AVERSION STRATEGIES

Three types of aversive conditioning strategies have been used in the treatment of cigarette smoking: electric shock, imaginal stimuli (e.g., covert sensitization), and cigarette smoke itself. Because aversion strategies are discussed more fully in another chapter in this volume, we limit our discussion to methods involving smoke aversion, as they have been used most frequently and have enjoyed the greatest measure of success.

Satiation

Satiation involves having a smoker double or triple her or his usual smoking rate for a specified number of days just prior to quitting. Satiation is carried out in the smoker's natural environment, which makes it more convenient but also more difficult to monitor compliance and possible stressful physiological effects.

Clinical trials of satiation with at least 1-year follow-up have produced quit rates ranging from 18 to 63%, with a median of 34.5% abstinence.[2] Multicomponent programs developed by Best[27] and Lando[28] have attained the most impressive outcomes.

Rapid Smoking

Rapid smoking has been the most extensively studied aversion method. In rapid smoking, the participant is instructed to puff rapidly—every 6–8 seconds—and to continue puffing until it is no longer bearable. Programs usually administer two or three trials at six to eight treatment sessions in the clinic or laboratory.

A successful series of early studies by Lichtenstein and colleagues notwithstanding,[29,30] Schwartz[2] concludes that results are better when rapid smoking is combined with other procedures. Such studies, with at least 1-year follow-up, have yielded cessation rates ranging from 7 to 52%, with a median of 30.5% abstinence.[2] However, the best multicomponent programs involving rapid smoking have attained quit rates of about 50% at 6- and 12-month follow-ups.[27,31,32]

Side Effects of Rapid Smoking

Practical drawbacks exist to the use of rapid smoking, as the procedure greatly intensifies the naturally harmful effects of smoking. Cardiovascular complications remain the major concern, as cardiac irregularities on electrocardiogram (ECG) readings have been reported, though they have not led to any significant clinical symptoms.[14]

Overall, rapid smoking appears safe for young, healthy adults; however, procedures for medical screening and selection of patients should be followed.[33] Similar procedures should be followed for satiation. Given these limitations, we recommend that rapid smoking and satiation be considered only after nonaversive alternatives have proven unsuccessful.

Reduced-Smoke Aversion Techniques

Investigators have sought variations of rapid smoking, which would minimize its risk while retaining its therapeutic effectiveness. Regular-paced aversive smoking,[29,31] smoke holding,[34] and rapid puffing[35] are promising alternatives, which have produced long-term outcomes that are only moderately less successful than rapid smoking, when combined with other behavioral procedures.[2,12]

NICOTINE FADING

Nicotine fading is a nonaversive procedure that addresses both pharmacological and psychological factors. The nicotine-fading rationale is that cigarette smoking is physically addicting for many smokers and that gradually reducing their dependence on nicotine will reduce the intensity of their withdrawal symptoms at quit date, thus making quitting less difficult. Participants work toward a target quit date by switching brands to progessively lower nicotine-content cigarettes over a period of several weeks. Participants frequently report mild withdrawal symptoms throughout the brand-switching phase, suggesting a diffusion of the definite withdrawal effects that would ordinarily be experienced had they quit cold turkey from their regular brand.

Nicotine fading may also involve the self-monitoring of estimated nicotine and tar levels during the fading process. After self-recording their smoking rate, participants can calculate and plot their estimated intake of nicotine and tar each day. This self-monitoring of nicotine and tar provides participants with positive feedback regarding their efforts because these levels invariably go down if they follow the basic brand-changing instructions. Compliance with this procedure has been observed to increase participants' self-efficacy in their ability to quit. Given the high correlation ($r = .96$) between the tar and nicotine content of cigarette brands,[36] self-monitoring may also be limited to nicotine reductions alone.

In the first study, Foxx and Brown[37] combined nicotine fading and self-monitoring of estimated nicotine and tar intake and compared it with its two component procedures and a control. At 18-month follow-up, 4 of the 10 nicotine-fading–self-monitoring participants remained abstinent, as compared to none in the self-monitoring only condition, and 1 of 10 in the nicotine-fading only and control conditions.

Subsequent studies by Brown and Lichtenstein at the University of Oregon produced mixed results. One study produced modest outcomes with nicotine fading and no incremental effect of adding anxiety-management training.[38] A clinical-trials evaluations of a combined nicotine-fading and relapse-prevention maintenance procedure produced 46% abstinence at 6-month follow-up,[39] but a subsequent controlled study[40] failed to replicate this result.

Lando and colleagues conducted three nicotine-fading studies with large sample sizes and at least 1-year follow-ups. Abstinence rates of about 45% have been achieved when nicotine fading has been combined with a smoke-holding and a maintenance procedure,[41] and with a procedure to enrich group cohesiveness.[42] In a statewide field application of smoking cessation, between 75 and 80% of participants chose nicotine fading over satiation, and good long-term outcomes were produced.[43]

One drawback of nicotine fading is that it is not applicable for smokers who are already on the lowest nicotine-content brands. Furthermore, some prospective quitters may find that smoking reduced-nicotine brand ciga-rettes is aversive or may have a strong desire to quit right away, without undergoing a fading process over several weeks. Finally, it should be noted that actual reductions in nicotine intake may be less than those suggested by the published nicotine yield of the cigarette brand, as smokers may compensate by smoking more cigarettes or changing the topography of their smoking behavior. However, participants can be cautioned about this possibility and advised to keep such changes to a minimum.

Clinical trials of nicotine fading with at least 1-year follow-up have yielded quit rates ranging from 7 to 46%, with a median of 25% abstinence.[2] The best multicomponent programs involving nicotine fading have pro-duced quit rates of 40% or better at long-term follow-up,[37,41,42] These success rates are among the highest for nonaversive procedures.[44] As a nonaversive approach with good face validity, nicotine fading represents a more acceptable treatment opinion to most smokers,[43] and we recommend its use prior to consideration of aversive strategies.

Maintenance

Because the majority of treated smokers will quit initially but resume smoking within several months of treatment termination,[45] maintenance is a critical issue for smoking-cessation programs. Increased attention to this area in recent years has resulted in a better understanding of the factors associated with relapse. However, despite a large number of studies intended to develop effective maintenance strategies, significant advances in this area have been elusive. We focus on several of the more frequently employed maintenance strategies, and on two more recent approaches that appear promising.

COPING SKILLS

The coping-skills approach assumes that the individual lacks the bahavioral and cognitive skills necessary to become a permanent nonsmoker. Marlatt and Gordon[22,46] have proposed a cognitive-behavioral model of relapse that has stimulated a considerable amount of research. Although relapse prevention is covered elsewhere in this volume, it would be neligent not to acknowledge the role that this model has played in current thinking on cessation-treatment techniques.

Relapse-prevention theory proposes that the ability to cope with high-risk situations determines an individual's probability of maintaining abstinence. Successful coping in high-risk situations leads to an increased sense of self-efficacy,[8] but failure to cope initiates a chain of events in which diminished self-efficacy may lead to a slip, and perhaps to a full-blown relapse. In these instances, participants are taught to avoid both self-defeating attributions and the resulting negative emotional reactions (i.e., the abstinence violation effect) that promote continued smoking.[22,46]

Based on strategies suggested by Marlatt and Gordon,[46] Brown and Lichtenstein[39] developed a relapse-prevention program consisting of five components: identification of high-risk situations, coping rehearsal, avoiding the abstinence violation effect, life-style balance, and self-rewards. In two different trials of this program in combination with nicotine fading, one yielded 46% abstinence at 6 months,[39] and the second, only 19% abstinence at 1 year.[40]

Hall and colleagues[31] combined rapid smoking with a relapse-prevention program that focused on coping strategies, as well as commitment in maintaining abstinence. Coping skills addressed both withdrawal symptoms and situational factors related to relapse, and physiological feedback was provided. The program achieved an abstinence rate of 52% at 1-year follow-up, but subsequent studies with and without the addition of nicotine gum produced more variable results.[47,48]

Glasgow and Lichtenstein[44] reviewed a number of other studies, which found no effect for maintenance procedures based on relapse-prevention theory, although there is evidence that less-dependent smokers are more likely to benefit from this approach. The relapse-prevention model continues to focus attention on the central role of coping in maintaining long-term abstinence, and it will continue to stimulate research on relapse and its determinants.

Social Support

The role of family and peer influences in successful smoking cessation has been well documented.[49] Social support could be a source of motivation for quitting and of positive reinforcement for successfully maintaining abstinence. Social support might also provide a buffer against the stress of quitting or other stressful events that might precipitate a relapse.

Several early studies evaluating the efficacy of buddy systems produced equivocal results.[2] More recent investigations have focused on the role of spousal social support in smoking cessation. Spousal or partner support has been found to be related to long-term abstinence.[50,51,52] Several studies have also found that social factors can serve to either precipitate relapse or enhance coping.[23,50,53] Smokers with friends and spouses who either have never smoked or were ex-smokers were more likely to achieve long-term abstinence than those whose social networks included smokers.[50,54]

However, despite persuasive evidence for the role of social support in successful cessation, interventions designed to enhance social support have generally met with negative results.[55,56,57] Lichtenstein, Glasgow, and Abrams[58] summarize the similarities among the results from their respective research programs in this area and conclude that social support deserves further consideration in smoking-cessation programs.

CONTINUED TREATMENT CONTACT

Numerous studies have evaluated the efficacy of simply extending treatment contact by adding booster sessions, and they have generally shown poor results.[14,44] Telephone support for the maintenance of nonsmoking may also be provided through regular phone contacts by the therapist. Unfortunately, the results of such interventions have generally been negative, and in some instances, participants have fared worse than if contacted less frequently or not at all.[14]

One positive finding in this area was serendipitous,[59] in that weekly therapist phone contacts were originally conceived of as a control condition for two experimental maintenance strategies. At 2-year follow-up, the therapist contact group had the highest rate of abstinence.[60] A subsequent attempt at replication yielded a significant effect of therapist phone contact at 6 months, but not at 1-year follow-up.[61]

CUE EXPOSURE

Several studies of active smokers have found that smoking-related stimuli can elicit increases in peripheral vasconstriction, as well as increases in blood pressure and urges to smoke.[7,62] Abrams and colleagues[63] found that increases in urge, anxiety, and heart rate in response to a smoking confederate were greater for smokers who had relapsed than for never-smoked control subjects. Successful quitters had intermediate levels of reactivity. However, there appears to be considerable interindividual variation in the patterning of smoking cues related to reactivity, and the kinds of responses that have been elicited by cues also vary greatly.[7]

There are several studies currently underway that may further elucidate that relationship between smoking cue reactivity and relapse. At present, there is evidence to suggest that substance-use cues are present in a percentage of smoking relapses.[7] Thus, in vivo or imaginal exposure to physical smoking cues may become an important adjunct to relapse-prevention programs for some smokers.

EXERCISE

There has been considerable interest recently in the role that physical activity may play in preventing relapse. Because vigorous exercise is incompatible with stimultaneous smoking, exercise can serve as a substitute behavior following cessation. Exercise may also be a good alternative to restrained eating or dieting for individuals who are concerned about postcessation weight gain. In addition, exercise may moderate mood changes such as depression and anxiety, and therefore it may serve to attenuate nicotine withdrawal.[23,26,64]

Only three studies to date have examined the contribution of physical exercise to smoking cessation. Of the two that did not find increased cessation among individuals who were in exercise conditions, one was plagued by low compliance with the exercise regimen,[65] and the other by the lack of a formal cessation component.[66]

Marcus and colleagues (unpublished data), in the most comprehensive study to date, provided sedentary female smokers with either a smoking-cessation program alone, or a cessation program plus 15 weeks of supervised exercise. At 3-month follow-up, 3 of 10 had remained continuously abstinent in the exercise group, while none of the 10 participants in the cessation-only group had done so. Although the sample size was small, this study provides preliminary evidence for the role of exercise training as a behaviorally oriented relapse-prevention strategy. Additional attention to exercise as a maintenance procedure for smoking cessation is clearly warranted.

Pharmacological Adjuncts to Treatment

Pharmacological management may be an essential smoking-cessation component for some smokers.[12,67] There has been renewed interest in treatment that target both the pharmacological and psychological aspects of tobacco dependence. We consider recent developments in this area to be quite promising, yet we only touch on them briefly, as they are discussed in several other chapters in this volume.

When combined with a cognitive–behavioral relapse-prevention program, nicotine polacrilex (gum) has produced higher abstinence rates than placebo gum,[12,67,68] but it may be more effective in increasing short-term abstinence, rather than long-term outcome.[12,47,67,69]

There is also good evidence that the efficacy of nicotine gum is enhanced when combined with behavioral treatment approaches. Goldstein and colleagues[70] compared cognitive–behavioral relapse prevention to a health education–support maintenance condition, and a fixed versus an ad lib schedule of nicotine gum delivery. At 6-month follow-up, there were no differences for schedule of gum delivery, but behavioral treatment plus gum was superior to health education–support plus gum (36.7 vs. 17.5%). Two other studies have demonstrated that nicotine gum was more effective when combined with behavioral treatment than when combined with nonspecific interventions.[15,47]

The nicotine transdermal patch is an alternative nicotine replacement system, which may provide more stable infusion of nicotine and better adherence than the gum. Initial results have been promising,[71] and additional clinical trials are currently underway. Other pharmacological agents that hold promise for use in smoking cessation include clonidine hydrochloride[16,72,73] and antidepressants such as doxepin[74] and fluoxetine[67].

Other Clinical Concerns

WEIGHT GAIN

Smoking cessation is associated with weight gain of 6.40 pounds and increases in caloric intake of 200–350 calories per day.[75,76] The issue of cessation-related weight gain clearly has implications for treatment outcome. Fear of weight gain may be a barrier to quitting for some individuals.[77]

Although some investigators have postulated that weight gain among recent quitters may cause relapse, two studies have found that postcessation weight gain predicted abstinence rather than recidivism.[78,79] Hall and colleagues[78] hypothesized that individuals in their study who did not gain weight may have actively deprived themselves of food, thus increasing the reinforcing properties of smoking, as well as the probability of relapse. An important aspect of smoking-cessation treatment for such individuals may be to learn adaptive, alternative means of coping that will minimize their sense of deprivation. In addition, it may also be prudent to focus on the preoccupation and concerns about weight gain.

NEGATIVE AFFECT

A number of investigations have focused on the relationship between negative affect and the processes of smoking cessation and relapse. Stress has been found to be a major obstacle to successful cessation and has been one of the most frequently reported reasons for relapse.[22,23,53,80] In a study of stress and coping in smokers who have recently quit, successful ex-smokers were found to be more skillful at coping and showed less anxiety while describing how they would respond to stressful situations, compared to relapsers.[26]

Other studies have examined the relationship between smoking and depression.[7,80] Glassman and colleagues[73] found that over 60% of individuals who presented for formal smoking-cessation treatment had a history of major depression, and that nondepressed patients with a history of depression were less successful than nondepressed patients without a depressive history. When smokers with a history of depression attempt cessation, they often develop depressive symptoms.[81] Depressed smokers are also more likely to relapse.[82] Nicotine may serve to medicate the depression by regulating neuroendocrine function.[80,83]

Because some smokers use nicotine to regulate affect, successful smoking-cessation outcome may be dependent on skills training for affect regulation. Teaching smokers adaptive means of moderating negative mood states may facilitate successful quitting and relapse prevention.[80] Incorporation of pharmacological agents such as nicotine polacrilex or antidepressants into cessation treatment may be particularly important for smokers with a history of depression. Several studies investigating these strategies are currently underway.

Summary and Concluding Remarks

Cigarette smoking kills. This fact is increasingly being recognized by smokers, who are quitting in large numbers. Yet cigarette smoking is very difficult to give up and is now generally accorded its place along with the other drug addictions. Unidimensional theories of cigarette smoking have given way to integrative theories, which acknowledge that complex inter-actions among pharmacological and psychosocial variables make smoking behavior so tenacious.

We know that most smokers who quit do so on their own, without participating in formal smoking—cessation programs. Those smokers who do enroll in cessation programs have made more prior quit attempts, are heavier smokers, and are undoubtedly unable to quit on their own. The smoking rate among those with less formal education, in blue-collar occupations, and from black, Hispanic, or other ethnic minority groups remains elevated, yet this population is less likely to avail themselves of formal smoking-cessation programs.

The challenge for the health-care professions to promote smoking cessation is twofold: First, dissemination of broad-scale, community inter-ventions is essential, to reach the greatest possible number of smokers; second, there is a need for more effective, clinic-based cessation procedures tailored for those smokers who require and seek out these services.

The first goal can best be achieved through the dissemination of self-help materials and minimal interventions by physicians and other health-care personnel, in hospitals, at the worksite, in the media, and through com-munity organizations. Because quitting smoking is best viewed as a process, frequently involving three or four unsuccessful attempts prior to suc-ceeding, motivating smokers to initiate and sustain quit attempts is a worthwhile goal. Finally, population-based interventions must also target high-risk, underserved groups, such as blue-collar workers and members of ethnic minorities.

The focus of this chapter has been the behavioral treatment of cigarette smoking in the clinic setting, and thus has been most relevant to the second goal. There is clearly a large subgroup of heavily dependent smokers who cannot quit on their own, and who will not be successful with minimal-intervention strategies. New treatment strategies are needed to assist these individuals. Furthermore, the development and evaluation of effective treatment methods had traditionally been derived from clinic-based research and subsequently transferred to larger-scale applications. This kind of technology transfer will likely continue as new treatment approaches emerge.

A social learning perspective is believed to be the most applicable and to provide the best framework for recommendations on implementing smoking-cessation programs. We advocate a multicomponent approach consisting of three interrelated phases of treatment: preparation, quitting, and maintenance.

While behavioral approaches derived from clinic trials have been moderately successful, the changing characteristics of future clinic participants will require that novel treatment strategies be developed. Pharmacological adjuncts to behavioral treatments appear promising, particularly for the more dependent smoker. Nicotine-replacement products, clonidine, and several antidepressants have all provided cause for cautious optimism. Interventions to increase motivation and readiness for change are needed to augment existing approaches. While there is a great need for more research, we should not be deterred from implementing our available knowledge. Behavioral approaches still appear to be the most useful, and certainly the most accountable, means now available for the modification of cigarette smoking.

Acknowledgments. We would like to thank David B. Abrams for his support and useful suggestions concerning this chapter, Raymond Niaura and Bess H. Marcus for their helpful comments and contributions to an earlier draft, and Alice Baker for her secretarial assistance with the manuscript.

References

1. U.S. Department of Health and Human Services. Reducing the health consequences of smoking: 25 Years of progress (a report of the Surgeon General). Rockville, MD: Public Health Service, Office on Smoking and Health, 1989.
2. Schwartz JL. Review and evaluation of smoking cessation methods: The United States and Canada, 1978–1985. NIH Publication No. 87-2940. Bethesda, MD: U.S. Department of Health and Human Services, Public Health Service, National Institutes of Health, National Cancer Institute, Division of Cancer Prevention and Control, 1987.
3. Fiore MC, Novotny TE, Pierce JP, et al. Methods used to quit smoking in the United States: Do cessation programs help? JAMA 1990; 263: 2760–2765.
4. Pierce JP, Fiore MC, Novotny TE, Hatziandreu EJ, Davis RM. Trends in smoking in the United States: Projections to the year 2000. JAMA 1989; 261: 61–65.
5. Cohen S, Lichtenstein E, Prochaska JO, et al. Debunking myths about self-quitting: Evidence from 10 prospective studies of persons who attempt to quit smoking by themselves. Am Psychol 1989; 44: 1355–1365.

6. Killen J, Fortmann S, Telch M, Newman B. Are heavy smokers different from light smokers? A comparison after 48 hours without cigarettes. JAMA 1988; 260: 1581–1585.

7. Abrams DB, Emmons KM, Niaura RS, Goldstein MG, Sherman CB. Tobacco dependence. In: Nathan PE, Langenbucher JW, McCrady BS, Frankenstein W, eds. The annual review of addictions treatment and research. Vol. 1. New York: Pergamon Press, 1990.

8. Bandura A. Self-efficacy: Toward a unifying theory of behavioral change. Psychol Rev 1977; 84: 191–215.

9. Prochaska JO, DiClemente CC. Stages and processes of self-change of smoking: Toward an integrative model of change. J of Consult Clin Psychol 1983; 5: 390–395.

10. DiClemente CC, Prochaska JO. Processes and stages of self-change: Coping and competence in smoking behavior change. In: Shiffman S, & Wills T, eds. Coping and substance use. Orlando, FL: Academic Press, 1985: 319–341.

11. American Psychiatric Association. Diagnostic and statistical manual of mental disorders. 3rd ed, rev. Washington, DC: Author, 1987.

12. U.S. Department of Health and Human Services. The health consequences of smoking: Nicotine addiction (a report of the Surgeon General). Rockville, MD: Public Health Service, Office on Smoking and Health, 1988.

13. Kozlowski LT, Wilkinson DA, Skinner W, Kent C, Franklin T, Pope M. Comparing tobacco cigarette dependence with other drug dependencies: Greater or equal "difficulty quitting" and "urges to use," but less "pleasure" from cigarettes. JAMA 1989; 261: 898–901.

14. Lichtenstein E, Brown RA. Current trends in the modification of cigarette dependence. In: Bellack AS, Hersen M, Kazdin AE, eds. International handbook of behavior modification and therapy. New York: Plenum, 1982.

15. Killen JD, Maccoby N, Taylor CB. Nicotine gum and self-regulation training in smoking relapse prevention. Behav Ther 1984; 15: 234–248.

16. Wei H, Young D. Effect of clonidine on cigarette cessation and in the alleviation of withdrawal symptoms. Brit J Addict 1988; 83: 1221–1226.

17. Pechachek TF, Danaher BG. How and why people quit smoking: A cognitive–behavioral analysis. In: Kendall PC, Hollon SD, eds. Cognitive–behavioral interventions: Theory, research, and procedures. New York: Academic Press, 1979.

18. Fishbein, M. Consumer beliefs and behavior with respect to cigarette smoking: A critical analysis of the public literature. In: Federal Trade Commission, report to Congress: Pursuant to the Public Health Cigarette Smoking Act, for the year 1976. Washington, DC: Federal Trade Commission, May 1977.

19. Lichtenstein E, Brown RA. Smoking cessation methods: Review and recommendations. In: Miller WR, ed. The addictive behaviors: Treatment of alcoholism, drug abuse, smoking, and obesity. Oxford: Pergamon Press, 1980.

20. Velicer W, DiClemente C, Prochaska J, Brandenburg N. A decisional balance measure for predicting smoking cessation. J of Pers and Soc Psychol 1985; 48: 1279–1289.

21. Levinson BL, Shapiro D, Schwartz GE, Tursky B. Smoking elimination by gradual reduction. Behav Ther 1971; 2: 477–487.

22. Marlatt GA, Gordon JR, eds. Relapse prevention. New York: Guilford Press, 1985.

23. Shiffman S. Relapse following smoking cessation: A situational analysis. J of Consult Clin Psychol 1982; 50: 71–86.
24. Lichtenstein E, Mermelstein RJ. Review of approaches to smoking treatment: Behavior modification strategies. In: Matarazzo JD, Weiss SM, Herd JA, Miller NE, Weiss SM, eds. Behavioral health: A handbook of health enhancement and disease prevention. New York: Wiley, 1984.
25. Shiffman S. Coping with temptations to smoke. In: Shiffman S, Wills T, eds. Coping and substance abuse. Orlando, FL: Academic Press, 1985.
26. Abrams DB, Monti PM, Pinto RP, Elder JP, Brown RA, Jacobus SI. Psychological stress and coping in smokers who relapse or quit. Health Psychol 1987; 6: 289–303.
27. Best JA, Owen LE, Trentadue L. Comparison of satiation and rapid smoking in self-managed smoking cessation. Addict Behav 1978; 3: 71–78.
28. Lando H. Successful treatment of smokers with a broad-spectrum behavioral approach. J of Consult Clin Psychol 1977; 44: 361–366.
29. Lichtenstein E, Harris DE, Birchler GR, Wahl JM, Schmahl DP. Comparison of rapid smoking, warm, smoky air, and attention placebo in the modification of smoking behavior. J of Consult Clin Psychol 1973; 40: 92–98.
30. Schmahl DP, Lichtenstein E, Harris DE. Successful treatment of habitual smokers with warm, smoky air and rapid smoking. J of Consult Clin Psychol 1972; 105–111.
31. Hall SM. Rugg D. Tunstall C, Jones R. Preventing relapse to cigarette smoking by behavioral skill training. J of Consult Clin Psychol 1984; 52: 372–382.
32. Brandon TH, Zelman DC, Baker TB. Effects of maintenance sessions on smoking relapse: Delaying the inevitable? J of Consult Clin Psychol 1987; 55: 780–782.
33. Lichtenstein E, Glascow RE. Rapid smoking: Side effects and safeguards. J of Consult Clin Psychol 1977; 45: 815–821.
34. Kopel SA, Suckerman KR, Baksht A. Smoke holding: An evaluation of physiological effects and treatment efficacy of a new nonhazardous aversive smoking procedure. Paper presented at the annual meeting of the Association for Advancement of Behavior Therapy, December, 1979, San Francisco, CA.
35. Erickson LM, Tiffany ST, Martin EM, Baker TB. Aversive smoking therapies: A conditioning analysis of therapeutic effectiveness. Behav Res and Ther 1983; 21: 595–611.
36. Russell MAH, Wilson C, Patel UA, Feyerabend C, Cole PV. Plasma nicotine levels after smoking cigarettes with high, medium, and low nicotine yields. Brit Med J 1975; 2: 414–416.
37. Foxx RM, Brown RA. Nicotine fading and self-monitoring for cigarette abstinence or controlled smoking. J of Applied Behav Anal 1979; 12: 111–125.
38. Beaver C, Brown RA, Lichtenstein E. Effects of monitored nicotine fading and anxiety management training on smoking reduction. Addict Behav 1981; 6: 301–305.
39. Brown RA, Lichtenstein E. Effects of a cognitive–behavioral relapse prevention program for smokers. Paper presented at the annual meeting of the American Psychological Assication, September 1980, Montreal.
40. Brown RA, Lichtenstein E, McIntyre KO, Harrington-Kostur J. Effects of

nicotine fading and relapse prevention on smoking cessation. J of Consult Clin Psychol 1984; 52: 307–308.

41. Lando HA, McGovern PG. Nicotine fading as a nonaversive alternative in a broad-spectrum treatment for eliminating smoking. Addict Behav 1985; 10: 153–161.
42. Etringer BD, Gregory VR, Lando HA. Influence of group cohesion on the behavioral treatment of smoking. J of Consult Clin Psychol 1984; 52: 1080–1086.
43. Lando HA. Long-term modification of chronic smoking behavior: A paradigmatic approach. Bull of the Soc of Psychol in Addict Behav 1986; 5: 5–17.
44. Glasgow RE, Lichtenstein E. Long-term effects of behavioral smoking cessation interventions. Behav Ther 1987; 18: 297–324.
45. Hunt WA, Bespalec DA. An evaluation of current methods of modifying smoking behavior. J of Clin Psychol 1974; 30: 431–438.
46. Marlatt GA, Gordon JR. Determinants of relapse: Implications for the maintenance of behavior change. In: Davidson PO, Davidson SM, eds. Behavioral medicine: Changing health lifestyles. New York: Brunner/Mazel, 1980.
47. Hall SM, Tunstall C, Rugg D, Jones RT, Benowitz N. Nicotine gum and behavioral treatment in smoking cessation. J of Consult Clin Psychol 1985; 53: 256–258.
48. Hall SM, Tunstall C, Ginsberg D, Benowitz NL, Jones RT. Nicotine gum and behavioral treatment: A placebo controlled trial. J of Consult Clin Psychol 1987; 55: 603–605.
49. Colletti G, Brownell K. The physical and emotional benefits of social support: Applications to obesity, smoking and alcoholism. In: Hersen M, Eisler R, Miller P, eds. Progress in behavior modification. Vol. 13. New York: Academic Press, 1982.
50. Horwitz MB, Hindi-Alexander M, Wagner TJ. Psychosocial mediators of abstinence, relapse, and continued smoking: A one-year follow-up of a minimal intervention. Addict Behav 1985; 1: 29–39.
51. Mermelstein R, Cohen S, Lichtenstein E, Baer JS, Kamarck T. Social support and smoking cessation and maintenance. J of Consult Clin Psychol 1986; 54: 447–453.
52. Coppotelli HC, Orleans CT. Partner support and other determinants of smoking cessation maintenance among women. J of Consult Clin Psychol 1985; 53: 455–460.
53. Ockene JW, Benfari RC, Nuttall RL, Jurwitz I, Ockene IS. Relationship of psychosocial factors to smoking behavior change in an integrative program. Prev Med 1982; 11: 13–28.
54. West DW, Graham S, Swanson M, Wilkinson G. Five year follow-up of a smoking withdrawal clinic population. Am J of Public Health 1977; 67: 536–544.
55. McIntyre-Kingsolver K, Lichtenstein E, Mermelstein RJ. Spouse training in a multicomponent smoking-cessation program. Behav Ther 1986; 51: 67–74.
56. Malott JM, Glasgow RE, O'Neill HK, Klesges RC. Co-worker social support in a worksite smoking program. J of Applied Behav Anal 1984; 17: 485–496.
57. Abrams DB, Pinto RP, Monti PM, Jacobus S, Brown RA, Elder JP. Health education vs. cognitive stress management vs. social support training for

relapse prevention in worksite smoking cessation. Paper presented at the annual meeting of the Society of Behavioral Medicine, March, 1985, New Orleans, LA.

58. Lichtenstein E, Glasgow RE, Abrams DB. Social support in smoking cessation: In search of effective interventions. Behav Ther 1986; 17: 607–619.

59. Colletti G, Kopel SA. Maintaining behavior change: An investigation of three maintenance strategies and the relationship of self-attribution to the long-term reduction of cigarette smoking. J of Consult Clin Psychol 1979; 47: 614–617.

60. Colletti G, Stern L. Two-year follow-up of a nonaversive treatment for cigarette smoking. J of Consult Clin Psychol 1980; 48: 292–293.

61. Colletti G, Supnick JA. Continued therapist contact as a maintenance strategy for smoking reduction. J of Consult Clin Psychol 1980; 48: 665–667

62. Niaura RS, Rohsenow DJ, Binkoff JA, Monti PM, Pedraza M, Abrams DB. Relevance of cue reactivity to understanding alcohol and smoking relapse. J of Abn Psychol 1988; 97: 133–152.

63. Abrams DB, Monti PM, Carey KB, Pinto RP, Jacobus SI. Reactivity to smoking cues and relapse: Two studies of discriminant validity. Behav Res and Ther 1988; 26: 223–25.

64. Shiffman S. Coping with temptations to smoke. J of Consult and Clin Psychol 1984; 52: 261–267.

65. Russell PO, Epstein LH, Johnston JJ, Block DR, Blair E. The effects of physical activity as maintenance for smoking cessation. Addict Behav 1988; 13: 215–218.

66. Taylor CB, Houston-Miller N, Haskell WL, DeBusk RF. Smoking cessation after acute myocardial infarction: The effects of exercise training. Addict Behav 1988; 13: 331–335.

67. Goldstein MG, Niaura R, Abrams DB. Medical and behavioral treatment of nicotine dependence. In: Stoudemire A, Fogel BS, eds. Advances in medical–psychiatric practice. Washington, DC: American Psychiatric Press, in press.

68. Hughes JR, Miller SA. Nicotine gum to help stop smoking. JAMA 1984; 252: 2855–2858.

69. Harackiewicz JM, Blair LW, Sansone C, Epstein JA, Stuchell RN. Nicotine gum and self-help manuals in smoking cessation: An evaluation in a medical context. Addict Behav 1988; 13: 319–390.

70. Goldstein MG, Niaura R, Follick MJ, Abrams DB. Schedule of nicotine gum administration and smoking cessation treatment outcome. Am J of Psychi 1989; 146: 56–60.

71. Abelin T, Muller P, Buehler A, Vesanen K, Imhof PR. Controlled trial of transdermal nicotine patch in tobacco withdrawal. Lancet 1989; 1: 7–10.

72. Ornish SA, Zisook S, McAdams LA. Effects of transdermal clonidine treatment on withdrawal symptoms associated with smoking cessation. Arch of Internal Med 1988; 148: 2027–2031.

73. Glassman AH, Stetner F, Walsh BT, et al. Heavy smokers, smoking cessation and clonidine: Results of a double-blind, randomized trial. JAMA 1988; 259: 2863–2866.

74. Edwards NB, Murphy JK, Downs AD, Ackerman BJ, Rosenthal TL. Doxepin as an adjunct to smoking cessation: A double-blind pilot study. Am J of Psychi 1989; 146: 373–376.

75. Klesges RC, Meyers AW, Klesges LM, Vasque ME. Smoking, body weight,

and their effects on smoking behavior: A comprehensive review of the literature. Psychol Bull 1989; 106: 204–230.

76. Rodin J. Weight change following smoking cessation: The role of food intake and exercise. Addict Behav 1987; 12: 303–317.

77. Klesges RC, Brown K, Pascale RW, Murphy M, Williams E, Cigrang JA. Factors associated with participation, attrition, and outcome in a smoking cessation program at the workplace. Health Psychol 1987; 7: 575–589.

78. Hall SM, Ginsberg D, Jones RT. Smoking cessation and weight gain. J of Consult Clin Psychol 1986; 54: 342–346.

79. Streator JA, Sargent RC, Ward DC. A study of factors associated with weight change in women who attempt smoking cessation. Addict Behav 1989; 14: 523–530.

80. Carmody TP. Affect regulation, nicotine addiction, and smoking cessation. J of Psychoactive Drugs 1989; 21: 331–342.

81. Glassman AH, Covey LS, Stetner F. Smoking cessation and depression. Presented at the annual meeting of the American Psychiatric Association, May, 1989, San Francisco, CA.

82. Hall SM. Smoking, sweets, and sadness: Dependence, treatment failure, and regulatory systems. Paper presented at the annual meeting of the American Psychological Association, August 1988, Atlanta.

83. Hughes JR. Clonidine, depression and smoking cessation. JAMA 1988; 254: 2901–2902.

10
Recovery-Oriented Nicotine Addiction Therapy

TERRY A. RUSTIN

Recovery-Oriented Nicotine Addiction Therapy is an integrated psycho-therapeutic approach to the treatment of nicotine addiction. It uses 12-step concepts as a basis for treatment of nicotine addiction in the same way that alcoholism treatment incorporates the philosophy of Alcoholics Anonymous (AA) into alcoholism treatment; it embraces 12-step principles, but it is not a 12-step program. This chapter presents the theoretical and practical applications of this methodology; as yet, no controlled studies of the method exist.

Recovery-Oriented Nicotine Addiction Therapy is appropriate for patients who (a) are significantly addicted to nicotine, (b) have been unable to maintain abstinence from tobacco by simpler means, and (c) are willing to commit to a program of self-discovery, which will require an investment of time and effort. Previous experience with either 12-step recovery or addiction to another substance is not necessary for success.

In Recovery-Oriented Nicotine Addiction Therapy, the therapeutic professional strives to achieve the following treatment goals:

1. The patients will accept that they are addicted to a mind- and mood-altering chemical and will recognize how this addiction has altered and controlled their behavior.
2. The patients will understand that they are no longer able to control or predict their use of mind- and mood-altering chemicals and that complete abstinence from these chemicals is the only tenable option.
3. The patients will discover that they are not at fault or to blame for having an addiction, but that they now have the responsibility for maintaining their recovery.
4. The patients will identify the self-defeating behaviors that have repeatedly put them in situations where relapse is unavoidable and failure in life is inevitable.
5. The patients will learn and demonstrate specific skills for maintaining abstinence.

6. The patients will develop a plan for continued abstinence, which includes lifestyle changes, continued self-improvement, and a connection with a group of similarly addicted recovering individuals working together to maintain abstinence.

These are the same treatment goals that addiction treatment professionals apply to patients addicted to alcohol, heroin, cocaine, and other chemicals. In recovery-oriented treatments, the addiction is considered a primary, chronic, progressive disease with biological, genetic, psychological, and spiritual components, regardless of the specific chemicals involved. Treatment focuses on acceptance of the illness and taking personal responsibility for recovery through action. What data there are suggest that a recovery-oriented approach succeeds more often than other approaches, including treating the addiction as secondary to a psychiatric illness, insight-oriented therapy, medication alone, and no treatment.[1]

Recovery-oriented treatment programs utilize 12-step concepts, and at times, the distinction between recovery groups and therapy becomes unclear. AA describes itself as a fellowship of men and women who have joined together to share their experience, strength, and hope, in order to recover from their addiction and to assist others in doing so. Elsewhere in this volume (Chapter 27), Jay L. describes Nicotine Anonymous, a 12-step program that has adapted AA concepts to recovery from smoking dependence and nicotine addiction. In all 12-step programs, all members are seen as equals, and sharing is a two-way process.

Treatment is a professionally led encounter between an authority ("the therapist"), who is presumed to know the answers, and an individual seeking help ("the patient"), who accepts the authority of the other. The two are not seen as equals, and the help-giver is not expected to discuss the helpgiver's personal issues or even to answer any personal questions.

The goal in 12-step recovery programs is a spiritual recovery based on abstinence; the goal in therapy is to discover the truth about one's life. These two are not mutually exclusive and may be synergistic, but they are different. Qualified therapists recognize these differences and observe the boundaries.[2]

Recovery-Oriented Nicotine Addiction Therapy and Nicotine Anonymous (NA) are complementary; having been through treatment, patients are advised to attend NA meetings to further their recovery, and an individual unable to maintain abstinence through NA might seek professional assistance as well. The two programs, however, are distinct in the same way that AA and alcoholism treatment are different.

Recovery-Oriented Nicotine Addiction Therapy relies on cognitive dissonance to achieve the aforementioned six goals.

The Theory of Cognitive Dissonance

The Theory of Cognitive Dissonance was first advanced by Leon Festinger in 1957 as a way to explain and predict changes in human behavior.[3] Human beings, said Festinger, strive for consistency in their attitudes and behavior; any inconsistency (called "Dissonance") causes "psychological discomfort," which the individual seeks to resolve. Dissonance can exist between two attitudes, or between an attitude and a behavior that is inconsistent with that attitude. As the strength of the dissonance increases, the dissonant attitude becomes more likely to change.

The theory goes on to state that small rewards for behavior change produce stronger and more long-lasting attitude changes than large rewards, and behavior changes in response to the threat of small punishments produce stronger and more long-lasting attitude changes than behavior changes in response to the threat of severe punishments.

An ambivalent individual suffers constant dissonance, believing one way (e.g., "smoking is harmful") and behaving another way (e.g., "I am smoking"). When the individual resolves the dissonance through a change in behavior ("I choose not to smoke"), they become *consonant*. However, when this change occurs with minimal reward, new dissonance develops ("I like smoking, but I didn't smoke—and for what?") This dissonance is resolved by a change in attitude ("I prefer not to smoke.") Festinger, in 1957, even used the dissonance of a cigarette smoker to illustrate his theory. Twenty or more times each day, the smoker experiences dissonance: "I want to quit, yet I am lighting up another cigarette."

Dissonant smokers try to avoid dealing with their conflicts and to rationalize their behavior; nicotine, a mood enhancer, tends to quell this dissonance and is thus reinforcing. In Recovery-Oriented Nicotine Addiction Therapy, patients complete a series of exercises in the patient guide[4] that amplify this dissonance; the group process underscores the conflict and keeps the patient working. Change is achieved as the individual resolves the dissonance by reducing tobacco use.

Application to Patient Treatment

I have described the application of these techniques in detail elsewhere[5] and mention them here briefly.

The group spends the first 20 minutes of a $1\frac{1}{4}$-hour session sampling the mood and progress of the group via open-ended questions and group process in the style of Yalom.[6] Having identified a central issue, we then devote about 20 minutes to a didactic discussion of that issue, relating it to each patient. We then engage the group in a process discussion for about 20 minutes. In the final 15 minutes, we elicit goals that each patient will work on for the next session. I have used several other methods, both more and less sophisticated, to present the same information, but this format has been the most successful.

We have offered treatment primarily to outpatients, in small-group sessions, held twice a week for $1\frac{1}{4}$ hours each session, over a 12-week period. We have previously tried a more intensive schedule of 3 hours each night, three nights a week for 3 weeks. This intensive schedule was disastrous. It did not allow the patients sufficient time to grieve the loss of their tobacco, to put into action the skills they were learning, or to gradually detoxify themselves. A program of at least 8 weeks appears necessary. Sixteen weeks might produce better abstinence rates, but less compliance, because most patients have been unwilling to commit to such an extended program.

We have also tried running groups in which we did not ask for a commitment to come every week. My impression is that patients did about as well in these low-structure groups as in a more structured system. However, some weeks, no one showed up, and some weeks, everyone did, making it difficult to run such a program.

We have tried both open-ended groups (in which patients come into the program as they present themselves for treatment and agree to attend a given number of sessions) and closed-ended groups (in which the patients all start and end together.) Each has advantages and disadvantages.

With a *closed-ended group*, the facilitator can design a firm, comfortable structure, with certain topics slated for each session. There is little chaos and little confusion. There is considerable peer pressure to continue through the course of treatment and to complete assignments as they are given. Patients are expected to progress together, all quitting at about the same time, all completing the program and graduating from treatment on the same day. In many ways, closed-ended groups become more like an academic course than a therapy group.

Unfortunately, the rigidity of the closed-ended structure serves the facilitator's needs more than those of the patient. It assumes that a group of motivated patients of just the right size will appear, eager for treatment, at just the right moment. Program managers would love potential patients to be this compliant and well-organized, but unless the pool of potential patients is overwhelmingly large (as in a company of 3,000 employees), a closed-ended program is impractical. In addition, it allows little latitude if patients drop out because new patients cannot be added, even if they want to join.

Open-ended groups admit patients as they present themselves for treatment. Thus, there will be some patients in each group who are brand new, some who have been in the group for a while, and some who are completing the program. Each session must then engage and appeal to patients in each stage of treatment—no easy task. Rather than rely on a rigid structure, open-ended groups deal with the issues present in the room at the

TABLE 10.1. Patient characteristics predicting success or failure in Recovery-Oriented Nicotine Addiction Therapy.

Consistent with success
  Verbal
  Gregarious
  Compliant
  Other-centered
  Codependent
  Smokes to control or deal with dysphoric feelings
  Has failed at single-intervention treatments (injections, acupuncture, hypnosis, aversion therapy)
  35 Years and older
  In recovery from another chemical (alcohol, heroin, cocaine)
  Has suffered significant consequences
  Strong superego
  Depressed affect without major depression
Predictive of failure
  Highly independent
  Concrete
  Impatient
  Smokes mostly in response to withdrawal symptoms
  25 years and younger
  Has suffered few losses
  Narcissistic
  Antisocial
  Schizophrenic or other major mental disorders
  Clinically depressed

time, with advanced patients helping newcomers and much of the work done by each patient independently between groups.

This system is comparable to that usually employed in addiction treatment centers, where patients are admitted whenever they are willing. As in the treatment of other addictions, engaging patients when their motivation is highest improves the success of both the patient and the program.

Adolescents, whose damage from smoking has been minimal, do not do well in these groups. Patients with serious mental disorders (schizophrenia, major depression, bipolar illness) appear to self-medicate with cigarettes and also respond poorly (see Table 10.1). As with most smoking-cessation programs, success is related to motivation, willingness, and the extent of the consequences of smoking.

Smokers uniformly believe they would be better off not smoking, and most express a desire to quit, but they do not step forward to do so unless they are coerced in some way. DiClemente and Prochaska[7] have described this process, which they call "stages of change." When smokers have no interest in quitting or no plan to quit, they are in the stage of Precontemplation. When they are considering quitting but have no firm plans, they are in the stage of Contemplation. When they have made a decision to quit but have taken no action, they are in the Determination stage. When they have actually done something about quitting, they are in the stage of Action. When they have achieved their goal and are stable, they are in the Maintenance stage.

These authors have also described the protracted process of moving from contemplation through determination and into action.[8] We cannot expect potential patients, however much in need of our services, to volunteer for treatment at their first opportunity, or to progress on any set schedule. A program offering Recovery-Oriented Nicotine Addiction Therapy must commit itself to months of planning and promotion and must look to the future.

In Recovery-Oriented Nicotine Addiction Therapy, the structure resides in the mind of the therapist, not on paper. Highly structured groups, while less chaotic and easier to facilitate, do not reflect accurately the process of recovery, which requires resolution of ambivalence. Patients stand a better chance of maintaining abstinence if they face their ambivalence and resolve it themselves than if the facilitator resolves it for them.

This form of therapy is a psychotherapy program focused on nicotine-addiction treatment. Patients who can quit via information alone, medication alone, or less intensive methods, ought to do so. This methodology requires a significant investment of time and effort and is therefore appropriate only for those who have been unable to maintain abstinence by less intensive means and who are willing to engage in treatment (see Table 10.2).

Elements of Recovery-Oriented Nicotine Addiction Therapy Programs

Reasons for Wanting to Quit

The program's initial project asks, "What is a good reason for *you* to stop smoking?" The facilitator accepts any reason offered by the patient for wanting to quit smoking as being legitimate. This nonthreatening attitude sets the tone for the group and communicates that each individual's goals are honored, and each person's experience is respected.

Each patient is then asked to elaborate on her or his reasons, making them as specific and personal as possible. The facilitator describes four types of reasons, asks each member of the group to identify the reasons they gave as one of the four, and encourages them to make their reasons more personal.

The first kind of reason is *someone else's reasons*. The facilitator tells the group members the following:

People have been telling you that you ought to quit smoking for so long now that you think their reasons are your reasons. You might quit for someone else's rea-

TABLE 10.2. Structure of Recovery-Oriented Nicotine Addiction Therapy programs.

Characteristic	Better	Worse
Setting	Group	Individual
Location	Outpatient	Inpatient
Admissions	Open-ended	Closed-ended
Size	8–11 Participants	> 12 Participants
Session length	$1-1\frac{1}{4}$ Hours	< 1 Hour
Session frequency	1–2 Times/week	> 2 Times/week
Program length	10–14 Weeks	< 8 Weeks

sons, but you will not stay quit for someone else's reasons. We need to go beyond these reasons and discover your own reasons for wanting to quit.

Patients often bring up such "someone else's reasons" as the mess created by cigarettes and the effects of environmental smoke. The facilitator will point out that "Other people cannot change us, and whenever one person attempts to impose their needs on another, resentments develop. Thus, if we quit for someone else, we may harbor resentments, and will probably start smoking again."

The second kind of reason is *housekeeping reasons*. These are perfectly good reasons, but they will not have enough impact on the patient's life-style to really make much of a difference. Housekeeping reasons often center around money. Patients may consider the $700 they spend each year on cigarettes to be a substantial amount of money. If so, the facilitator would point out that $700 is not enough money to affect their life-style, and thus is not a significant issue. "If I offered to give you $700 to not smoke for the next 365 days, would you accept it?" the facilitator will ask. When phrased in this way, the patients will realize that their cigarettes have been more important to them than money, and that they will need to find other reasons to quit. The chemical is more important to any addicted person than is money.

The third type of reason is *sensible reasons*. These are reasons that no one would argue with, that make perfect sense, but that have not yet been sufficiently strong to make the addict change—such as the effects of smoking on the smoker's health.

"Someone else's reasons" provoke resentment; "housekeeping reasons" produce guilt; "sensible reasons" cause anxiety. None of them elicit change. Only *personal reasons*, reasons which reflect each person's true self, can elicit lasting change. Having dealt with the other three reasons, personal reasons come more easily. Patients will speak of relatives who died of emphysema, recalling their wheezing and their suffering. They will speak about feeling ashamed when children ask them why they still smoke. They will describe their desperate attempts to quit and their feelings of failure when they relapse.

Observe the cognitive dissonance at work: As the dissonance between the patients' behavior and beliefs increases, their beliefs change to fit their behavior. They then start choosing not to smoke some of the cigarettes they do not need in order to stay out of withdrawal and the ones to which they are less highly conditioned. According to the Theory of Cognitive Dissonance, this behavior change confirms the validity of the attitude change, which will subsequently create further behavior change.

The facilitator asks the patients to follow each of their reasons for change with a positive statement, beginning, "when I am a nonsmoker". Through this process, the patient confronts the pain of the past and expresses hope for the future. Smokers coming for treatment are embarrassed by their smoking; ending this project with a message of hope helps relieve their shame.

As the session nears its end, we ask each patient to set a goal for the following session. At this point, the facilitator is willing to accept any commitment, however small, and discourages goals that seem excessive.

Working on motivations for change engages the client, models the accepting attitude of the facilitator, begins the process of self-selected goal setting, and identifies ambivalence. The facilitator strives to clarify, personalize, and make more specific the motivations for change described by clients, ending with their statements of hope for the future.

Nicotine Is Addicting

Acceptance by patients that their chemicals are addicting and that they are addicted is central to any recovery-oriented method. Smokers may acknowledge that they have developed physical dependence on nicotine, but they usually do not consider nicotine to be equivalent to drugs like heroin or cocaine. They say "I know I'm hooked" in the same superficial way that cocaine addicts say, "Sure, anybody who uses cocaine has got a problem." "I know I'm hooked" can be a defense against truly experiencing the pain of knowing that one's life is completely controlled by an addicting substance. Successful recovery demands more.

Reaching beyond the cognitive level to a personal level of acceptance requires more than just *information*. Adequate *information* about the dangers of tobacco has been available to smokers since 1964,[9] but information alone has not been sufficient for most smokers to quit. If information alone were sufficient, the patient would not be seeking our help.

Informing patients about the addictive nature of nicotine helps them recognize the importance and the difficulty of achieving long-lasting change. This process emphasizes the similarity between nicotine and other addicting chemicals, and each group member's specific addictive behaviors. As before, their dissonance is maximized, and their ambivalence is left unresolved.

Acceptance

The First Step of all 12-step programs focuses on acceptance: "We admitted we were powerless over alcohol—that our lives had become unmanageable" (p. 59).[10] The word "admitted" has taken on new meaning over the years, with the step now meaning much more than a grudging admission that a problem exists, but a sense of recognition, both a comfort with and a release of guilt over past behavior. With drugs such as alcohol, cocaine, and heroin, the consequences of the addiction are so severe that the powerlessness and unmanageability cannot be denied. With nicotine, however, few patients can see the degree to which their lives have been controlled by the drug. Recovery-Oriented Nicotine Addiction Therapy avoids AA jargon, including the terms *powerless* and *unmanageable*, except with patients in recovery from another drug, where AA language can actually help. Instead, the facilitator keeps these concepts in mind while focusing the group's attention on how nicotine controls their behavior (powerlessness) and how it has ruled their lives (unmanageability).

Patients resist dealing with these issues, which intensify their sense of loss of control. This resistance is a powerful tool, which the facilitator uses to recognize the heart of the problem.

Times I Want a Cigarette

Patients identify as many triggers to smoking as they can, such as "when I finish a meal," or "when I feel guilty," or "when I first wake up in the morning." As before, the facilitator probes for more personal detail, more depth, more intensity; each trigger should yield five or more specifics. Then, an alternative to smoking can be deduced for each one. For some, these will be behavioral: "When I want a cigarette after I finish a meal, instead of smoking, I will brush my teeth right away." For some, they will be emotional: "When I feel guilty, instead of smoking, I will recognize what I did that was contrary to my values and will resolve to change that behavior." For some, they will be pharmacological: "When I want a cigarette when I wake up in the morning, instead of smoking, I will chew a quarter of a piece of Nicorette gum for 1 minute." Because not every solution fits every situation, we encourage patients to figure out several potential strategies to deal with each trigger, so that they will be prepared for a variety of circumstances.

Each trigger can often be traced back in time, revealing its logical antecedents. "I want a cigarette when I get into my car to drive home" is preceded by "I want that cigarette as I am walking across the parking lot," "I begin to crave the cigarette as I am leaving the elevator," and "I actually start thinking about lighting up as the clock approaches 5:00." With each such stage, the patient can plan a different set of alternatives.

Pain and Pleasure

Nicotine and cigarettes have served smokers well for many years. Patients have relied on tobacco to solve problems, to succeed, to enact a life role, to deal with dysphoric feelings, and to help them feel better. There is no point in trying to talk them out of this past pleasure, to attempt to convince them that they did not enjoy smoking, or that there were no advantages to smoking. Instead, we seek to help patients *accept* the pleasure they got from smoking, and recognize that the actual and potential consequences of smoking now exceed its advantages.

The facilitator takes a nonjudgmental attitude, helping the patient understand that their previous behavior was not bad or stupid, but that it had benefits at one time and now causes problems. The natural tendency is to avoid or reduce pain; the facilitator concentrates on the pain, makes it explicit, and intensifies the ambivalence, which increases the cognitive dissonance. This increases the patient's motivation to change.

Cigarettes Are Your Best Friend

Not only have cigarettes given these patients much pleasure, but they have also actually become companions and friends, often their best friends. While human friends have their own agendas and are often fickle, cigarettes are constant and predictable. Human friends may not be available in times of stress, but cigarettes always are. Friends die or move out of town, but cigarettes are available everywhere.

Many patients come to rely on cigarettes as they would an intimate companion or lover, sharing secrets and private moments. When they receive bad news, they turn to cigarettes for relief instead of friends or family. When they recognize how they have made their cigarettes their friends and lovers, they can become overwhelmed with emotion; some react with anger, others with disgust, others with shame, as in this poem written by a patient:

There she was
All wrapped in a gown of
Silver accentuated by strips of blue,
Adorned with an emerald . . .
I smiled with wild anticipation
Not a word was spoken as I removed her silver top
Panting rapidly
I gently stroked every inch of her lovely white body
While inhaling her aromatic fragrance
Lighting her fire with mad passion
Sucking on her orifice
Tasting her sweet addictive juices.
I felt my hormones and adrenalin
Coursing through my body.

I had to have her again and again.
After a while my craving was satisfied.
And she lay exhausted,
Broken in the ash tray.

For many smokers, cigarettes start out as a companion, become a friend, then a lover, and then like a part of their body. Recognizing this, we give patients time to grieve the loss of their cigarettes, allowing them to reduce their smoking at their own pace. This also favors resolution of their dissonance through action, with minimal reward. We tell patients the following:

Recovery is a process, not an event. Recovery is in the journey; it is not the destination . . . the day you snuff out your last cigarette is an important point on the journey, but it is just one more point. Whether you actually stop smoking today, tomorrow, or 6 months from now is not that important. Our goal is that when you quit, you will *stay quit.*

Through this project, often one of the most powerful of all, patients come to realize that their reliance on cigarettes as a friend, lover, and intimate part of themselves shows how *unmanageable* their lives have become.

Rituals, Roles and Automatic Smoking Behaviors

Smokers, more than other addicts, develop complex rituals around their drug use. While a cocaine addict might use crack 4 times a day, a nicotine addict may use 40 or more cigarettes a day. While other addicts must be secretive about purchasing and using drugs, nicotine addicts can smoke legally and in public. Smokers develop fascinating idiosyncrasies around their cigarette use, which we use to help patients recognize how completely nicotine controls their lives.

After introducing the concept of ritual use of tobacco, the group explores their ritual behaviors: opening packs, holding a cigarette, puffing in a certain way, putting it out, and so on. These rituals help them feel secure, but they also perpetuate their smoking and demonstrate their powerlessness over smoking.

Smoking behavior eventually becomes automatic, another sign of unmanageability. Patients work in the group, to describe and understand their automatic smoking behaviors, and to find techniques for interrupting them.

Cigarettes allow patients to play some specific life roles they would have difficulty playing without cigarettes. The facilitator describes how Lauren Bacall and Humphrey Bogart used their cigarettes as part of their roles. We ask patients to investigate which roles they use cigarettes to help them play, such as "the sophisticate," or "the tough guy." Similarly, we look at how advertising creates an image for each brand of cigarette:

Think of the brands you have smoked. What image comes to mind? For the price of a pack, you can buy into that image. . . . If that's what you are like, you don't need a cigarette to prove it, and if you are *not* like that, a four-inch piece of compost won't change you.

During these sessions, the facilitator focuses the group on how rituals, automatic smoking, and cigarette-related roles demonstrate their powerlessness over tobacco.

Feelings

Nicotine effectively disguises feelings, although most smokers are unaware that the drug does so. It is not until they have quit smoking for a while that they discover how they have medicated anxiety, anger, resentment, rejection, guilt, shame, depression, fear, boredom, worry, grief, or embarrassment by smoking. As they cut down, they become more aware, and their progress increases, but their fear of progress also increases.

Many therapists avoid this issue because there is no ready answer for these emerging feelings, and the patients would rather not deal with their dysphoria either. We make these feelings explicit by asking, "What feelings do you cover up by smoking? What feelings have you experienced today that you would rather not have to feel? If you did not smoke, what did you do with the feelings? What will you do with these feelings when you are a nonsmoker?" Opening up these issues results in some clients requiring therapy subsequently, usually for treatment of depression or alcoholism.

Smokers commonly use tobacco to deal with anxiety, so we make this an explicit issue, identifying causes of anxiety in each patient's life. We then trace these situations back to their antecedents, recognizing how they use tobacco in each instance to deal with the anxiety. Then, the facilitator and the group help each other find specific measures to deal with anxiety in each situation. As the patients reduce their use of tobacco, more and more anxiety becomes apparent, which gives the facilitator and the group an opportunity to identify these problems and to find specific solutions as they arise.

Goodbye Letters

The Fourth Step of the AA program asks people to make a "searching and fearless moral inventory" of themselves; in the Fifth Step, they are instructed to admit "to God, to ourselves, and to another human being the exact nature of our wrongs" (p. 60).[10] In practice, AA members may spend years working on the Fourth Step; many find that they are as much changed by working on this step as they are by getting sober. To complete the Fifth step, they then get together with another person, usually a cleric or a sponsor, to present themselves and their understanding of their recovery.

In Recovery Oriented Nicotine Addiction Therapy, patients write a series of letters to achieve the same recovery goals. They summarize what they have learned about themselves and their addiction and their recovery in a letter to tobacco, which starts, "Goodbye, Tobacco." In this letter, they acknowledge the advantages they received from smoking, the difficulty they will have in staying clean, and their hope for the future. In their second letter, "Hello, Me," they describe the changes they see themselves having made and their goals for further improvement.

Patients read these letters in a group session a week or so after they have smoked their last cigarette. We do not recommend that they do this right after their last cigarette (for one thing, it may not have been their last one); a week or so of struggling with abstinence improves their letters. Their book[4] contains examples of letters and suggestions for writing them.

Reading the letters in group can be a powerful emotional experience, but not one that every patient wishes to have. Only about half the group members actually complete this project while coming to group, but some will do so on their own, after the group sessions are over.

Relapse-Prevention Planning

From the beginning of the treatment process, we deal with relapse issues. Patients are asked to recall periods of abstinence and to identify factors responsible for their relapse. They list situations, feelings, and individuals that make them want to smoke more, or that might make them more likely to smoke after they have quit. They make both specific plans for dealing with pressures to relapse and specific plans to manage an actual relapse.

We always refer to these events as "relapses," not "slips," or "lapses." We identify a relapse to patients in this way:

When we smoke again after having not smoked for a while, we have "relapsed." *Relapse* means that our addiction has taken hold again. It means that there were some things we needed to be doing to stay clean that we stopped doing. The relapse starts when it becomes *possible* to smoke again, before the smoke hits our lungs. When our behavior changes so that smoking is possible, we are "building up to smoke."

In writing their relapse-prevention plan, patients develop the skills necessary to prevent a relapse or to interrupt a relapse in progress. The plan is action-oriented. Patients identify specific problems and solutions, and they practice these while in treatment. We hope that patients will quit smoking in the middle of treatment so that they will have opportunities to practice these behaviors while still coming to group.

The Twelfth Step of AA states, "Having had a spiritual awakening as a result of these steps, we tried to carry this message to alcoholics, and to practice these principles in all our affairs" (p. 60).[10] Carrying the message of recovery to those who continue to suffer has great value for all patients who have achieved abstinence; the danger is that they will become so self-righteous that they will become intolerable to others. Therefore, we include a discussion of "the kind of nonsmoker I will be" in the relapse-prevention plan.

Amends

At an advanced stage of recovery, patients are ready to look at the wreckage around them and to make amends for the damage caused by their smoking. We do this in group, in a manner derived from the Eighth and Ninth Steps of AA: "(We) made a list of all persons we had harmed, and became willing to make amends to them all," and "(We) made direct amends to such people wherever possible, except when to do so would injure them or others" (p. 60).[10]

We ask patients to list those whom they might have harmed in some way because of their smoking, suggesting a long list of possible people and situations. The patient brings the list to group and discusses the situations with the group. This is an opportunity to deal with shame, guilt, and honesty—to face the truth of the past and set out a new course for the future. The groups have been uniformly supportive and loving, and most patients feel a tremendous relief from working on this project.

Separation

As patients leave the group, or as a closed-ended group prepares to terminate, we enact a brief ceremony of completion, with the patients expressing what they are taking with them and what they have gotten from each group member. They focus on skills they have learned and their commitment to continued recovery.

Summary

Recovery Oriented Nicotine Addiction Therapy utilizes the 12-step concepts of acceptance, powerlessness, and unmanageability over a chemical, of relief of shame, of taking of personal responsibility for recovery, and of abstinence as a goal. It employs the power of cognitive dissonance to elicit change, relying on the strength of a group to keep the process going. Written materials support the work of a trained facilitator, usually in an outpatient setting.

While working with patients, the group facilitator keeps in mind the six goals of addiction-recovery programs listed at the beginning of this chapter. The facilitator takes an attitude of acceptance and encouragement, where confrontation is kept to a minimum and is tempered with attention to the patients' personal goals (see Table 10.3). The facilitator

TABLE 10.3. Patient and facilitator behaviors predictive of success and failure in Recovery-Oriented Nicotine Addiction Therapy.

Consistent with success
  Patient behaviors
    Making a commitment to complete the course of treatment
    Spending more time with friends who are staying abstinent
    Becoming receptive to new information
    Working on every project
  Facilitator behaviors
    Taking an attitude of acceptance
    Having patience with slow progress
    Maintaining appropriate expectations of the patients
    Giving many examples of success
    Providing many practical solutions to the everyday problems encountered by patients
    Regularly offering medication for detoxification
Predictive of failure
  Patient behaviors
    Demanding immediate success
    Unwillingness to connect with other group members
    Inconsistent attendance at group meetings
    Setting unattainable goals
  Facilitator behaviors
    Only providing information without providing therapy
    Only providing detoxification without providing therapy
    Telling the patients how to succeed on the basis of the facilitator's own recovery instead of guiding the patients to the discovery of their own solutions
    Threats, promises, or pleading as the primary motivator
    Using 12-step jargon with a nonrecovering clientele
    Allowing the patient to retain an attitude of being "special" or "different from the others"
    Providing examples of the consequences of smoking without examples of benefits of abstinence

regularly makes references to the similarities between nicotine addiction and other drug addictions, without using 12-step jargon.

Recovery Oriented Nicotine Addiction Therapy provides a method for treating the physical, mental, emotional, and spiritual components of nicotine dependency. While not appropriate for every smoker, it offers those willing to engage in the process an opportunity for a significant life-changing experience.

References

1. Muhleman D. 12-Step study groups in drug abuse treatment programs. J of Psychoactive Drugs 1987; 19(3): 291–298.
2. Zweben JE. Recovery-oriented psychotherapy: Facilitating the use of 12-step programs. J of Psychoactive Drugs 1987; 19(3): 243–250.
3. Festinger L. A theory of cognitive dissonance. Palo Alto, CA: Stanford University Press, 1957.

4. Rustin T. Quit and stay quit: Medical treatment program for smokers. Houston: Discovery Publishing, 1989.
5. Rustin T. Facilitator's guide to Quit and stay quit. Houston: Discovery Publishing, 1989.
6. Yalom ID. The theory and practice of group psychotherapy, 3rd ed. New York: Basic Books, 1985.
7. DiClemente CO, Prochaska JO, Gilbertini M. Self-efficacy and the stages of self-change of smoking. Cognitive Ther and Res 1985; 9: 181–200.
8. Prochaska JO, DiClemente CO. Toward a comprehensive model of change. In: Miller WR, Heather N, eds. Treating addictive behaviors. New York: Plenum, 1986: 3–27.
9. U.S. Department of Health, Education and Welfare. Smoking and health: A report to the Surgeon General of the Public Health Service, PHS Publication No. 1103. Washington, DC: U.S. Department of Health, Education and Welfare, Public Health Service, Center for Disease Control, 1964.
10. Alcoholics Anonymous. The Big Book. 3rd ed. New York: Alcoholics Anonymous World Services, 1976.

11
Counterconditioning Methods

JAMES W. SMITH

Behavior-modification therapy for the treatment of addictions has been used in one form or another for centuries. For example, the ancient Romans attempted to treat alcoholism by inducing a distaste for alcohol by placing a dead spider or other unpleasant item in the bottom of a wine goblet to be discovered by the drinker upon draining the cup.[1] As tobacco use began to become popular, some nations attempted to intervene by royal decree. Increasingly severe penalties were imposed, including, in some cases, execution for a third offense. Though effective in eliminating further tobacco use by the executed individual, this crude form of behavior-modification therapy was ultimately ineffective in stemming the tide of nicotine dependence.

More refined and experimentally based forms of aversion therapy for this dependence were developed in the 1960s and early 1970s. These approaches evolved along several lines:

1. Noxious smoke techniques
2. Faradic (electric shock) based aversive techniques
3. Taste aversion techniques
4. Covert sensitization
5. Combinations of the preceding techniques

Noxious Smoke Techniques

A substantial body of literature has been published on treatment approaches in which the various aspects of tobacco smoke are used as aversive stimuli. These approaches are generally based on the concept that greater effectiveness is achieved when the behavior to be eliminated is closely related to the aversive stimulus.[2] Examples of these techniques include focused smoking (including smoke holding, taste satiation, and rapid puffing), warm smoky air blown into the face of the subject, rapid smoking, satiation, and others (including combinations of these techniques).

Focused Smoking

Focused smoking, also known as "normal paced aversive smoking," involves having the subjects smoke at their usual rate (puffs per minute). At the same time, they are instructed to focus on the negative sensations associated with smoking (light-headedness, tiredness, nausea, burning sensation, coughing, breathing discomfort).[3] This technique was originally used as a "placebo control" for comparison to other aversion techniques but was noted to have some effectiveness. Lichtenstein, Harris, Birchler, Wahl, and Schmahl[4] reported that it was effective only for short-term cessation. Hackett and Horan[5,6] reported abstinence rates of 40% and 56% at 6- to 9-month follow-up in two small studies. However, in a study with chronically ill subjects with significant medical reasons to stop smoking, the technique was ineffective.[7] There are several variations of focused smoking. These include "taste satiation," "smoke holding," and "rapid puffing."

TASTE SATIATION

Tori[8] reported the results of a *taste-satiation* procedure. It requires the subjects initially to close their eyes and focus on the sensations in their lungs, throat, and mouth. After 5 minutes, they light a cigarette and swish the smoke around the mouth for 30 seconds while breathing through the nose. The smoke is then exhaled, following which the sequence is repeated with modifications. After 20 seconds of mouth holding, the subjects are instructed to focus attention on their lungs and to inhale. This is followed by exhalation through the nose. This sequence is repeated with a 5-minute rest period between cigarettes. Inhalations are limited to four or five per cigarette. Four to five cigarettes are usually smoked in each treatment session. The session is terminated when the subject reports loss of desire to continue. Treatment sessions were conducted for 5 consecutive days. Five weekly posttreatment hypnotherapy sessions were also included. Tori reported that 68% of the subjects were abstinent at 6-month follow-up.

SMOKE HOLDING

A *smoke-holding* procedure was reported by Kopel, Suckerman, and Baksht.[9] It closely resembles the taste-satiation procedure except that no smoke inhalation occurs. They reported a 6-month abstinence rate of 33%. In a later study, Walker and Franzini[10] reported a smoking rate of 39% of baseline at the 3-month follow-up (compared to 57% for a second group treated with focused smoking).

RAPID PUFFING

Perhaps the most simple variation of focused smoking is *rapid puffing* (or *quick puff*). In this technique, the cigarette is puffed (but not inhaled) rapidly. The smoke is hot and unpleasant tasting.[11] Erickson, Tiffany, Martin, and Baker[12] compared the results of rapid puffing, rapid smoking, and nonaversive counseling in 25 volunteer male and female smokers. All subjects were abstinent at the conclusion of six therapy sessions. At the 12-month follow-up, rapid-smoking treatment resulted in 70% abstinence, rapid puffing resulted in 33 hr ⅓% abstinence, and behavioral counseling achieved the lowest rate—14.3% abstinence.

Powell and McCann[13] reported the results of a somewhat more complex rapid-puffing procedure. Their *pinky-puffing and smoke signaling* procedure requires the subjects to puff a cigarette without inhaling. The cigarette is held between the last two fingers of their nonsmoking hand. It is puffed on the side of the mouth opposite that on which cigarettes are usually smoked. The subjects are required to puff quickly without inhaling with the intention of producing a hot sensation around the lips and an accumulation of smoke in the eyes. At the same time, additional aversive stimuli are presented. These include

1. A large ash tray placed in front of the subject, which is filled with cigarette litter
2. Cigarette filters coated with a bitter-tasting antinailbiting solution
3. A tape recording playing loud "white noise"
4. Presentation of a slide show depicting smoking-induced diseased organs, interspersed with magazine advertisements for cigarettes

They reported 100% abstinence rates in the immediate posttreatment period, 76.5% at 6 months, and 63% at 1 year posttreatment. These 1-year results were based on self-reports of subjects contacted by mail or telephone with responses from all but one subject (98%), who was arbitrarily classified as smoking. The study also included an introductory meeting and four consecutive treatment meetings held 1 week later. All subjects were treated as a group. At the end of the treatment phase, subjects were randomly assigned to one of three maintenance conditions. These consisted of a 4-week support group, offering the opportunity to discuss feelings and thoughts, a 4-week telephone contact system, which enabled subjects to call one another, and a no-contact control group. The small number of recidivists in each group precluded posttreatment smoking rates being used to demonstrate differential effects due to support treatment. The authors did, however, show that the support group subjects gave a significantly higher rating for program satisfaction than did the other two groups.

Warm Smoky Air to the Face

Wilde[14] reported that successful results were obtained with a small group of subjects (seven) by blowing warm stale smoke at them while they were smoking at their normal rate. Subsequently, Wilde[15] reported that almost all of his subject relapsed. Franks, Fried, and Ashem[16] reported equivocal results using an improved smoke-blowing apparatus. Their study was troubled by a high attrition rate and lack of a control group.

In a replication of the Franks et al. study with the addition of a control group and a monetary deposit (which greatly minimized attrition), Grimaldi and Lichtenstein,[17] reported no significant differences among any of the groups (contingent-smoke group, noncontingent-smoke group, or attention-placebo group). Relapse rates were high, and none achieved 6 months of abstinence. With further refinement of the technique, Lublin and Joslyn[18] reported improved results with a group of heavy smokers. They massed sessions and required subjects to smoke rapidly (thereby apparently adding a rapid-smoking aversive component to the procedure). They also offered high levels of encouragement. They reported 21 treatment dropouts. However, of the 78 subjects who completed at least three treatment sessions, 40 stopped smoking entirely. One year later, 15 (19%) were still abstinent, and 16 (21%) were smoking at less than 50% of baseline.

In an attempt to distinguish between the treatment effects of warm smoky air and rapid smoking, Lichtenstein, Harris, Birchler, Wahl, and Schmahl[4] randomly assigned 40 subjects to the following treatment conditions:

1. Attention placebo
2. Warm smoky air only
3. Warm smoky air and rapid smoking
4. Rapid smoking only

In addition, three of the experimenters (graduate students) were randomly assigned to see each subject for an average of 7.2 sessions. The attention-placebo group subjects were told they would be helped to extinguish their desire to smoke and that the importance of not smoking between sessions was related to the extinction process. They were also given Bantron® pills (lobeline); all but one subject was abstinent at the end of the treatment period. Twenty-one of the 39 subjects contacted were still abstinent 6-months later (52% abstinence rate). Seven of the 10 attention-placebo group were again smoking at 6-months (30% abstinence). Only 12 of the 30 treatment subjects had returned to smoking (60% abstinence). There were no significant differences in outcome among the warm smoky air, warm smoky air plus rapid smoking, or rapid smoking only groups.

They concluded that the smoke-blowing apparatus and rapid smoking have no additive effect and that they are virtually interchangeable. It should be noted, however, that this study had much better outcomes associated with the warm smoky air technique than was found by Wilde;[15] by Franks, Fried, and Ashem;[16] and by Grimaldi and Lichtenstein.[17] The authors gave no explanation for this marked difference, which leaves one to wonder whether other aspects of the procedure may have accounted for the good results.

Rapid Smoking

EFFICACY

Lichtenstein and his colleagues at the University of Oregon have published extensively on the *rapid-smoking* technique, in which the subject is required to puff and inhale normally from a cigarette once every 6 seconds. The subject uses her or his own brand of cigarettes. The treatment session continues for approximately 5 minutes or until the subject indicates that further inhalations cannot be tolerated (e.g., because of nausea). After a 5-minute rest period, the subject smokes a second cigarette in the same manner. This is followed by a second 5-minute rest period, after which the subject is encouraged (but not required) to smoke a third cigarette in the same way. Timing of treatment sessions in different reports have varied from consecutive days to weekly intervals.[4,19]

Rapid smoking is one of the most widely researched and widely employed treatment approaches.[20] The procedure grew out of the warm smoky air aversive technique, and the early studies combined the two. Initial outcome reports were very encouraging. Six-month abstinence rates of 60% or higher were reported by Lichtenstein's group.[4,21] These results were particularly striking when compared to other outcome studies of the day. Hunt and Bespalec[22] reported a 30% abstinence rate in 89 programs offering a variety of approaches. Of particular interest is the fact that this figure was applied to the subjects who were abstinent at the end of treatment, rather than to the total group of subjects who started treatment.

Subsequent studies indicate that the initial striking results did not hold up over longer follow-up periods. Lichtenstein and Rodrigues[19] determined, through telephone interviews with participants in four rapid-smoking/blown-smoky-air aversion treatment protocols for dependent smokers, that 34% reported abstinence at 2- to 6-year posttreatment follow-up. Lando and McGovern[23] reported a 46% abstinence rate for 24 subjects at 12-month, 24-month, and 48-month posttreatment follow-up intervals, after participating in a similar aversion (and support) treatment protocol. Of particular interest in this report is their conclusion that the relapse curve appeared to level off by 1-year posttreatment. At that point, subjects who resumed smoking were replaced by an equal number of subjects who resumed abstinence. Danaher[24] reviewed 22 rapid-smoking studies, 14 of which allowed comparison with a placebo control or alternative treatment. In 10 of these, rapid smoking produced a higher long-term abstinence rate, however, in no study did these increases reach statistical significance. Perhaps the most extensive review of the procedure is that of Schwartz;[25] in an analysis of 49 rapid-smoking studies, the range of quit rates was 6% to 67%. The median quit rate for 1-year studies was 25%. In studies in which rapid smoking was the principal component of treatment, the median quit rate was also 25%. Studies that had quit rates above 50% combined rapid smoking with other techniques, such as covert sensitization, self-control, relaxation, and relapse-prevention training.

Lichtenstein and Danaher[3] suggest that two processes may underlie the efficacy of rapid smoking. The first is satiation, both physiological and psychological, which may temporarily reduce the attractiveness of cigarettes. The second involves cognitive rehearsal of the unpleasant experiences of treatment. The therapy may provide the subject with unpleasant experiences, which can later be reinstated cognitively as a means of counteracting future smoking urges.

SIDE EFFECTS OF RAPID SMOKING

Concerns have been voiced about potential risks involved in rapid-smoking approaches.[26] The possibility of nicotine poisoning was raised, but a direct comparison of blood-nicotine levels under regular and rapid-smoking conditions showed that nicotine poisoning was unlikely.[27] There is little doubt, however, that rapid-smoking procedures are associated with an increased heart rate, increased nicotine levels, increased carboxyhemoglobin, and blood gas changes.[27,28] Hall, Sachs, and Hall[29] reported on 24 healthy male cigarette smokers undergoing rapid-smoking treatment. After analyzing physiological measurements (electrocardiogram, arterial blood gases, and vital signs), they concluded that "rapid smoking was found to be safe for healthy subjects."

Poole, Sanson-Fisher, German, and Harker[30] studied the effects of 6 to 12 rapid-smoking aversion therapy sessions on the blood pressure, pulse rate, and cardiac functioning of 58 male and female smokers. They noted no evidence of a cumulative effect in the temporary treatment-related rise in pulse and blood pressure. The appearance of some T-wave flattening and S–T depression were not considered to represent a significant risk from such treatment. Glasgow, Lichtenstein, Beaver, and O'Neil[31] reported that such acute negative subjective reactions to rapid-smoking treatment as dizziness, tingling, and vomiting are apparently more related to relatively harmless temporary increases in carboxyhemoglobin levels then to any more harmful consequences of nicotine poisoning.

Most studies of side effects have been carried out on healthy subjects. This did nothing to ease concerns about unhealthy subjects, who may form a sizable proportion of smoking-treatment applicants. Hall, Sachs, Hall, and Benowitz[32] studied the effects of rapid smoking on a group of patients with cardiac and pulmonary disease. The patients were monitored medically under baseline, exercise, normal-smoking, and rapid-smoking conditions. There was no evidence of myocardial ischemia during rapid smoking. In fact, a smaller number of subjects had premature ventricular contractions (PVCs) during rapid smoking (29%) than with normal smoking (60%) or with treadmill exercise (59%).

Satiation

The satiation technique requires the subject to increase the number of cigarettes smoked without changing the pace of smoking. Most studies require the subject to double or triple the number of cigarettes smoked at baseline. Many studies had the subjects smoking at home,[25] though Lando and Davison[33] had subjects undertake satiation in the laboratory. The latter condition, of course, allows for greater reliability in establishing compliance to the study protocol. Although early reports were optimistic,[34] subsequent studies did not support that optimism.[35,36] In the five studies where satiation was the principal component of treatment, quit rates ranged from 15% to 35%[37] Most studies using satiation combine the technique with others (e.g., self-control, desensitization, contracting, group support, and rapid smoking). It is not possible to determine how much of the treatment results are from satiation and how much are the result of the other techniques. Eleven of these studies with 6-month follow-ups had a median quit rate of 38%. Twelve studies with 1-year follow-up had a median quit rate of 34.5%.[25]

Although there are some similarities between satiation and rapid smoking, satiation appears to be less effective. Lichtenstein and Danaher[3] proposed that the difference was due to a greater treatment time with rapid smoking. They also point out that there was minimal interpersonal persuasiveness in the satiation studies. They emphasize the value of "a warm, contingently persuasive interpersonal context" in a treatment program. Schwartz[25] also points out that in satiation procedures, there is less emphasis on "cognitive focusing and revivification." With rapid smoking, subjects are instructed to focus on negative experiences during the smoking procedure and immediately thereafter. Satiation, particularly out of the laboratory setting, does not generally include such specific instructions and thus may not induce generalization or maintenance.

Chain-Smoking

A form of satiation that includes a variation of rapid smoking aversion is chain-smoking. In this procedure, the subject smokes at a normal pace but smokes continuously (*chain-smokes*) for an extended period of time. Marrone, Merksomer, and Salzberg[38] reported on 32 smokers divided into three groups (control, chain-smoking for 10 hours, and chain-smoking for 20 hours). The setting was a motel room. At 4-month follow-up, the 20-hour group had significantly more abstinent subjects (6 out of 10). The

10-hour and control groups were nearly identical, having 2 and 1 abstinent subjects, respectively.

Young,[39] in a laboratory setting, gave twice-weekly chain-smoking treatments for 6 weeks. The subjects chain-smoked eight cigarettes. Pardoxical results were found, in that control subjects did better than chain-smoking subjects.

Faradic Shock

Azrin and Holz[40] defined *punishment* not in the terms non behaviorists commonly associate with the word (e.g., retribution for a socially unacceptable act), but in behavioral terms, as a decrease in the probability of a response (e.g., smoking) as a consequence of that response being followed by a punishing stimulus. In the field of behavior modification, the use of electric shock as a punishing stimulus for reducing the rate of undesirable behavior has been used extensively. Electric shock is a widely used noxious stimulus in smoking studies. Its convenience and precise timing of application within a treatment conditioning paradigm no doubt contribute to its frequent use.[41] When used in cigarette-smoking studies, reports on success rates have been mixed. Koenig and Masters[42] found that a shock-punishment group did not differ significantly from either a systematic-desensitization group or supportive-counseling group in reducing smoking rate. Mees[43] and Ober[44] reported that electric shock was no more effective than other kinds of treatment for reducing cigarette smoking. Carlin and Armstrong[45] attempted to assess the importance of attitudinal variables in aversive conditioning. They reported no differences in mean percentage of smoking reduction during 4 treatment days among shock conditioning, pseudoconditioning, and control groups. All groups, however, reduced smoking (to about 50% of baseline). No long-term follow-up data were reported. These studies and others[46] suggest that *office-bound* (i.e., in the clinician's office) electric shock treatment has little effectiveness.[41]

In contrast, Gendreau and Dodwell[47] reported that the smoking rate of a shock-treated group was significantly less than a control group. They used volunteer male prison inmates ($n = 9$) and administered increasingly strong shocks, which were terminated by the subject extinguishing his cigarette. The four control subjects were treated the same in all respects except that they were given subliminal shock. Three shock treatment subjects were still abstinent 250 days after treatment. The general applicability of this study is limited by the samll number of subjects.

In a similar study, McGuire and Vallance[48] reported that 6 of 10 persons were nonsmokers 1 month after treatment, which consisted of electric shocks following cigarette inhalations. A more systematic study[49] demonstrated that the rate of smoking decreased as the intensity of shock increased. They used a special cigarette pack that automatically delivered a shock when opened. Of interest is the fact that it was found that the greater the intensity of the shock, the less time the subjects wore the apparatus. That is, they appeared to develop an aversion to the apparatus, a factor that may limit the usefulness of self-administered aversive stimuli in various behavior-modification approaches.

Steffy, Meichenbaum, and Best[50] extended the aversion-conditioning paradigm to include both overt and covert verbalizations of smoking, as well as the actual act of smoking. They reported that the group receiving shocks for smoking in an escape–avoidance paradigm while covertly imagining themselves in smoking situations were smoking less at the 2- and 6-month follow-ups than the overt verbalization groups and an insight therapy.

Chapman, Smith, and Layden[51] pointed out that none of the preceding studies employed one of the most effective designs for eliminating a behavior. They noted that animal research indicates that the most efficient method for eliminating the target behavior is to follow every instance of the behavior with a strong aversive stimulus while offering an alternative nonpunished response.[40] In their study, the nonpunished response consisted of putting down the cigarette, moving the hand away from it or, in general, any act that could be construed as the opposite of a smoking act.

Chapman, Smith, and Layden[51] used five consecutive daily electric shock treatments and self-management training with two groups of smokers ($n = 23$) who had smoked 14 to 60 cigarettes from 4 to 48 years. Group I received 2 weeks of posttreatment therapist monitoring, and Group II received 11 weeks of monitoring. Only 1 subject in each group failed to stop smoking by the end of the 5 days of treatment. Follow-up at 1, 3, 6, and 12 months showed longer cessation of smoking in Group II. Six of 11 (54%) of them were still nonsmokers at 12 months, compared to 3 of 12 subjects (25%) in Group I. They concluded that electric-shock punishment combined with self-management training is effective for eliminating smoking in most subjects, and posttreatment therapist monitoring is important in maintaining long-term abstinence.

Smith[11] reported on a commercial stop-smoking program (Schick) based on the Chapman, Smith, and Layden[51] original study. The treatment used 5 days of electric-shock counterconditioning, combined with a noxious-smoke technique (quick puff). It also included an educational and counseling component during the initial counterconditioning phase and a 6-week support phase with weekly support group meetings. An additional innovation was one booster counterconditioning treatment in the second week. Of the 327 clients contacted at least 1 year later (mean of 13.7 months), 52% were still abstinent. The importance of the home environment was highlighted by this study. Of those returning to a nonsmoking home, over 60% of the clients remained nonsmokers. Of those who returned to a smoking household, 70.2% returned to smoking.

This study, though included in the section on faradic shock, also includes one of the noxious-smoke techniques, as well as posttreatment support. It therefore also qualifies as a combination treatment study (see the later section on combined treatments). It is impossible to determine the precise contribution of any one element of the treatment protocol to the outcome, a situation that is true of a great many of the smoking studies.

Covert Sensitization

Cautela[52,53,54] pioneered some of the important concepts in covert sensitization, particularly the importance of cognitive antecedents and consequences of a behavior. The objective of covert sensitization is to produce avoidance behavior through the use of the subjects' imagination.[25] Cautela[53] points out that the process is a type of punishment paradigm because the smoker is instructed to imagine a noxious sensation while associating cigarettes with aversive thoughts (e.g., imagining preparing to smoke, then imagining experiencing nausea and vomiting). Relief is then provided by instructing the subject to imagine feeling better as he or she turns away from the cigarette. Subjects are given training in the laboratory and are generally instructed to carry out the procedure in the natural environment. This procedure, in general, used the principles advocated by Chapman, Smith, and Layden,[50] associating the unwanted behavior with an aversive stimulus while offering an alternative nonpunished response.

Reviews of the procedure indicate that, used alone, there appears to be little, if any, beneficial effect.[3,25,55] A typical study is that of Lowe, Green, Kurtz, Ashenberg, and Fisher.[56] Covert sensitization was used in one of two self-control groups. Three clinic meetings per week were held for 3 weeks. The covert sensitization images included nausea and vomiting, coughing and choking. The subjects also practiced situations and aversive scenes of their own choosing. They were further urged to use covert sensitization in their natural setting as a way to control smoking urges. The procedure also included 10 maintenance sessions over a 90-day period. Thirty of 33 subjects attended at least half of the treatment sessions before quit dates. There were no statistically different abstinence rates between the two groups. In fact, there was a nonsignificant trend for the group *not* using covert sensation to do better (37% abstinence at 6 months vs. 29%).

Some authors report that combining covert sensitization with one or more other procedures results in better outcomes than with any of the procedures separately.[57,58] Tongas[59] assigned subjects to covert sensitization, rapid smoking, group therapy, or combined treatment. Nineteen treatment and maintenance sessions were given. Covert sensitization was given in five sessions. Home assignments were also given. At 2 years, covert sensitization and rapid smoking showed equal results (19% success), while the combined group showed 38% success.

In another study Severson, O'Neal, and Hynd[60] reported 50% success at 9-month follow-up for the combination treatment group, compared to 30% for rapid smoking alone and 11% for covert sensitization alone. In contrast, in a similar study, Barbarin[61] reported no difference between combined treatment and covert sensitization alone. Both had success rates of only 7%.

In his review, Schwartz[25] notes that of 10 covert sensitization studies with at least a 6-month follow-up, the median quit rate was 25.5%. He further states "It should be noted that the quit rates were low when covert sensitization was used alone, and when covert sensitization was combined with other procedures, it added little to the effectiveness. (p. 81)"

Taste Aversion

When the mouth and tongue have been exposed to silver acetate, the taste of tobacco smoke is altered so that the majority of individuals perceive it as bitter and unpleasant. This principle has been used in attempts to reduce or eliminate smoking. The bitter taste response is experienced by approximately 85% of individuals and lasts up to 3 hours.[62]

Silver acetate deterrent therapy is reviewed in Chapter 12. More extensive studies utilizing silver acetate in combination with other aversive procedures, such as smoke holding, rapid puffing, rapid smoking, or faradicshock aversion, have not been reported. The simultaneous application of a variety of aversive techniques using different sensory pathways might offer better results than when only a single technique is applied.

Combination Treatments

Because smoking is a complex, multidetermined, and multidimensional behavior, many researchers have developed treatment programs that combine several therapeutic components. Indeed, in virtually all clinical treatment programs, more than one therapeutic component is included (e.g., education and support), along with the therapeutic element being emphasized (e.g., rapid smoking).[20] A number of the studies use rapid smoking, or some variant of the procedure, with self-management strategies (e.g., self-monitoring, stimulus control, problem solving, and other coping strategies). Other components may include contingency contracting,[63] relaxation training,[24] stress management,[64] and others.[20] Lando[65] reported on one of the early combination programs using satiation (for 6 days) as a component, combined with discussions about the learned basis of smoking. Control subjects received the same 6 days of treatment but did not receive the maintenance component (discussions). Results were encouraging, in that 76% of the combined treatment group were abstinent at 16 months, compared to 35% for the controls. Best[66] also reported encouraging results with rapid smoking, combined with components tailored to the subjects' locus-of-control scores, attitude-change techniques, and stimulus control. At 6 months, 50% of the subjects were abstinent.

Less encouraging results were reported by Danaher,[24] who compared rapid smoking alone with rapid smoking plus self-control. At 13-week follow-up, the rapid smoking (only) group had a higher abstinence rate (35%) than the combination group (21.4%). Possible explanations for this negative effect have been offered by Danaher[24] and by Collette, Payne, and Rizzo.[20] These primarily deal with errors in technique (e.g., timing of the presentation of the self-control technique, an overload of skills presented, lack of follow-through in the use of skills presented).

Elliot and Denny[67] reported significantly higher abstinence rates (45%), at 6-month follow-up, in the combination group than in the rapid smoking only group (17%). The combination group included rapid smoking, covert sensitization, applied relaxation, systematic desensitization, self-reward and self-punishment, cognitive restructuring, behavioral rehearsal, and emotional role-playing. Other researchers have found encouraging results when combining rapid smoking with other components. Many of these other techniques are described in detail elsewhere in Chapters 9, 10, 13, 20, 25, 26, and 27 of this volume.

In summary, it can be said that counterconditioning aversive techniques of a wide variety have been used in smoking-cessation treatments. Used in isolation, without some sort of support and/or other relapse-prevention strategy, they, like any other unitary approach, do not appear to be associated with long-term success. However, when used with these abstinence-maintenance approaches, they seem to be associated with significantly improved long-term abstinence rates.

References

1. Rackham H. Pliny's natural history: Books I–II. Cambridge, MA: Harvard University Press, 1938.
2. Wilson GT, Davison GC, Aversion techniques in behavior therapy: Some theoretical and metatheoretical considerations. J of Consult and Clin Psychol, 1969, 33: 327–329.
3. Lichtenstein E, Danaher BG, Modification of smoking behavior: A critical analysis of theory, research, and practice. In Hersen M, Eisler RM, Miller PM, eds. Progress in behavior modification. Vol. 3. New York: Academic Press, 1976: 79–132.
4. Lichtenstein E, Harris DE, Birchler GR, Wahl JM, Schmahl DP. Comparison of rapid smoking, warm, smoky air, and attention placebo in the modification of smoking behavior. J of Consult and Clin Psychol 1973; 40: 92–98.
5. Hackett G, Horan JJ. Focused smoking: An unequivocally safe alternative to rapid smoking. J of Drug Educ 1978; 8: 261–265.

6. Hackett G, Horan JJ. Partial compound analysis of a comprehensive smoking program. Addict Behav 1979; 4: 259–262.
7. Lichtenstein E. The smoking problem: A behavioral perspective. J of Consult and Clin Psychol 1982; 50(6): 804–819.
8. Tori CD. A smoking satiation procedure with reduced medical risk. J of Clin Psychol 1978; 34: 574–579.
9. Kopel SA, Suckerman KR, Baksht A. Smoke holding: An evaluation of physiological effects and treatment efficacy of a new nonhazardous aversive smoking procedure. Paper presented at the 13th Annual Meeting of the Association for Advancement of Behavior Therapy, San Francisco, 1979.
10. Walker WB, Franzini LR. A comparison of low-risk aversion group treatments for smoking cessation. Paper presented at the 16th annual convention of the Association for Advancement of Behavior Therapy, Los Angeles, 1982.
11. Smith JW. Long term outcome of clients treated in a commercial stop smoking program. J of Subst Abuse Treat 1988; 5: 33–36.
12. Erickson LM, Tiffany ST, Martin EM, Baker TB. Aversive smoking therapies: A conditioning analysis of therapeutic effectiveness. Behav Res and Ther 1983; 21: 595–611.
13. Powell DR, McCann BS. The effects of a multiple treatment program and maintenance procedures on smoking cessation. Prevent Med 1981; 10: 94–107.
14. Wilde GJS. Behavior therapy for addicted smokers. Behav Res and Ther 1964; 2: 107–110.
15. Wilde GJS. Letter to the editor. Behav Res and Ther 1965: 2: 313.
16. Franks CM, Fried R, Ashem B. An improved apparatus for the aversive conditioning of cigarette smokers. Behav Res and Ther 1966; 4: 301–308.
17. Grimaldi KE, Lichtenstein E. Hot smoky air as an aversive stimulus in the treatment of smoking. Behav Res and Ther 1969; 4: 275–282.
18. Lublin I, Joslyn L. Aversive conditioning of cigarette addiction. Paper read at the meeting of the American Psychological Association, Los Angeles, September, 1968.
19. Lichtenstein E, Rodrigues MRP. Long-term effects of rapid smoking treatment for dependent cigarette smokers. Addict Behav 1977; 2: 109–112.
20. Colletti G, Payne TJ, Rizzo AA. Treatment of cigarette smoking. In: Nirenberg, TD, and Maisto, SA (eds.) Development in the assessment and treatment of addictive behaviors. Norwood, New Jersey: Ablex Publishing Corporation, 1987, p. 245.
21. Schmahl DP, Lichtenstein E, Harris DE. Successful treatment of habitual smokers with warm, smoky air and rapid smoking. J of Consult and Clin Psychol 1973; 39: 105–111.
22. Hunt WA, Bespalec DA. An evaluation of current methods of modifying smoking behavior. J of Clin Psychol 1974; 30: 431–438.
23. Lando HA, McGovern RG. Three-year data on a behavioral treatment for smoking: A follow-up rate. Addict Behav 1982; 7: 177–181.
24. Danaher BG. Rapid smoking and self-control in the modification of smoking behavior. J of Consult and Clin Psychol 1977; 45: 1068–1075.
25. Schwartz JL. Review and evaluation of smoking cessation methods: The United States and Canada 1978–1985. Bethesda, MD, National Institutes of Health, 1987.

26. Horan JJ, Lindberg SE, Hackett G. Nicotine poisoning and rapid smoking. J of Consult and Clin Psychol 1977; 45: 344–347.
27. Russell MAH, Raw M, Taylor C, Feyerabend C, Saloojee Y. Blood nicotine and carboxyhemoglobin levels after rapid-smoking aversion therapy. J of Consult and Clin Psychol 1978; 46: 1423–1431.
28. Sachs DPL, Hall RG, Hall SM. Effects of rapid smoking: Physiologic evaluation of a smoking-cessation. Annals of Internal Medicine 1978; 88: 639–641.
29. Hall RG, Sachs DPL, Hall SM. Medical risk and therapeutic effectiveness of rapid smoking. Behav Ther 1979; 10: 249–259.
30. Poole AD, Sanson-Fisher RW, German GA, Harker J. The rapid-smoking technique: Some physiological effects. Behav Res and Ther 1980; 8: 581–586.
31. Glasgow RE, Lichtenstein E, Beaver C, O'Neil K. Selective reactions to rapid smoking and normal paced aversive smoking. Behav Res and Ther 1981; 6: 53–59.
32. Hall RG, Sachs DPL, Hall SM, Benowitz NL. Two year efficacy and the safety of rapid smoking therapy in patients with cardiac and pulmonary disease. J of Consult and clin Psychol 1984; 52: 574–581.
33. Lando HA, Davison GC. Cognitive dissonance as a modifier of chronic smoking behavior. J of Consult and Clin Psychol 1975; 43: 750.
34. Resnick JH. Effects of stimulus satiation on the overlearned maladaptive response of cigarette smoking. J of Consult and Clin Psychol 1968; 32: 500–505.
35. Claiborn WI, Lewis P, Humble S. Stimulus satiation and smoking: A revisit. J of Clin Psychol 1972; 28: 416–419.
36. Sushinsky LW. Expectation of future treatment, stimulus satiation, and smoking. J of Consult and Clin Psychol 1972; 39: 343.
37. Schwartz JL, Dubitzky M. The results of helping people fight cigarettes. California's Health 1967; 24: 78–83.
38. Marrone RL, Merksomer MA, Salzberg PM. A short duration group treatment of smoking behavior by stimulus saturation. Behav Res and Ther 1970; 8: 347–352.
39. Young FD. The modification of cigarette smoking by oversatiation and covert behavior rehearsal. Doctoral Dissertation for University of Windsor, Canada, 1973.
40. Azrin NH, Holz WC. Punishment. In: Honig WK, ed. Operant behavior: Areas of research and application New York: Appleton-Century-Crofts, 1966: 380–447.
41. Lichtenstein E, Keutzer CS. Modification of smoking behavior: A later look. In: Pulin RD, Fensterheim H, Lazarus AA, Franks GM (eds.) Advances in behavior therapy, 1969. New York: Academic Press, 1971: 61–75.
42. Koenig KP, Masters J. Experimental treatment of habitual smoking. Behav Res and Ther 1965; 3: 235–243.
43. Mees HL. Placebo effects in aversive control: A preliminary report. Paper presented at the joint meeting of the Oregon–Washington State Psychological Associations, Ocean Shores, Washington, May, 1966.
44. Ober DC. Modification of smoking behavior. J of Consult and Clin Psychol 1968; 32: 543–549.
45. Carlin AS, Armstrong HE Jr. Aversive conditioning: Learning or dissonance reduction? J of Consult and Clin Psychol 1968; 32: 674–678.

46. Engeln RG. A comparision of desensitization and aversive conditioning as treatment methods to reduce cigarette smoking. Doctoral dissertation for Washington State University, Department of Psychology, 1969.
47. Gendreau PE, Dodwell PC. An aversive treatment for addicted cigarette smokers: Preliminary report. Can Psychologist 1968; 9: 28–34.
48. McGuire JR, Vallance M. Aversion therapy by electric shock: A simple technique. Brit Med J 1964; 1: 151–153.
49. Powell JR, Azrin N. The effects of shock as a punisher for cigarette smoking. J of Applied Behav Anal 1968; 1: 63–71.
50. Steffy RA, Meichenbaum D, Best JA. Aversion and cognitive factors in the modification of smoking behavior. Behav Res and Ther 1970; 8: 115–125.
51. Chapman RF, Smith JW, Layden TA. Elimination of cigarette smoking by punishment and self-management training. Behav Res and Ther 1971; 9: 255–264.
52. Cautela JR. Covert sensitization. Psychol Rep 1967; 20: 459–468.
53. Cautela JR. Treatment of smoking by covert sensitization. Psychol Rep 1970; 26: 415–420.
54. Cautela JR. Covert extinction. Behav Ther 1971; 2: 192–200.
55. Schwartz JL, Rider G. Review and evaluation of smoking control methods: The United States and Canada. Washington, DC: U.S. Department of Health Education and Welfare, Bureau of Health Education. Center for Disease Control, Public Health Service, 1978: 87.
56. Lowe MR, Green L, Kurtz SMS, Ashenberg ZS, Fisher EB. Self-initiated cue extinction, and covert sensitization procedures in smoking cessation. J of Behav Med 1980; 3: 357–372.
57. Wagner JK, Ragg RA. Comparing behavior modification approaches to habit decrement smoking. J of Consult and Clin Psychol 1970; 34: 258–263.
58. Sachs LB, Bean H, Morrow JE. Comparison of smoking treatments. Behav Ther 1970; 1: 465–472.
59. Tongas PN. The Kaiser-Permanente smoking control program: Its purpose and implication for an HMO. Professional Psychol 1979; 10: 409–418.
60. Severson HH, O'Neal M, Hynd GW. Cognitive coping strategies and aversive counterconditioning in the modification of smoking behavior. Paper presented at the annual meeting of the Western Psychological Association, Seattle, 1977.
61. Barbarin OA. Comparison of symbolic and overt aversion in the self-control of smoking. J of Consult and Clin Psychol 1978; 46: 1569–1571.
62. Fey MS. The role of smoking deterrent lozenges. In: Helping smokers to quit. Vol. 1. Morris Plains, NJ: New Life Products Corporation, 1989: 1.
63. Spring FL, Sipich JF, Trimble RW, Goeckner DJ. Effects of contingency and noncontingency contracts in the context of a self-control-oriented smoking modification program. Behav Ther 1978; 9: 967–958.
64. Beaver C, Brown RA, Lichtenstein, E. Effects of monitored nicotine fading and anxiety management training on smoking reduction. Addict Behav 1981; 6: 301–305.
65. Lando HA. Successful treatment of smokers with a broad-spectrum behavioral approach. 1977; 45(3): 361–366.
66. Best JA. Tailoring smoking withdrawal procedures to personality and motivational differences. J of Consult and Clin Psychol 1975; 43: 1–8.
67. Elliot CH, Denny CH. A multiple-component treatment approach to smoking reduction. J of Consult and Clin Psychol 1978; 46: 1330–1339.

12
Silver-Acetate Deterrent Therapy: A Minimal-Intervention Self-help Aid*

MICHAEL FEY, MARK HOLLANDER, and NORMAN HYMOWITZ

Cigarettes are among this nation's most heavily advertised products, and they have the dubious distinction of being the only product that, when used as directed, kills the people who use it.[1] What may even be worse, there is a substantial body of knowledge suggesting that cigarettes may also be harmful to nonsmokers.[2]

The adverse health effects of cigarette smoking and other forms of tobacco use have been described and documented in a series of Surgeon General reports dating back to 1964.[2] One of the past Surgeon Generals of the United States considered cigarette smoking to be the single most important preventable cause of death and disability in our society, and he issued the challenge of creating a smoke-free society by the Year 2000.[2] Preventing the onset of smoking in young people and helping current smokers to quit represent important health priorities for the nation. This chapter focuses on cessation.

The process of helping smokers to stop smoking is a complicated one, and it is made more difficult by the sheer numbers of people affected. Approximately 50 million Americans smoke cigarettes, and many more use other tobacco products.[2] This nation's poor and undereducated are disproportionately represented among the ranks of current smokers,[3] relatively more of today's smokers may be classified as heavy smokers (>25 cigarettes/day) than in the past,[2] and it is now recognized that cigarette smoking is an addiction.[4] The task of meeting the Surgeon General's Year 2000 goal is a formidable one.

When smokers seek formal assistance in stopping smoking, their chances of kicking the habit are modest, at best.[5] From a public-health perspective, the value of group or individual smoking-cessation therapy is compromised by the small number of smokers who can be accommodated, the high cost

---

*Preparation of this manuscript was supported in part by a Small Business Innovative Research (SBIR) Grant Number 1 R43 HL42738-01 to Michael Fey and subcontract to Norman Hymowitz.

of treatment, and the relatively modest outcomes produced. For those who succeed in quitting smoking, the chances of remaining abstinent are low. One-year outcome data for a variety of labor-intensive treatment programs hover around 20–30%.[5]

While there are no doubt many smokers who benefit from formal smoking-cessation treatment, public-health considerations demand a different approach. Examination of the experience of the millions of Americans who have quit smoking in the past is instructive.[6] More than 90% of them quit smoking on their own, without the aid of a formal program. When current smokers are asked about the kind of help they want to quit smoking, the vast majority say they prefer to try to quit smoking on their own.[7] They ask for minimal-intervention self-help aids. Given the magnitude of the smoking problem in the United States, as well as around the globe, it behooves the medical, behavioral, and public-health communities to encourage and facilitate the process of self-initiated quitting and to provide cessation aids that can be used with little or no professional supervision.

From a public-health point of view, it is important to reach large numbers of smokers, even though the clinical impact may be less than what can be obtained with a more intensive intervention. Compare, for example, the importance, from a public-health point of view, of a labor-intensive group program for 20 smokers, which yields a relatively high 12-month quit rate of 50% to that of, say, a mass-media campaign, which reaches 25,000 smokers and results in a 12-month quit rate of only 3–5%. Clearly, the mass-media campaign is more effective from a public-health perspective.

Examples of minimal interventions that are aimed at helping smokers quit smoking on their own are the use of self-help booklets and biblio-therapy (e.g., Glasgow et al.[7]), external cigarette filters,[8] mass-media campaigns,[9] brief physician interventions (e.g., Kottke et al.[10]), worksite competitions and incentives,[11] and community-based education and in-tervention (e.g., Farquhar et al.[12]). Each represents relatively cost-effective approaches that can affect a large number of smokers. Their aim is to accelerate the process of self-initiated quitting and to provide aids to cessation, which smokers can put into use on their own.

Silver-Acetate Products

Silver-acetate products (gum, lozenge, spray) represent another self-help aid that may have an important role to play in the antismoking arena. Available commercially in Europe as an over-the-counter (OTC) smoking deterrent for more than a decade, silver acetate was first introduced as a smoking-deterrent lozenge, Respaton,[13] and later, as a chewing gum, Tabmint.[14] In 1975, Woodcraft was issued the first United States patent incorporating silver salt as an antismoking ingredient in a chewing gum form. A sprayable composition containing silver acetate was patented by Beskin in 1988.

Essentially, the silver interacts with smoke from cigarettes, and, presumably, other compounds that are smoked, to cause a noxious metallic taste. The aversive taste causes smokers to discard the cigarette, and repeated aversive conditioning encounters lessens the urge to smoke. Like disulfiram (Antabuse) therapy for alcoholics, smokers are encouraged to chew the gum to deter smoking.

There are limits to the amount of silver acetate that people can safely ingest. A scientific panel to the Food and Drug Administration (FDA)[15] found 6-mg silver-acetate products (chewing gum) to be safe at recommended usage levels (i.e., do not exceed six times per day, every 4 hours, for a 3-week period). Silver-acetate products are currently listed as Category III drugs, meaning that the FDA requires more information to demonstrate safety and efficacy.

The only safety concern cited by the scientific panel was the potential for *argyrism*, a permanent, but otherwise harmless discoloration of skin, which could occur after extended usage. Malcolm et al.[16] also reported cases of nausea, heartburn, abdominal cramps, skin rash, and oral complaints (dry mouth, bad taste with food) in subjects who used Tabmint® for 3 weeks.

Jensen et al.[17] studied serum concentrations and accumulation of silver in skin during 3-month treatments of 6 Tabmints per day. Serum concentrations of silver rose after chewing gum use had started, and concentrations quickly returned to normal after use had ceased. The number of silver granules in skin biopsies, observed by autometallography, increased after the gum had been used for 12 weeks. None of the 21 subjects under study developed clinical signs of silver poisoning (*argyria*).

When used as directed, silver-acetate products are safe, and there have been no adverse reports following years of smoking-deterrent usage in Europe. Two cases of argyria associated with deterrent use reported in the literature are for individuals who consumed massive amounts of the product. In one case, a nurse consumed 32 Respaton lozenges daily for 6 months.[18] In another case, an Englishman took 6 Respaton lozenges per day for 2 years.[19] Cases such as these, fortunately, are few and far between. Argyria is unlikely to occur at oral cumulative doses lower than 3.8 grams. This is the equivalent of approximately 633 doses of a 6.0-mg product. This is far in excess of the 126-piece limit of 6-mg silver-acetate product recommended by the FDA.

From a behavioral point of view, the rationale for silver-acetate smoking deterrence is sound because aversive conditioning procedures, such as rapid smoking, have been found to be among the most successful quit-smoking therapies.[5] From a public-health perspective, OTC smoking deterrents meet many of the requirements for an effective quit-smoking aid. They can be used by large numbers of smokers, either alone or in combination with bibliotherapy, physician advice, or even as part of a broader antismoking effort.

Several studies in Europe and one in the United States provide some clinical support for the efficacy of the silver-acetate-based products, although considerably more research is required before their true value can be measured. Rosenberg[14] evaluated the effects of Tabmint on smoking cessation in a double-blind placebo-controlled trial. At the end of 2 weeks, 11 of 30 subjects (37%) in the Tabmint condition, and 5 of 30 subjects (17%) in the placebo condition reported that they quit smoking. Thus, Tabmint more than doubled the quit rate obtained in the control groups. Unfortunately, the author did not report follow-up data, nor did he use an objective measure of smoking status.

Arvidsson[20] similarly evaluated the efficacy of Tabmint in a double-blind placebo-controlled study. Again, smokers were instructed to use the gum for 2 weeks. At the end of the second week, subjects in the silver-acetate condition smoked an average of 10.6 cigarettes per day; those in the control group smoked an average of 18.4 cigarettes per day. Actual quit rate data were not reported. Follow-up data and objective verification of smoking status also were lacking.

Using a somewhat different approach, Schmidt[21] recruited 1000 subjects through a special media campaign. In a double-blind fashion, 500 subjects were assigned randomly to Tabmint and 500 to placebo. Four to 5 weeks after treatment onset, the participants received a questionnaire to determine their smoking status. Complete data were obtained and analyzed for 619 subjects, approximately half in each experimental condition. Thirty-one percent of smokers in the Tabmint condition and 24.9% of smokers in the placebo group reported that they quit smoking. The difference between the two groups was not statistically significant, although the observed differences were in the direction that favored active ingredient.

This study is of particular interest because of its true public-health approach. The gum, placebo as well as Tabmint, served as a stimulus for self-initiated smoking cessation, influencing a large number of smokers to quit smoking on their own. Unfortunately, follow-up data and objective measures of cigarette smoking were lacking. Moreover, it is likely that the actual quit rates were much more modest because a high proportion of participants who did not return their questionnaires probably were still smoking.

The most thorough study of silver acetate gum as a deterrent to smoking was reported by Malcolm et al.[16] In a double-blind controlled study, subjects using silver acetate for 3 weeks had a smoking-cessation rate of 11%. Placebo subjects had a smoking-cessation rate of 4%. Without further treatment, the group using silver acetate revealed a 7% non-smoking rate at 4 months, compared with a 3% nonsmoking rate for the placebo group. Blood carboxyhemoglobin levels served as an objective measure of smoking status.

The between-group differences reported by Malcolm et al.[14] at 3 weeks achieved statistical significance. Those at 4 months did not, although more than twice as many smokers in the Tabmint group were abstinent, compared with those in the placebo group. In view of the fact that most quitters relapse within 3 months of treatment,[22] the follow-up data are encouraging. Further clinical evaluation of the long-term efficacy of silver acetate is required, to evaluate its impact on smoking cessation and public-health potential.

One shortcoming presented by the aforementioned silver-acetate smoking-deterrent products is the restrictions placed on their usage due to the potential for argyria. It might be advantageous, for example, to use the product for 3 weeks to quit smoking and to use additional product on an as-needed basis to prevent recidivism. Studies are underway in this direction.

In 1989, a United States patent was awarded, specifying a wide range of antismoking oral compositions containing a silver compound and a sweetener, in which the silver compound was present in amounts ranging from 0.1 to 2.5 mg, and with a ratio of sweetness intensity based on sucrose to silver compound content of 100:1 to 2500:1. Relatively small doses of silver compounds are effective as smoking deterrents if applied at the time of smoking and confined to the oral mucosa. Sweeteners improve consumer acceptance of silver acetate, which imparts a bitter taste when not in the presence of smoke.

The lozenge form is probably the most effective delivery of the drug. In a consumer home use test, a 2.5-mg lozenge gave an average smoking deterrent duration of 2 hours after usage, as compared to 1 hour for a 6-mg gum. The lozenge probably bathes the mouth with a uniform and consistent supply of silver ions as it dissolves, whereas the gum releases silver complex ion more rapidly. Further, the lozenge can be expelled at any time by the smoker after an effective deterrent taste response, which would reduce the amount of silver intake. The 2.5-mg lozenge also offers a potentially longer consumer usage period if a scientific panel's recommended limit to the FDA of 756 mg is adopted. The guidelines would permit the use of 302 pieces of the 2.5-mg lozenge. A clinical evaluation of the effectiveness of the 2.5-mg lozenge for smoking cessation and relapse prevention currently is in progress.

Discussion

Cigarette smoking was relatively unknown in this country at the turn of the 20th century, as was death from lung cancer, heart disease, and chronic obstructive lung disease.[2] All of this has changed, as mass-production techniques and persuasive advertising led to a dramatic increase in the per capita consumption of cigarettes during the course of this century. Heart disease, lung cancer, and nonneoplastic bronchopulmonary disease have reached epidemic proportions in our society, and new information on the health consequences of smoking continue to accumulate.[2]

Cigarette smoking is now one of this country's foremost health problems, and helping smokers to stop smoking is a high public-health priority. Self-help aids such as silver-acetate smoking-deterrent gums and lozenges have an important place in the antismoking arena. As OTC self-help quit-smoking aids, they can be used by large numbers of smokers with little, if any, professional supervision or assistance.

At this time, the efficacy of silver-acetate deterrent therapy for smoking cessation is undertermined. While available studies suggest modest efficacy for short-term initial cessation, long-term outcome data are lacking. Future studies should be directed toward determining long-term effectiveness and toward identifying conditions under which the effects of deterrent therapy can be maximized. For example, the effectiveness of the product may be different for a smoker who uses it after seeing it on display in a pharmacy, compared to another smoker who uses it on the advice of his or her personal physician.

Recent refinements in silver-acetate product development by Michael Fey are particularly intriguing. The 2.5-mg silver-acetate lozenge has obvious advantages over the 6-mg lozenge, with respect to safety and ease of usage. The lower-dose lozenge also has potential for counteracting tendencies toward relapse, perhaps the most difficult problem in clinical practice and in the smoking-cessation literature. Product efficacy for initial cessation and relapse prevention would represent a major contribution to the antismoking literature. Research currently underway at the New Jersey Medical School addresses these issues.

References

1. Warner KE. Selling smoke: Cigarette advertising and public health. Washington, DC: American Public Health Association, 1986.
2. U.S. Department of Health and Human Services Reducing the health consequences of smoking: 25 Years of progress. DHHS Publication No, (CDC)89-8411. Washington, DC: U.S. Department of Health and Human Services, Public Health Service, Office on Smoking and Health.
3. Novotny, TE, Warner KE, Kendrick JS, Remington PL. Smoking by blacks and whites: Socioeconomic and demographic differences. Am J of Public Health 1988; 78: 1187–1189.
4. U.S. Department of Health and Human Services. The health consequences of smoking: Nicotine addiction (a report of the Surgeon General). USDHHS Publication No. (CDC)88-8406. Washington, DC: U.S. Department of Health and Human Services, Public Health Service, Centers for Disease Control, Center for Health Promotion and Education, Office on Smoking and Health, 1988.

5. Schwartz JL. Smoking cessation methods: The United States and Canada, 1978–1985. NIH Publication No, 87-2840. Washington, DC: U.S. Department of Health and Human Services, Public Health Service, 1987.

6. Fiore MC, Novotny TE, Pierce JP, Giovino GO, Hatziandrew EJ, Newcomb PA, Surawicz TS, Davis RM. Methods used to quit smoking in the United States. JAMA 1990; 263; 20: 2760–6765.

7. Glasgow RE, Schafer L, O'Neill HK. Self-help books and amount of therapist contact in smoking cessation programs. J of Consult and Clin Psychol 1981; 49: 659–667.

8. Hymowitz N, Lasser NL, Safirstein BH. Effects of graduated external filters on smoking cessation. Prev Med 1982; 11: 85–95.

9. Flay BR. Mass media and smoking cessation. A critical review. Am J of Public Health 1987; 77: 153–160.

10. Kottke TE, Brekke ML, Solberg LI, Hughes JR. A randomized trial to increase smoking intervention by physicians. JAMA 1989; 261: 2101–2106.

11. Kleges RC, Vasey MM, Glasgow RE. A worksite smoking modification competition: Potential for public health impact. Am J of Public Health 1986; 76: 198–200.

12. Farquhar JW, Wood P, Breitrose H, Haskell WL, Myer AJ, Maccoby N, Alexander JK, Brown BW Jr., McAllister AL, Nash JD, Stern MP. Community education for cardiovascular health. Lancet 1977; 1: 1192–1195.

13. Rosenberg A. An investigation into the effect on cigarette smoking of a new anti-smoking preparation. J of Intl Med Res 1974; 2: 310–313.

14. Rosenberg A. An investigation into the effect on cigarette smoking of a new anti-smoking chewing gum. J of Intl Med Res 1977; 5: 68–70.

15. Food and Drug Administration. Smoking deterrent drug products for over-the-counter human use: Establishment of a monograph. Federal Register 1982, 47: 490–500.

16. Malcolm R, Currey HS, Mitchell MO, Keil JE. Silver acetate gum as a deterrent to smoking. Chest 1986; 89: 107–111.

17. Jensen EJ, Rungby J, Hansen JC, Schmidt E, Pederson B, Dahl R. Serum concentrations and accumulation of silver in skin during three months treatment with an antismoking chewing gum containing silver acetate. Human Toxicol 1988; 7: 535–540.

18. MacIntyre D, Mclay ALC, East BW, Williams ED, Boddy K. Silver poisoning associated with an antismoking lozenge. Brit Med J 1978; 2: 1749–1750.

19. Shelton DR, Goulding R. Silver poisoning associated with an antismoking lozenge. Brit Med J 1979; 1: 267.

20. Arvidsson T. A double blind investigation of the effectiveness of Tabmint, an antismoking chewing gum. OTC 1982; Vol 3. 170–178.

21. Schmidt F. Tabmint cure by means of antismoking chewing gum: A double blind test. OTC, 1977; 170–178.

22. Hunt WA, Bespalec DA. An evaluation of current methods of modifying smoking behavior, J of Clin Psychol 1974; 30: 431–438.

13
Hypnosis in the Treatment of the Smoking Habit

Louis Jolyon West

The use of hypnosis to bring about significant changes in behavior was well developed in clinical practice by the end of the 19th century and up to World War I. Many so-called bad habits, including alcoholism, drug addiction, as well as a variety of undesirable (to the subject) sexual practices, were reported by Bramwell[1] in 1903 to have been cured with hypnotic suggestion. We are indebted to Gravitz[2] for recently bringing to light the publication in 1847 of a discussion by Morley about the use of hypnosis in treating nicotine habituation by Robbins in Massachusetts. Robbins used hypnotic suggestions of an aversive nature to control a female patient's appetite for certain foods that exacerbated her dyspepsia, and also for tea, coffee, and nicotine-containing snuff. The treatment was successful, and Robbins subsequently employed a similar strategy to rid a medical student of "an inveterate attachment to tobacco in its various shapes."

In the literature of the first two thirds of the 20th century, there are numerous anecdotal descriptions of hypnotherapy to overcome unhealthy habits. By the 1970s, hypnosis was one of many techniques in use to help people break the smoking habit. Schwartz evaluated the various types of smoking-cessation programs that were available in the United States and Canada from 1969 through 1977. Of 67 trials conducted during this period, two fifths had 6-month abstinence rates of at least 35%, one fifth had abstinence rates between 22 and 34%, and two fifths had rates below 22%. Twenty-seven percent had at least a 40% success rate at 6 months; and 18% had 50% success at 6 months. The best results were for programs employing group counseling, hypnosis, and the rapid-smoking aversion technique.[3]

There have been numerous studies employing hypnosis with individuals or groups in single sessions or multiple sessions, with or without behavioral counseling, and in various other combinations. In 1977, I reviewed the literature to that date.[4] In general, the goal of hypnotic interventions was total cessation of smoking, and results were presented in sharply defined categories of success or failure, rather than in categories rating degree of smoking reduction. On the whole, hypnosis was more effective than other single methods in comparable reports. However, the success rates varied between 15 and 90%, depending upon the sample, the length of follow-up, and many other variables. Hypnosis combined with individual counseling or psychotherapy appeared to be more effective than hypnosis alone. Multiple doctor–patient contacts, which employed hypnotic reinforcement of initial suggestions of abstinence, were more effective than a single session. However, some of the best success rates were obtained by Spiegel with brief hypnotherapy alone.[5-8]

Extended group hypnotherapy sessions, as described by Kline,[9] produced even better reported results. Kline had the best results from a 12-hour hypnotherapy program in which a total of 60 patients were treated in six groups. Patients were instructed to refrain from smoking during the 24 hours preceding the session. One year later, 53 (88%) were abstinent and 7 (12%) were smoking.[9] Kroger[10,11] combined a type of behavior modification with hypnotherapy and self-hypnosis, apparently to good effect in many cases, although his statistics are not reported. Various minor modifications of hypnotic technique in treatment of smoking were described by other competent practitioners.[12-14]

Uncontrolled Studies Since 1977

Jones[15] mailed a questionnaire to 185 consecutive patients at least 6 months after they completed a program of hynotherapy (for a variety of problems). Of these, 141 completed questionnaires were analyzed. Among 44 who had been treated for smoking, 34 (77%) had stopped initially, but 28 (63.6%) had resumed smoking again.[15]

Sheehan and Surman[16] presented follow-up data on 100 consecutive patients who undertook hypnotherapy to stop smoking. All patients were given direct suggestions to stop smoking and positive reinforcements and motivational instructions for stopping. While the patient was hypnotized, smoking behavior was paired with noxious imagery (e.g., the exhaust fumes of an automobile). At mean follow-up of 18 months, 21.3% were still abstinent. Of those who were smoking, 60% had reduced their consumption by at least 40%. The mean number of treatment sessions was one and a half.[16]

Tori[17] found that a *smoking-satiation procedure* (requiring subjects to hold smoke in their mouths, with occasional inhalations) suppressed habitual smoking as effectively as satiation by rapid smoking. In view of the high relapse rates that usually follow the single application of an aversive conditioning procedure, Tori then employed follow-up hypnosis and counseling sessions in order to assist subjects in maintaining smoking cessation. At the time of the 6-month follow-up contact, confirmed abstinence reports for 66% of all subjects who received treatment were obtained.[17]

A number of reports on hypnotic single-session cessation programs have not been so favorable. Ryde[18] obtained follow-up information from smokers who had received, over a 20-year period, one-session hypnotherapy treatment for smoking. Information on 3-month follow-up was available on 408 of the 605 smokers treated. Of those, 161 (39.5%) were still abstinent at 3 months. Information was available on 64 more patients at 6 months. Of those, 20 (31.3%) were not smoking.[18]

Wagner and colleagues[19] obtained an 18% abstinence rate at 1 year follow-up of patients undertaking a single session of group hypnosis. Of 783 who participated in one of four separate 90-minute sessions, 618 (79%) were able to be reached (returned questionnaires or responded to phone survey) for a 1-year follow-up. Of these, 113 (18%) were not smoking. When nonrespondents are included as failures, the abstinence rate was 14%.[19]

Neufeld and Lynn[20] presented the results of a single 2-hour group self-hypnosis smoking-cessation program in which 27 subjects attended one of six sessions sponsored by the American Lung Association. Components of treatment relied on techniques of visualization. At 3 months, the nonsmoking prevalence rate was 25.93%, and it was 18.52% at 6 months.[20]

The method of hypnosis used by the American Health Foundation is modified from Spiegel.[7] It is a one-session treatment, reinforced by self-hypnosis exercises performed several times daily for 1 or 2 weeks. Suggestions are tailored to the individual. Of the hour, 30 minutes are spent in individual history taking and counseling, 20 minutes are spent in hypnotic procedures, and 10 minutes are spent teaching the participant self-hypnosis. Shewchuk[21] compared hypnosis with other psychotherapeutic intervention strategies employed by the American Health Foundation (i.e., group counseling and individual counseling). After 1 year, all three programs had about the same success rate, 25%. When the manner of assignment to each treatment was studied, data after 1 year showed an approximately 17% success rate across treatments, independent of assignment method.[21]

Berkowitz and colleagues[22] treated 40 self-referred patients using Spiegel's single-treatment method.[7] They found a 6-month total abstinence rate of about 25%, which was comparable to Spiegel's success rate. They recommended that future studies should include nontreatment control groups to validate the effects of the hypnotic method for smoking cessation.[22]

Controlled Studies Since 1977

A number of recent studies have compared hypnosis with other smoking interventions. Pederson and colleagues[23] analyzed various combinations, of single-session group hypnosis, group counseling, and *rapid smoking* (a one-session aversion technique that requires cigarettes to be smoked according to a predetermined schedule and that results in physical discomfort). The combination of hypnosis and counseling produced the highest percentage of abstainers at 6 months, 56%. Surprisingly, only 13% of the smokers exposed to the rapid-smoking session together with hypnosis and counseling were abstinent at 6 months. However, 38% remained abstinent who participated in the rapid smoking and group counseling, but not the group hypnosis.[23]

In a nonrandomized study, Shewchuk and colleagues[24] compared group therapy, individual counseling, and hypnosis. Each of 571 smokers selected one of three methods of smoking cessation: group therapy, individual counseling, and hypnosis. After 1 year, all methods produced a success rate of approximately 20%. It was generally found that younger, more educated smokers chose hypnosis; older, more educated smokers chose group therapy; older, less educated smokers chose individual counseling; and the youngest and generally least educated smokers chose to become nonattenders and not take part in therapy.[24]

In several randomized controlled studies, hypnosis compared favorably with other interventions. Byrne and Whyte[25] analyzed four smoking-cessation programs:

1. Individual hypnotherapy in four sessions using hypnotic suggestion to associate smoking with discomfort and unplesant consequences
2. Behavioral self-management based on stimulus control and response substitution with deep muscle relaxation; self-paced with no therapist contact between intake and follow-up
3. Behavior modification using the same principles as in the second program, but in a structured program, in which groups of five subjects were paced by a psychologist
4. Behavior modification based on the same principles but with covert sensitization and more intensively arranged (six sessions consecutively), in groups of five, and directed by a psychologist.

The 274 regularly smoking volunteers were randomly assigned to one of the four programs. Subjects were reevaluated at 3, 7, and 12 months after completion of the program. Results were consistent with other studies that showed good short-term smoking cessation but with rather discouraging (only 31%) long-term effectiveness. (Other studies have reported long-term cessation at between 15% and 25%.) Relapse generally occurred 3 months after completing a program, and no single program was significantly superior to the others.[25]

Frank and colleagues[26] presented results of a study that compared hypnosis with and without behavioral therapy. In the initial study, 48 subjects were assigned to one of three treatments: two 1-hour hypnotic sessions, four hypnotic sessions with a booster, or two hypnotic and two behavioral sessions with a booster. The hypnotic sessions were scheduled once every 2 weeks, and the booster was 3 weeks after the last session. Another group of 15 subjects was later recruited to receive four hypnotic sessions (two per week) and a booster session. At the end of the treatments, 31% were abstinent. After 6 months, only 9% were still abstinent, and another 28% had reduced their smoking by 50%. There were no differences between groups regardless of the frequency, length between sessions, or addition of behavioral methods.[26]

Williams and Hall[27] compared single-session hypnosis with a placebo control condition and no treatment. Twenty of 60 volunteers for smoking cessation were assigned to single-session hypnosis, 20 to a placebo control condition, and 20 to a no-treatment control condition. Patients in the single-session hypnosis group were significantly more abstinent at posttest (40%) and, surprisingly, even more were abstinent at 48-week follow-up (45%) compared to the placebo and no-treatment control groups, in which no one was abstinent during the study. The hypnosis group had also reduced cigarette consumption significantly more than the other groups, which had no reductions.[27]

Hyman and coworkers[28] compared hypnosis with focused smoking, placebo, and no treatment. Several measures of smoking behavior were employed: estimated smoking rate, self-monitoring, and chemical analysis (i.e., thiocyanate blood levels). They achieved cessation rates of 11 to 15% but found no significant differences between treatments directly after treatment or at the 3- and 6-month follow-ups. The three measures of smoking behavior were all highly correlated.[28]

Javel[30] presented results of a study comparing 3-month success rates in three groups of 10 who received (1) full hypnotic induction plus suggestions, such as those of Stanton[29] and Spiegel[7]; (2) suggestions alone; or (3) no treatment. After 3 months, the success rates for each group were 60%, 40%, and 0%, respectively. However, perhaps because of the small sample size, the advantage offered by full induction was not statistically significant (chi square = .8); either therapy was better than none.[30]

Jeffrey and coworkers[32] evaluated a brief group-treatment package that included hypnotic induction for maintenance of smoking cessation. The five-session program included a 48-hour pretreatment abstinence period, four 1-hour sessions of cognitive and behavioral maintenance strategies as appropriate, and 15 minutes of suggestions as described by Crasilneck,[31] Spiegel,[7] and Stanton[29]. Thirty-five subjects entered the program and were compared with a control group of 30 on the waiting list for treatment. Twenty-two subjects completed the protocol. Of these, 11 (50%) were not smoking at 3-month follow-up, compared with none (0%) of the controls.[32]

In another study, Jeffrey and Jeffrey[33] compared exclusion therapy (48 hours of pretreatment abstinence combined with a five-session group hypnosis and behavioral program) or identical treatment that only encouraged but did not require pretreatment abstinence. Forty-nine subjects (40.8%) did not complete the protocol; there was no difference in completion rate of each group. All remaining subjects were abstinent at the completion of treatment. At 1-month follow-up, 30 (88.2%) exclusion, and 24 (64.9%) nonexclusion subjects were abstinent. At 3 months, 24 (70.6%) exclusion and 20 (54.1%) nonexclusion subjects were abstinent.[33]

Kaufert and coworkers[34] examined the predictive value of health beliefs in determining success of alternate modalities of smoking cessation. Volunteers were randomized either to a control group or to one of three cessation programs that used behavior modification, health education, or hypnosis. A questionnaire was used to document health beliefs, demographic characteristics, and smoking history. Blood samples were taken before and after the completion of intervention programs, to measure changes in serum thiocyanate as a check on reported smoking behavior. A follow-up questionnaire was used to assess smoking behavior after 6 months. Statistically significant decreases in serum thiocyanate levels followed participation in each of the three programs. Factor analysis and reliability tests were used to identify four scales reflecting major variable dimensions in the health belief model. Significant correlations between change in serum thiocyanate and two of the scales (general health concern and perceived vulnerability) were found only for the group randomly assigned to the health education intervention program.[34]

Lambe and coworkers[35] conducted a randomized controlled trial of hypnotherapy for smoking cessation. In the hypnosis group, 21% of patients quit smoking by the 3-month follow-up, compared with 6% in the control group. However, by 6 months, there were no significant differences between the two groups. At 1 year, 22% in the hypnosis group and 20% in the control group had quit.[35]

Rabkin and colleagues[26] conducted a randomized trial of 168 volunteers, comparing smoking-cessation programs that used behavior modification, health education, or hypnosis, compared with a control group. Follow-up data 3 weeks after completion was available on 140 subjects. Each program showed significant reductions both in reported cigarette consumption and in serum thiocyanate levels, compared to their entry levels and to the control group. However, there were no significant differences among the hypnosis, health education, or behavior-modification groups with respect to the proportion who reported quitting smoking, the number of cigarettes smoked, or the degree of change in serum thiocyanate levels. Reported cigarette consumption ascertained 6 months later again showed no significant differences among these three approaches. Factors such as subject age, age at starting cigarette smoking, educational level, marital status, and spouse or partners smoking did not identify subgroups with differences between treatment responses. Thus, hypnosis, health education, and behavior modification were each effective (and, in this study, equally effective) programs for changing cigarette smoking.[36]

Response Prediction

Because of the high relapse rates, many studies have been conducted to determine differences between those who successfully quit and those who relapse. In the study by Lambe and coworkers that compared hypnotherapy for smoking cessation with a control, the only significant predictor of success was having a college education.[35] Javel's[30] comparison of full hypnotic induction plus suggestion, suggestion alone, or no treatment found no significant differences in 3-month success rates for full hypnotic induction versus suggestion alone, although both therapies were better than none. Demographic and historical factors that may have decreased success appeared to be (1) having had a mother who smoked and (2) the absence of a smoking-related illness.[30]

Frank's study[26] that compared hypnosis with and without behavioral therapy indicated no difference in smoking cessation 6 months after treatment regardless of the frequency, length between sessions, or addition of behavioral methods. Successful subjects were more educated, less able to use their imagination, and had fewer smokers at home.[26]

Horwitz and colleagues[37] examined psychosocial mediators of abstinence, relapse, and continued smoking following a minimal intervention. Subjects particpated in a single-session group hypnosis treatment for smoking cessation. Questionnaires completed by participants (both prior to treatment and at a 1-year follow-up obtained information on health locus of control, health beliefs, social support, use of nonsmoking areas, and objection to another person's smoking. Ex-smoker, recidivist, and continuing smoker groups were defined using follow-up data from 219 participants (70 males and 149 females). The results show that the three smoking status groups could be discriminated. Ex-smokers actively coped with smokers in their environment, avoided other smokers in public places, and received considerable support from spouses and friends after treatment. In contrast, recidivists did not actively cope with smokers, were more likely to participate in additional hypnosis treatments, and felt their health was most contingent on fate or on "powerful others." It was concluded that posttreatment factors are more important for long-term maintenance of nonsmoking than entry characteristics of participants. Recommendations included the incorporation of coping skills training into cessation programs and the restriction of smoking in the ex-smokers' environments to prevent relapse.[37]

Hypnotic Susceptibility

Clinicians have addressed the issue of susceptibility to hypnosis as one factor in the success or failure of hypnotherapy. Hypnotizability is a complex subject. Schubert[38] looked at the relationship between hypnotizability and abstinence in their comparison of hypnotherapy with systematic relaxation. In this study, 87 volunteers who wanted to quit cigarette smoking were assigned randomly to each group: the experimental hypnosis group, the comparison relaxation group, or the waiting-list control group. Subjects in the treatment groups had four weekly 50-minute, individual sessions. Four months after the completion of treatment, they were administered a questionnaire and a hypnotic susceptibility scale. Subjects in the hypnosis group who were in the upper two thirds in terms of hypnotic susceptibility had reduced their cigarette consumption substantially more than subjects in the relaxation group who were in the upper two thirds of the group in terms of hypnotic susceptibility. Thus, the hypnotic state appears to be most therapeutic for more hypnotizable individuals, especially those who can enter medium or deep states of hypnosis.[38]

Perry and Mullen[14] studied the effects of hypnotic susceptibility in reducing smoking behavior that is treated by a hypnotic technique. At the first of two sessions, susceptibility was evaluated unobtrusively. At the second session, subjects were taught Spiegel's self-hypnotic method to stop smoking. At the end of a 3-month follow-up period, 7 of 54 volunteers were completely abstinent (13%), while 31% had reduced smoking by 50% or more. Of the 7 totally abstaining subjects, 1 was high, 1 was low, and 5 were medium in terms of susceptibility, which is not unlike the distribution of hypnotic susceptibility in the general population. However, it was found that significantly more subjects of higher susceptibility reduced smoking by 50% or more than did less susceptible subjects.[14]

Frankel and Orne[39] compared hypnotizability ratings of 24 phobic patients interested in the therapeutic use of hypnosis, but for whom smoking was not a problem, with ratings of an equal number of non-phobic smokers keen to quit smoking through hypnosis. The mean Stanford Hypnotic Susceptibility Scale score of the phobics was 8.08 on a 12-point scale. The mean of the smokers was 6.08. The difference (namely, that phobics were more hypnotizable than smokers) was significant beyond the .01 level (two-tailed). Thirty percent of smokers were essentially nonresponsive. No phobics were nonresponsive.[39]

Baer and colleagues[40] studied the relationship between hypnotic susceptibility and treatment outcome in 137 patients who had been hypnotized for smoking cessation using a standardized techique. Subjects were followed up at a point between 3 months and 3 years after treatment. Hypnotic ability was assessed by the Stanford Hypnotic Clinical Scale (SHCS) at the time of treatment. Results indicated that low hypnotizables (SHCS = 0–1) had abstinence rates of only 20% at 1 week after treatment. Medium-to-high hypnotizables (SHCS = 2–5) stopped smoking at significantly higher rates than low hypnotizables, with 1-week abstinence rates of approximately 60–70%, and long-term abstinence rates in the 20–30% range after 1 year. Abstinence rates did not significantly differ between medium and high hypnotizables. The authors concluded that low hypnotic susceptibility indicates a poor prognosis for smoking cessation. Conversely, hypnosis produces results at least equal to other treatment modalities for medium and high hypnotizables. Regarding the potential risks of hypnosis, one must weight these against the known risks of cigarette smoking.[40] Following a review of 16 studies published between 1970 and 1980, Agee[41] analyzed the factors most likely to be involved in a successful smoking-cessation program. He employed hypnosis in single sessions, multiple sessions, and group sessions. Results were evaluated on five methodological variables (client vs. solicited volunteers; group vs. individual therapy; training in self-hypnosis vs. no training; one session vs. multiple sessions; and individualized vs. standardized suggestions). The roles of susceptibility, motivation, therapist, telephone contact, and individualization were also examined. Agee's concluding recommendations for a successful smoking-cessation program were the following: several hours of treatment, support from the therapist, individualized suggestions, and most importantly, a client who is motivated to stop smoking.[41]

Discussion

Hypnosis can be useful in treatment of the smoking habit. However, its usefulness may not be easy to document in well-controlled studies, compared with other methods that are more easily standardized. Accomplished clinicians, with much experience in employing hypnosis for a variety of conditions, both psychiatric and medical, are very familiar with some of the variables that impede standardization.

Consider, for example, the matter of hypnotizability. While this quality may be related to one or more fundamental psychobiological characteristics, it is not in itself highly predictable. Even the most sophisticated tests of hypnotizability are useful only up to a point. A subject may be more hypnotizable by one method than another, by one person than another, for one purpose than another, or at one time than another. Knowing of this variability, one would be unwise to discard hypnotherapy as a technique to achieve smoking cessation—especially in a case with serious health implications—merely on the basis of a failed attempt at trance induction. Indeed, for a given patient, superior results might be achieved without ever suggesting a trancelike state, or even eye closure.

The key phrase here is "a given patient." All of the master hypnotists in the modern era have been able to modify their technique constantly, as dictated by the unfolding picture of the patient's state and the dynamic interplay of rapport between clinician and subject.

It is not possible to describe all the modifications of hypnotic technique that may be appropriate in various cases. For the clinician, it is often the case that a given session is different—at least in some details—from any other in her or his experience. It is certainly not uncommon to begin along one line, only to shift to another—or even several others—before the session is ended.

In this connection, it must be emphasized that most of the variability derives from individual differences among patients: their personalities, their illnesses, their expectations or mental sets, their apprehensions, and of course their attitudes toward smoking. In regard to the last variable, it should be noted that hypnosis can sometimes be most useful if it is not aimed directly at cessation of the habit—or at least not immediately in the course of therapy. For example, hypnotic age regression to the time of first smoking may reveal a completely unexpected and useful approach to the case.

Some patients want to feel in control at all times; others wish to be passive in relation to the therapist. Some need a primary focus on the purely medical aspects of the need to stop smoking; others are more motivated by aesthetic, interpersonal, or social considerations. Some who are highly resistant to the therapist as a parental or authority figure will be surprisingly cooperative with the therapist as a coach. In certain cases, it may prove useful to supplement hypnotherapy with the use of medication, or environmental manipulation, or prescribed fitness regimens, or group therapy, or all or even none of these modalities.

In my experience, the best chance for success is to look upon hypnosis as one of many resources available to the clinician in his or her efforts to help the tobacco habitué. If such a person comes to me for hypnotherapy, I try (not necessarily in so many words) to convey the following message: "If you want to stop smoking, I'll help you. If other approaches have failed and you now what to try hypnosis, we'll try it. If at first we don't succeed, we'll try again. If a single method doesn't work, we'll try more than one in combination. If you don't give up, I won't. Sooner or later, we shall succeed."

By using such an approach and accepting each patient for the duration of his or her struggle with the smoking habit rather than just for hypnotherapy alone, I believe that hypnosis can be employed to maximum advantage, and that most applicants for treatment can be freed from their dependency on tobacco.

References

1. Bramwell JM. Hypnotism: Its history, practice and theory. New York: Julian Press, 1903.
2. Gravitz MA. Early uses of hypnosis in smoking cessation and dietary management: A historical note. Am J of Clin Hypn 1988; 31(1): 68–69.
3. Schwartz JL. Review and evaluation of methods of smoking cessation, 1969–77: Summary of a monograph. Public Health Rep 1979; 94(6): 558–563.
4. West LJ. Hypnosis in treatment of the tobacco smoking habit. In Jarvik ME, Cullen JW, Gritz ER, Vogt T, West LJ, eds. Research on smoking behavior.

NIDA Research Monograph No. 17. Washington, DC: U.S. Government Printing Office, 1977.

5. Dengrove E. A single-treatment method to stop smoking using ancillary self-hypnosis: Discussion. Intl J of Clin Exper Hypn 1970; 18(4): 251–256.

6. Nuland W. A single-treatment method to stop smoking using ancillary self-hypnosis: Discussion. Intl J of Clin Exper Hypn 1970; 18(4): 257–260.

7. Spiegel H. A single-treatment method to stop smoking using ancillary self-hypnosis. Intl J of Clin Exper Hypn 1970; 18(4): 235–250.

8. Wright ME. A single-treatment method to stop smoking using ancillary self-hypnosis: Discussion. Intl J of Clin Exper Hypn 1970; 18(4): 261–267.

9. Kline MV. The use of extended group hypnotherapy sessions in controlling cigarette habituation. Intl J of Clin Exper Hypn 1970; 18(4): 270–282.

10. Kroger WS, Fezler WD. Hypnosis and behavior modification: Imagery conditioning. Philadelphia: Lippincott, 1976.

11. Kroger WS, Libott RY. Thanks, Doctor, I've stopped smoking. Springfield, IL: Thomas, 1967.

12. Hall A, Crasilneck HB. Development of a hypnotic technique for treating chronic cigarette smoking. Intl J of Clin Exper Hypn 1970; 18(4): 283–289.

13. Nuland W, Field PB. Smoking and hypnosis: A systematic clinical approach. Intl J of Clin Exper Hypn 1970; 18(4): 290–306.

14. Perry C, Mullen G. The effects of hypnotic susceptibility on reducing smoking behavior treated by an hypnotic technique. J of Clin Psychol 1975; 31(3): 498–505.

15. Jones OL. A study of hypnotherapy in general practice. Practitioner 1986; 230(1413): 275–280.

16. Sheehan DV, Surman OS. Follow-up study of hypnotherapy for smoking. J of the Am Soc of Psychosomatic Dentistry and Med 1982; 29(1): 6–16.

17. Tori CD. A smoking satiation procedure with reduced medical risk. J of Clin Psychol 1978; 34(2): 574–577.

18. Ryde D. Hypnotherapy and cigarette smoking. Practitioner 1985; 229(1399): 29–31.

19. Wagner TJ, Hindi-Alexander M, Horwitz MB. A one-year follow-up study of the Damon Group Hypnosis Smoking Cessation Program. J of the Okla State Med Assoc 1983; 76(12): 414–417.

20. Neufield V, Lynn SJ. A single-session group self-hypnosis smoking cessation treatment: A brief communication. Intl J of Clin Exper Hypn 1988; 36(2): 75–79.

21. Shewchuk LA. Smoking cessation programs of the American Health Foundation. Prev Med 1976; 5(3): 454–474.

22. Berkowitz B, Ross-Townsend A, Kohberger R. Hypnotic treatment of smoking: The single-treatment method revisited. Am J of Psychi 1979; 136(1): 83–85.

23. Pederson LL, Scrimgeour WG, Lefcoe NM. Incorporation of rapid smoking in a community service smoking withdrawal program. Intl J of Addict 1980; 15(5): 615–629.

24. Shewchuk LA, Dubren R, Burton D, Forman M, Clark RR, Jaffin AR. Preliminary observations on an intervention program for heavy smokers. Intl J of Addict 1977; 12(2–3): 323–336.

25. Byrne DG, Whyte HM. The efficacy of community-based smoking cessation strategies: A long-term follow-up study. Intl J of Addict 1987; 22(8): 791–801.

26. Frank RG, Umlauf RL, Wonderlich SA, Ashkanazi GS. Hypnosis and behavioral treatment in a worksite smoking cessation program. Addict Behav 1986; 11(1): 59–62.
27. Williams JM, Hall DW. Use of single session hypnosis for smoking cessation. Addict Behav 1988; 13(2): 205–208.
28. Hyman GJ, Stanley RO, Burrows GD, Horne DJ. Treatment effectiveness of hypnosis and behaviour therapy in smoking cessation: A methodological refinement. Addict Behav 1986; 11(4): 355–365.
29. Stanton HE. A one-session approach to modifying smoking behavior. Intl J of Clin Exper Hypn 1978; 26: 22–29.
30. Javel AF. One-session hypnotherapy for smoking: A controlled study. Psychol Rep 1980; 46: 895–899.
31.· Crasilneck HB, Hall JA. Clinical hypnosis: Principles and applications. New York: Grune & Stratton, 1975.
32. Jeffrey TB, Jeffrey LK, Greuling JW, Gentry WR. Evaluation of a brief group treatment package including hypnotic induction for maintenance of smoking cessation: A brief communication. Intl J of Clin Exper Hypn 1985; 33(2): 95–98.
33. Jeffrey LK, Jeffrey TB. Exclusion therapy in smoking cessation. A brief communication. Intl J of Clin Exper Hypn 1988; 36(2): 70–74.
34. Kaufert JM, Rabkin SW, Syrotuik J, Boyko E, Shane F. Health beliefs as predictors of success of alternate modalities of smoking cessation: Results of a controlled trial. J of Behav Med 1986; 9(5): 475–489.
35. Lambe R, Osier C, Franks P. A randomized controlled trial of hypnotherapy for smoking cessation. J of Fam Pract 1986; 22(1): 61–65.
36. Rabkin SW, Boyko E, Shane F, Kaufert J. A randomized trial comparing smoking cessation programs utilizing behavior modification, health education or hypnosis. Addict Behav 1984; 9(2): 157–173.
37. Horwitz MB, Hindi-Alexander M, Wagner TJ. Psychosocial mediators of abstinence, relapse, and continued smoking: A one-year follow-up of a minimal intervention. Addict Behav 1985; 10(1): 29–39.
38. Schubert DK. Comparison of hypnotherapy with systematic relaxation in the treatment of cigarette habituation. J of Clin Psychol 1983; 39(2): 198–202.
39. Frankel FH, Orne MT. Hypnotizability and phobic behavior. Arch of Gen Psychi 1976; 33(10): 1259–1261.
40. Baer L, Carey RJ Jr, Meminger SR. Hypnosis for smoking cessation: A clinical follow-up. Intl J of Psychosom 1986; 33(3): 13–16.
41. Agee LL. Treatment procedures using hypnosis in smoking cessation programs: A review of the literature. J of the Am Soc of Psychosomatic Dentistry and Med 1983; 30(4): 111–126.

14
The Treatment of Smoking and Nicotine Addiction with Acupuncture

STUART KUTCHINS

Acupuncture has a functionally important and practically expanding role to play in the treatment of a variety of addiction disorders. Much of the serious attention recently given to acupuncture has been in relation to its use in treatment of substance abuse. Indeed, it appears that 20 years of success in treatment of substance abuse may prove more effective in creating paths to institutional acceptance of acupuncture in America than all the successes of the previous 20 centuries.

While much of the recent public notice given to acupuncture treatment of addictive disorders has focused on its remarkable success in drug detoxification or "detox" (i.e., the treatment of addiction to so-called hard drugs such as heroin, cocaine, and methadone),[1-6] there have also been reports of success in treatment of alcoholism and nicotine dependency,[5,7-14] (Although the terms *nicotine dependency* and *habitual smoking* are used interchangeably here, in the interests of easier reading, they actually indicate somewhat different aspects of this complex disorder.)

Good results have been reported for treatment of nicotine addiction using several acupuncture treatment approaches, including innovations in needle placement and stimulation techniques.[9-14] This suggests that a competent practitioner may be able to choose from among a variety of strategies and to select the particular methodology especially suited to her or his style of treatment and the specific needs of individual patients.

Evaluating Competency

One of the fundamental concerns regarding the use of acupuncture treatment in a conventional medical setting or in cooperation with practitioners of modern biomedicine is the potential for cooption and the erosion of the distinction between Oriental and Western medicine. It should be borne in mind that acupuncture is a medical art and science with a distinct theoretical base. The tendency among some Westerners to regard Oriental medicine as no more than a set of techniques to be plugged into the biomedical armamentarium is to demean the practice of medicine in general and to degrade a millenia-old healing art to a bag of tricks; the concomitant dismissal of Oriental medical philosophy is a form of intellectual jingoism that speaks ill of those who indulge in it.[15]

Not to put too fine a point on it, the best results in treatment can be expected only when the practitioner is adequately trained and is competent to design and execute treatments that factor in the specific needs of individual patients. To deny patients adequate care from a competent professional acupuncturist is as irresponsible as to permit a briefly trained technician to prescribe antibiotics to patients who present with acute infections—it is not that there could not be an encouraging level of success, it is just that many of the failures would be tragic and unnecessary.

Professional credentialing of acupuncturists in the United States has developed rapidly in the past few years. Professional acupuncturists are licensed in about 20 jurisdictions at the time of this writing, the requirements for licensure varying from state to state. However, a national board of examiners in acupuncture, the National Commission for the Certification of Acupuncturists (NCCA), was jointly chartered by the national professional association and the national educational association in 1982. Since 1985, the NCCA has offered national board examinations to qualified candidates at two or three sites each year.

Eligibility for candidacy for national certification is determined by factoring a number of criteria such as professional education, formal training and professional practice. Candidates are required to successfully complete a course in clean procedure now administered by the National Council of Acupuncture Schools and Colleges and to pass the certification examinations. The current examination program consists of both written and practical tests based on behaviorally defined criteria of professional competence. Examinations have been offered in the Chinese and Korean languages, as well as in English.

To date, about 2400 acupuncturists have been certified as "Diplomates in Acupuncture of the NCCA." National certification or use of the national board examination is either accepted or required for licensure as a professional acupuncturist in over 90% of the licensing jurisdictions in the United States.[16]

Credentialing in acupuncture education has also proceeded apace. The National Accreditation Commission of Schools and Colleges of Acupuncture and Oriental Medicine (NACSCAOM), chartered in 1982 by the National Council of Acupuncture Schools and Colleges, has accredited eight institutions offering 3-year programs at the Masters degree level in acupuncture and Oriental medicine. Four more schools are presently in candidacy status. The NACSCAOM has been approved by the U.S. Department of Education and, more recently, has been recognized by the Committee on Post-Secondary Accreditation.

Treatments Versus Treatment Programs

The concept of *treatment* is not entirely adequate in dealing with addictive disorders. It is far more fruitful to think in terms of *treatment programs*, analyzing the needs of the particular patient to determine the components of an adequate program. In general, it is abundantly obvious that addictive behavior is a multidimensional problem with causal factors best described as physiological, psychological, neurological, social, and cultural. In specific cases, any number of these factors may be significantly operative, and long-term success in treatment will ultimately depend on how adroitly the operative causal factors are accounted for in the treatment program.

Even at the first level of analysis, the problem we are addressing combines physiological (nicotine dependency), neuromotor (habitual smoking), and psychosocial (the role of being a smoker) elements. While this is generally true of addictive disorders and substance abuse, the difficulty of the smoker's plight is especially complicated by the fact that the specific behaviors associated with the addiction are intimately interwoven into the very fabric of the habitual smoker's public and private life. Alcohol abuse and eating disorders may in some percentage of cases become similarly tightly wound into the addict's behavior, but it is rare for anything to rival the mechanics of smoking in pervading the minute details of moment-to-moment living. Furthermore, unlike the situation typical of many other addictions, the activities surrounding smoking may well figure into the addict's management of his or her perceived *normality*, the presentation of a self as well-adjusted not only to a special (similarly addicted) group, but also to society at large.

In the present author's practice, clients seeking treatment for smoking addiction are encouraged to participate in the analysis of the dimensions of their smoking problem and to formulate their own treatment program, of which the acupuncture treatment is a part. It is emphasized that overcoming nicotine addiction is an important opportunity for the client to assume more personal control over her or his own life, and clients are encouraged to regard self-determination and personal choice as important aspects of good health. While there is no attempt to downplay the importance of acupuncture or any other expert intervention in accomplishing the goal, clients are encouraged to regard the healing program as belonging to them rather than to the practitioners. Clients who depend on the practitioner to cure them seem to do less well than those who seek help in healing themselves.

It must be recognized that smoking plays some positive role in the addict's life, and the treatment program should include new, more productive forms of support for what is otherwise sought from smoking. Each significant factor may call for addition of another element of support in the treatment program. For example, clients who feel overwhelmed by the onrush of stimuli may need to establish other forms of "times-out," such as following their breath, taking walks, repeating affirmations, and so on. Such clients might also be good candidates for biofeedback training.

Considerations of this sort may also be included in the design of the acupuncture treatment. Klate[17] uses a characterological analysis to determine the perceived needs for smoking and treats the systems that are associated with these problems, according to the Oriental medical tradition. For example, if smoking helps control anger, the Liver channel may be treated; if it is the client's method of dealing with worry, the Spleen channel may be treated; if it is part of the mechanism for knuckling down and getting things done (i.e., supporting praxis or will-power), then the Kidney channel may be treated; and so forth. Those untrained in traditional medicine, who may dismiss this aspect of the tradition as fanciful, are urged to consider that what is meant by "Liver," "Kidney," "Spleen," and so on, within the Oriental tradition is not identical to what these terms conventionally designate in the West. While knowing this will not eliminate the strangeness, one may be encouraged not to dismiss what one simply does not understand. The theoretical framework for this system of correspondences is well explained in introductory texts.[18-20]

Treatment Outcomes

Response to treatment may vary considerably. Some clients report immediate cessation of all interest in smoking, yet a few seem to experience little help from treatment. The most dramatic example of the instant-cure clients was a normally bright and alert client treated for hay fever, who reported that he stopped smoking spontaneously after a single treatment and did not notice the change until 2 days later. The most dramatic example of the intractably resistant to treatment was a man who reported that he had "kicked junk and booze" but could not give up cigarettes despite our best efforts. Most, of course, fall between the two extremes, reporting success based on the combination of their determination plus treatment plus the personal support systems we encourage them to set up.

Long-term abstention from smoking is a complex issue, subject to many mediating factors. Schwartz[21] performed a critical review of the published studies of acupuncture treatment for smoking cessation and concluded that there was generally inadequate long-term follow-up. Furthermore, in the studies where methodology was adjudged sound and long-term follow-up was performed, the outcomes were not promising. Leaving much unsaid about the evaluation of Schwartz's discussion, one must take note of his conclusion: "Acupuncture may handle the addictive component of smoking. If so the psychological and social aspects of smoking must also be handled."

Regarding acupuncture as the magic bullet that will kill the tobacco demon forever seems naïve. More realistically, evaluation of long-term outcome seems to reflect less on the efficacy of short-term treatment interventions than on the effectiveness of the entire package or program that the client commits to. While Schwartz regards the benefit of acupuncture treatment for smoking undocumented, there is a wealth of favorable clinical experience, both published[9-14] and unpublished, and there have been very encouraging reports of well-designed studies for acupuncture treatment of other forms of substance abuse.[1-8] In particular, the studies of Culliton's treatment of severe chronic alcoholics demonstrated significant reduction of craving, lower consumption, and less recidivism than in controls.[7,8]

While long-range outcomes may reflect more on the characteristics of the client and the whole treatment program, middle-range (second stage) outcomes are important to consider, as many apparent successes recidivate in the transition from withdrawing to stably recovered if there is inadequate follow-through. This second stage may be considered to begin at the close of withdrawal, in 1–2 weeks after the last cigarette was smoked, and to end at the time when the client no longer feels that she or he confronts nonsmoking as a difficult or unresolved issue. In our practice, we have come to relate follow-through with follow-up treatment at increasing intervals, sometimes spanning several months, particularly for clients whose treatment programs seem thin or whose support networks seem attenuated. Clinically, it may serve as a powerful incentive to sustain the great effort needed to reintegrate one's life as a nonsmoker. Some colleagues offer inexpensive or free follow-up treatment if at any time beyond the initial treatment program the client feels threatened with unmanageable craving, motivated at least in part by the conviction that knowing that help is available can itself be a significant aid to recovery.

In any event, for most clients, a multidimensional or multidisciplinary approach seems necessary. Even where acupuncture treatment alone is effective for first-stage withdrawal, many clients require other interventions (e.g., counseling or body-oriented therapy) in later stages, where suppressed feelings or unresolved psychological wounds reach a crisis.

It is worth adding that a few clients who had stopped smoking unassisted some months before initiating acupuncture treatment for apparently unrelated conditions were still suffering withdrawal symptoms (e.g., headache, irritability, insomnia) despite the fact that the so-called withdrawal period had long since elapsed. In these cases, the withdrawal symptoms have generally responded well to acupuncture treatment independently of whether the other presenting complaints proved tractable.

Treatment Methods

Acupuncture is the most widely known treatment method in the field of Eastern medicine. Many, though by no means all, of its practitioners are also trained in one or more of its other modalities—prescription of natural substances (Chinese medicine), myotherapy and physical therapy (*Tui Na,*

Shiatsu, bone-setting), physical exercise (*Tai Ji Chuan*, external *Qi Gong*), respiratory exercises and internal exercises (various meditative practices, including internal *Qi Gong*). This section focuses on treatment by acupuncture. While all of the other modalities may contribute to a successful treatment program, it is beyond the scope of this chapter to elaborate on their application. The skilled practitoner will readily perceive the appropriate indications and contraindications for their employment. Similarly, though some acupuncturists regard prescription of vitamin supplements, mineral supplements, homeopathic remedies, Western herbal remedies, and so on, as important elements of their treatment programs, such practices are not the unique province of this field and are left for others to describe.

Acupuncture treatment may be applied usefully to traditionally described points (herein called "body points") and/or to loci defined in specialized, more recently developed systems, such as the ear points (of auriculotherapy, developed principally by Paul Nogier of France[22,23]) or the hand points (of *Koryo Sooji Chim*, Korean hand acupuncture, developed by Tae Woo Yoo of Korea[24]). Based on personal interviews and review of the written literature, it appears that most practitioners prefer to combine traditional and specialized points, particularly auricular points.

Stimulation of the points may be variously accomplished by needle insertion, electrical current, laser beams, *moxibustion* (a form of heat treatment), application of magnets, or a combination of these methods. Most practitioners favor combined treatment of body points and auricular points and the use of needles, with or without electrical stimulation. Rarely are recommendations made for the use of *moxa* (the fibrous portion of dried foliage of Artemesia sinensis) in such treatments, perhaps because smoking generally fosters Yin-deficient (i.e., associated with drying of the body fluids) pathology. Our own preference is for needles alone, which has proven quite satisfactory in our experience; however, some practitioners prefer to use electrical stimulation. Molony[25] reports improved results in his practice with application of 4-Hz current.

Needles are usually left in place for 10–40 minutes. Many practitioners regard 20 minutes as an optimum, but some patients seem to benefit from longer treatments. There is little reason to assume that everyone will respond alike to any fixed interval. Some clients, when queried, will indicate either that they feel treatment is complete or that they would like it to go longer, but the opinions of various clients are not of equal value. Timing remains very much a matter of clinical judgment.

There are specific recommendations concerning the treatment of nicotine addiction that will prove useful in a great many cases. However, the skilled practitioner is encouraged not to fall into mechanical categorization of clients as merely smoking cases, but to remain alert to the specific condition of each person and to fashion treatments that will support the recovery of the clients' health in general. While some smokers present for treatment in states of relatively good health, smoking for many is only a part of a general picture of emotional or physiological disharmony. Many more are impelled to surrender their addiction only by the emergence of clinical or subclinical pathology.

In addition to treatment in the acupuncture clinic, it is common practice to provide means for ongoing stimulation of ear or hand points between treatments. This may be accomplished by taping down intradermal needles (or, less frequently, magnets, metallic pellets or herbal seeds) at auricular or hand points. Many, though by no means all, clients report added benefit from such treatment.

When this treatment is employed, these steps are followed to minimize the chances either of allergic inflammation from the adhesive or of infection: (1) The area is cleaned thoroughly with antiseptic (e.g., 70% isopropyl alcohol); (2) when it is dry, the area is painted with flexible collodion (e.g., Nu Skin®), on an area large enough to include the point and the covering tape, and it is permitted to dry; (3) sterile disposable needles are inserted, using sterile forceps; (4) the needles are then covered carefully with tape, sealing all the way around each needle. Hyapoallergenic tape is used. The needle should not hurt when pressed or when the area around it is moved. If it is painful at the time of insertion, it is best to wait a few minutes to recheck, as the soreness frequently subsides; if it is still painful, it should be removed and repositioned. Patients are cautioned not to put soap or alcohol on the ear or to rub it when it is wet. Needles are stimulated by lightly pressing and wiggling (not rubbing!) each point for 5–10 seconds three or four times per day routinely, and again whenever a strong urge to smoke arises. Needles are left in place up to a week, then removed and replaced (if necessary) on the opposite side. Of course, if there is any sign of infection or inflammation, the needles are immediately removed and the area treated appropriately.

Point Selection

In this matter and in all that follows in regard to treatment planning and execution, no claim is made that all successful methods are represented. The information selected for presentation is based on the combination of personal experience, discussions with colleagues, and published articles. It is readily admitted that there is a vast amount of valuable information that is beyond our personal knowledge.

Usually from 1 to 10 body points are selected, depending on the complexity of the condition, the age and strength of the patient, the strength of needle stimulation, and the frequency of treatment. To the body points may be added up to five auricular points, each insertion counting as one point, even where the same point is needled bilaterally.

Nomenclature of points is that given in *Acupuncture: A Comprehensive Text*.[18]

Principal Prescription

L-7 (LIEQUE)

L-7 (Lieque) is located in a little hollow on the radius, proximal to the styloid process, 1.5 *cun* (a unit of proportional measurement) proximal to the wrist crease.[18] This point is a very effective ingredient in treatment in almost all cases. In some cases, treatment of L-7 (Lieque) alone produces satisfactory results. Olms[13] reported an 84% success rate in the treatment of 535 addicts by needling a variant location of L-7 (Lieque), at the same level but slightly more dorsal than the position usually described. Whichever location is to be used, with this point as with all others, exactness of location is of great significance. As Olms remarks, needling even 1 or 2 mm off point may greatly diminish effectiveness. The unique effectiveness of this point may be due in part to its relationship to respiratory function, but the treatment of Lung ear points has also been extremely effective in treating all sorts of addictive disorders[1-8] and may well reflect on the role of the Lung (as understood in Oriental medicine) in the organization of human personality.

AURICULAR

The Lung points of the ear (located slightly above and below the center of the cavum concha)[18] seem to replicate in large measure the function of L-7 in treatment of smoking. Indeed, it is a principal point in the treatment of substance abuse in general.[26] The combination of the auricular points Lung, Sympathetic, and *Shenmen* is widely used in substance abuse and formed the basis of the successful treatment of alcoholism reported by Bullock et al.[7,8]

It should be noted that Nogier published an entirely dissimilar treatment plan, based solely on a different set of auricular points.[23] However effective it may be, it appears technically difficult to administer, and the requirement that the client abstain from smoking and taking other drugs for 6 hours before treatment seems impracticable.

Additional Prescription

In addition to the empirically derived treatment of the points discussed previously, there are two basic approaches to treatment construction— according to symptoms and according to traditionally described patterns of physiological disharmony. Analysis of the client's condition from one of these approaches should not by any means be thought to exclude the consideration of the other. We offer a few suggestions for treatment of each that accord with common treatment methods.[18,20,25,27,28]

BY PATTERN OF DISHARMONY

The concept of patterns of disharmony is specialized to traditional medicine, and there is no analog in modern biomedicine. Indeed, it runs counter to the flow of biomedical thought, as it procedes from the premise that an individual's health is more a matter of functional configuration than of the presence or absence of foreign pathogens. The organism is understood as a field of activity; the basis of existence is orderly flow and transformation, balance and harmony. Organs are viewed as matrices of psychophysical functions related to, but not identical to, specific anatomical structures. Pathology is described in terms of qualitative changes of activity. Such an approach has both strengths and weaknesses; it is not being held out as either superior or inferior to conventional biomedical thinking, but it is different. It is not possible here to explain these concepts properly and too few words may be worse than none at all. The interested reader is directed to some of the textbooks listed in the references section, for further information.[18–20,27]

A few of the patterns of disharmony that commonly appear in conjunction with habitual smoking are mentioned in the following list. Diagnostically significant symptoms and signs are given, to suggest the clinical picture of each pattern, but it should be appreciated that the exposition is necessarily oversimplified. These patterns may appear singly or in combinations. Some acupuncture points generally useful for treatment are listed, but the following list is meant to be suggestive rather than definitive:

Yin deficiency (afternoon fever, malar flush, heat in the palms and soles, night sweats, dry mouth and throat, yellow urine, dry stool, reddened tongue with little fur, thready and rapid pulse)—K-6 (*Zhaohai*), K-3 (*Taixi*), Sp-6 (*Sanyinqiao*), B-23 (*Shenshu*)

Lung Yin deficiency (subset of Yin deficiency; pattern as above plus dry, unproductive cough, scant production of sticky sputum, possibly streaked with blood)—select from the preceding points and from among L-5 (*Chize*), L-10 (*Yuji*), L-7 (*Lieque*), B-38 (*Gaohuang*), B-17 (*Geshu*)

Deficient Lung Qi (shortness of breath, weak cough, thin or clear sputum, weak voice, pallor, spontaneous perspiration, feel worse on exertion, weak pulse, pale tongue with thin white coat)—L-1 (*Zhongfu*), L-9 (*Taiyuan*), Sp-3 (*Taibai*), LI-4 (*Hegu*), S-36 (*Zusanli*), Co-6 (*Qihai*), Co-12 (*Zhongwan*), Co-17 (*Shanzhong*), B-13 (*Feishu*), B-20 (*Pishu*), B-21 (*Weishu*)

Constrained Qi (tightness in the chest, distension and pain, may feel better after activity, wiry pulse)—P-6 (*Neiguan*), Li-3 (*Taichong*), L-7 (*Lieque*), Co-17 (*Shanzhong*)

Liver Yang ascending (dizziness, headache, red face, bloodshot eyes, quick to anger, tinnitus, wiry, and rapid pulse, red tongue with thin yellow coating)—Li-2 (*Xingjian*), GB-34 (*Yanglingquan*), GB-20 (*Fengmen*), LI-11 (*Quchi*), K-3 (*Taixi*), B-18 (*Ganshu*), B-23 (*Shenshu*)

Deficient Heart blood (palpitations, insomnia, restlessness, nervousness, disturbing dreams, pale and lusterless face, pale tongue, thin and weak pulse)—H-7 (*Shenmen*), Gv-20 (*Baihui*), Gv-24 (*Shenting*), M-HN-3 (*Yintang*), Sp-6 (*Sanyinqiao*)

Auricular—selection as appropriate from among *Shenmen*, Heart, Spleen, Lung, Kidney, and Liver points.

BY SYMPTOM

Of course, the symptoms appear within the context of patterns of disharmony, diagnosis of which will lead to the most effective point selection. Nevertheless, in some cases, there are points that are very broadly effective. Choose from among the following points, combining them as appropriate with pattern-specific treatments given previously; the first two items are somewhat elaborated, to illustrate the process.

Nervousness, restlessness—general points: H-7 (*Shenmen*), P-6 (*Neiguan*), Co-14 (*Juque*), B-15 (*Xinshu*); add for constrained *Qi*: H-5 (*Tongli*), GB-40 (*Qiuxu*); add for deficient Yin: K-3 (*Taixi*), B-14 (*Jueyinshu*), B-23 (*Shenshu*), S-36 (*Zusanli*), Gv-20 (*Baihui*), M-HN-3 (*Yintang*), GV-24 (*Shenting*); add for deficient *Qi*: B-20 (*Pishu*), B-21 (*Weishu*)

Dizziness—Liver Yang rising: GB-20 (*Fengchi*), Liv-2 (*Xingjian*), K-3 (*Taixi*), B-18 (*Ganshu*), B-23 (*Shenshu*); deficient *Qi*: Gv-20 (*Baihui*), Gv-24 (*Shenting*), Sp-6 (*Sanyinqiao*), S-36 (*Zusanli*), Co-6 (*Qihai*), B-20 (*Pishy*); Phlegm: P-6 (*Neiguan*), S-40 (*Fenglong*), S-8 (*Touwei*)

Coughing—L-5 (*Chize*), L-1 (*Zhongfu*), K-6 (*Zhaohai*), L-6 (*Kongzui*), L-10 (*Yuji*), S-36 (*Susanli*), S-40 (*Fenglong*), Co-22 (*Tiantu*), Co-17 (*Shanzhong*), B-13 (*Feishu*), B-17 (*Geshu*)

Insomnia—H-7 (*Shenmen*), Sp-6 (*Zusanli*), N-HN-22 (*Anmian*), GB-12 (*Wangu*), B-15 (*Xinshu*)

Tightness in the chest—P-6 (*Neiguan*) , L-4 (*Xiabai*), Co-17 (*Shanzhong*), L-7 (*Lieque*), B-13 (*Feishu*), B-14 (*Jueyinshu*)

Headache—LI-4 (*Hegu*), Gv-24 (*Shenting*), GB-20 (*Fengchi*), M-HN-9 (*Taiyang*), S-8 (*Touwei*), GB-14 (*Yangbai*), M-HN-3 (*Yintang*)

Runny nose—LI-20 (*Yingxiang*), Gv-24 (*Shenting*), LI-4 (*Hegu*), B-2 (*Zanzhu*)

Regarding auricular points, there are a number of approaches to the addition of auricular points, some based on conventional theories of neurology and endocrinology, some on empirical investigation. Many practitioners favor treatment of such points as Mouth, Upper Jaw, Lower Jaw, *Shenmen*, Sympathetic, Brain, Occiput, Aggression. For patients who do not know what to do with their hands, the Brain Stem point may prove helpful.

Conclusion

Acupuncture treatment performed by competent professional acupuncturists can be expected to serve reliably as an important component of a program to overcome habitual smoking and nicotine dependency. It is essential that the program be adequate to each client's needs. Careful attention must be given to the analysis of the client's needs, realistic support sustems should be put in place, and the need for adequate follow-through should be emphasized. The client should occupy the central role in the treatment program and should bear primary responsibility and credit for its success. The course of treatment should be individuated to the client, based not only on empirically useful techniques for easing withdrawal, but also on the personal characteristics of the client and the specific symptoms manifested during treatment. Long-term outcomes ultimately rest with the client, but it is the practitioner's responsibility to direct each person to obtain all the help needed for long-term abstention.

Acknowledgments. Grateful acknowledgment is made of the invaluable assistance of Patricia Culliton, M.A., Dipl. Ac. (NCCA), Diane Polasky-Doggett, M.A., O.M.D., Dipl. Ac. (NCCA), David Molony, C.A., Dipl. Ac. (NCCA), Peter Eckman, M.D., Ph.D., M.Ac. (U.K.), Dipl. Ac (NCCA), and Jonathan Klate, B.Ac. (U.K.), Ph.D., Dipl. Ac. (NCCA). They supplied information, encouragement, suggestions, and corrections. What errors and omissions remain are solely the responsibility of the author.

References

1. Wen HL, Cheung SYC. Treatment of drug addiction by acupuncture and electrical stimulation. Asian J of Med 1973; 9: 138–141.
2. Wen HL, Teo SW. Experience in the treatment of drug addiction by electro-acupuncture. Mod Med Asia 1975; 11: 23–24.
3. Wen HL. Acupuncture and electrical stimulation (AES) outpatient detoxification. Mod Med Asia 1979; 15: 39–43.
4. Shakur M, Smith M. The uses of acupuncture in the treatment of drug addiction. Am J of Acupuncture 1979; 7: 223–228.
5. Smith MO, Squires R, Aponte J, Rabinowith N, Rodriguez RB. Acupuncture treatment of drug addiction and alcohol abuse. Am J of Acupuncture 1982; 10: 161–163.
6. Smith MO. Acupuncture treatment for crack: Clinical survey of 1,500 patients treated. Am J of Acupuncture 1988; 16: 241–246.

7. Bullock ML, Umen AJ, Culliton PD, Olander RT. Acupuncture treatment of alcoholic recidivism: A pilot study. Alcoholism (NY) 1987; 11: 292–295.

8. Bullock ML, Culliton PD, Olander RT. Controlled trial of acupuncture for severe recidivist alcoholism. Lancet 1989; 6: 1435–1438.

9. Sacks LL. Drug addiction, alcoholism, smoking, obesity treated by auricular staplepuncture. Am J of Acupuncture 1975; 3: 147–150.

10. Chen JYP. Treatment of cigarette smoking by auricular acupuncture: A report of 184 cases. Am J of Acupuncture 1979; 7: 229–234.

11. Requena Y, Michel D, Fabre J, Pernice C, Nguyen J. Smoking withdrawal therapy by acupuncture. Am J of Acupuncture 1980; 8: 57–63.

12. Choy DSJ, Lutzger L, Meltzer L. Effective treatment for smoking cessation. Am J of Med 1983; 75: 1033–1036.

13. Olms JS. Increased success rate using "Tim Mee" acupuncture point for smoking: 1981–1983—2282 cases. Intl J of Chinese Med 1985; 2: 360–365.

14. Dung HC. Clinical experiences in using acupuncture to help smoking withdrawal. Intl J of Chinese Med 1986; 3: 348–358.

15. Wolpe PR. The maintenance of professional authority: Acupuncture and the American physician. Social Problems 1985; 32: 409–423.

16. Certification examination for acupuncturists: Candidate handbook 1989. Available from the (NCCA), 1424 16th St., NW, Suite 501, Washington, DC 20036.

17. Klate J. Personal communication, August, 1990.

18. Bensky D, O'Connor J, transl. Acupuncture: A comprehensive text. Seattle, WA: Eastland Press, 1981.

19. Kaptchuk T. The web that has no weaver. New York: Congdon & Weed, 1983.

20. Deng LY, Gan YJ, He SH, Ji XP, Li Y, Wang RF, Wang WJ, Wang XT, Xu HZ, Xue XL, Yuan JL. Chinese acupuncture and moxibustion. Beijing: Foreign Languages Press, 1987.

21. Schwartz J. Evaluation of acupuncture as a treatment for smoking. Am J of Acupuncture 1988; 16: 135–142.

22. Nogier P. From auriculotherapy to auriculomedicine. Sainte Ruffine, France: Maisonneuve, 1983.

23. Nogier P. This much discussed anti-tobacco program. Auricular-Medicine and Acupuncture Physician 1975; 1: 14.

24. Yoo TW. Koryo hand acupuncture. Vol I. Seoul, Korea: Eum Yang Mek Jin Publishing, 1988.

25. Molony D. Personal communication, August, 1990.

26. Huang H, transl. Ear acupuncture. Emmaus, PA: Rodale Press, 1974: 242–245.

27. Eckman P, Kutchins S. Closing the circle—Lectures in the unity of Oriental medicine. Fairfax, CA: Shen Foundation, 1983.

28. Polasky-Doggett DH. Treatment of common disorders: an interdisciplinary approach (unpublished ms.) 540 Chama, N.E., suite 9, Albuguerque, NM 87108

15
Nicotine Gum*

MICHAEL G. GOLDSTEIN and RAYMOND NIAURA

This chapter provides a review of the use of nicotine gum, also known as "nicotine resin complex" and "nicotine polacrilex," as a treatment for nicotine dependence. After providing a rationale for the use of nicotine gum, we describe pharmacologic aspects of nicotine gum use, review the efficacy of nicotine gum treatment, discuss issues related to dose and schedule of administration, provide information on side effects and toxicity, review the potential for producing dependence on the gum, and provide guidelines for optimal use.

Rationale for Nicotine Gum Use

Jarvik and Henningfield have characterized the pharmacologic treatments for nicotine dependence using a typology that has been developed for treating other forms of drug dependence.[1,2] The four categories of pharmacologic treatment are (1) nicotine replacement or substitution, (2) blockade therapy, (3) deterrent therapy, and (4) nonspecific pharmacotherapy.[1,2] Nicotine gum is the most widely used form of nicotine relacement therapy. The primary principle of replacement therapy is to provide the patient with a more manageable and safer form of the drug during attempted abstinence to attenuate withdrawal symptoms and craving. Once these are controlled, the replacement drug is usually gradually withdrawn.[1-3] Nicotine replacement therapy with nicotine gum also provides an opportunity for the patient to develop strategies to deal with behavioral or learned components of the drug dependence while the physiologic need for the drug is controlled.[3] Because the method of administration of nico-

* This chapter was supported, in part by the National Institute on Drug Abuse, Grant No. DA05623 to Michael G. Goldstein and Raymond Niaura and The National Cancer Institute Cancer Prevention Research Consortium Grant No. PO1 CA50087 to James O. Prochaska, David B. Abrams, Wayne Velicer and Michael G. Goldstein.

tine with nicotine gum is sufficiently different from the method associated with cigarette smoking or other forms of tobacco use, the learned associations between cues associated with tobacco use and the physiologic effects of nicotine may be more easily broken.[3] For example, the use of nicotine gum over a prolonged period may decrease the craving that occurs when a patient talks on the telephone, an occasion previously associated with cigarette handling. Though nicotine gum was intended to be used as temporary relacement therapy, in some instances, patients remain on nicotine gum indefinitely. Because nicotine gum does not contain carbon monoxide, carcinogens, and other chemicals that are deleterious to health, its continued use is more desirable than the use of tobacco products.[3,4]

At the time of this writing, nicotine gum is the only form of nicotine replacement that has been approved for use by the United States Food and Drug Administration. It has been available for clinical use in the United States, by prescription only, since 1984.

Pharmacology of Nicotine Gum Use

Nicotine gum consists of nicotine bound to an ion exchange resin and incorporated into a gum base.[5] It is buffered with additives by the manufacturer to produce an alkaline pH, which facilitates absorption of nicotine through mucous membranes in the mouth.[2] Two-mg and 4-mg preparations are available in most countries, but only the 2-mg preparation is presently available for clinical use in the United States. Measurements of plasma levels of nicotine during cigarette smoking and nicotine gum chewing among regular heavy smokers indicate that nicotine levels are substantially lower while chewing 2-mg gum compared to levels achieved with smoking.[5,6] Though chewing 4-mg gum produced levels that were close to or equal to those achieved with ad libitum smoking in some studies,[6,7] levels were still substantially below those achieved during ad libitum smoking among heavy smokers in a recent well-standardized study.[5] Thus, with 2-mg gum use, it is very unlikely that *heavy smokers* (use of greater than a pack of cigarettes per day) will achieve true replacement of the nicotine levels they obtain from cigarette smoking. Incomplete replacement of nicotine in heavy smokers may limit the effectiveness of nicotine gum treatment in this population.

Chewing technique is an important determinant of the nicotine blood levels achieved with gum use. Extraction of nicotine from gum is highly dependent on the rate of chewing, and there is considerable variation among chewers in the amount of nicotine extracted from nicotine gum.[5,8,9] Buccal absorption of the gum is impaired if saliva is swallowed too quickly and, if the nicotine is swallowed, it undergoes first-pass metabolism in the liver, where it is converted to cotinine, an inactive metabolite.[5,8] Even when subjects are instructed to chew the gum slowly, 22% and 53% of the nicotine in the gum is swallowed during use of 2- and 4-mg gums, respectively.[5] Buccal absorption of nicotine is also effected by the pH of mouth fluids and is enhanced by an alkaline pH.[2] Therefore, acidity resulting from the recent ingestion of coffee, fruit juices, or other acidic beverages will decrease absorption of nicotine from nicotine gum. Because this fact is not well known, many patients are not instructed to avoid these beverages while chewing nicotine gum, thus limiting its potential usefulness.

The rate of rise of nicotine in the blood while chewing nicotine gum is also quite different than the rapid rise achieved with smoking.[10,11] While cigarette smoking produces boli of high concentrations of nicotine with each inhalation and peak blood levels within a few minutes, nicotine gum chewing produce a slow rise in blood-nicotine concentrations over the course of 20–30 minutes.[10,11] The very fast rate of nicotine delivery to the brain that occurs with cigarette smoking is thought to be a mediator of some of nicotine's neuromodulating effects,[2] whereas the slower rise in nicotine while chewing nicotine gum may not produce the same effects. This may help to explain why some patients continue to experience craving while chewing nicotine gum.[11] Moreover, the absence of a high peak in blood-nicotine levels when chewing nicotine gum may explain why individuals who smoke for stimulation appear to have greater residual withdrawal symptoms than other smokers when using nicotine gum during attempted abstinence from smoking.[12]

Efficacy of Nicotine Gum Treatment

Relief of Withdrawal Symptoms

Nicotine gum is effective in attenuating most nicotine withdrawal symptoms.[13-15] The gum appears to be most effective in suppressing anger, anxiety, and impatience during the withdrawal period and somewhat less effective in controlling restlessness, concentration difficulties and insomnia.[13-15] Nicotine gum's effects on craving and hunger are less consistent across studies.[13-15] Though several studies have found that nicotine gum reduces craving and hunger during abstinence from tobacco, the strength of this effect has not always been statistically significant in placebo-controlled trials.[13-15] Nicotine gum's limited effect on craving is not surprising, as craving is believed to be mediated by pharmacologic, psychologic, and behavioral aspects of drug dependence.[16,17]

Two recent well-controlled trials using 2-mg gum found that hunger was significantly decreased by active gum compared to placebo.[13,15] Active gum was effective in limiting both hunger and weight gain for the entire 10 weeks of gum treatment in one of these studies.[13,18] However, at 6-month follow-up, there was no difference in weight gain between the two treatment groups, suggesting that nicotine gum use delays rather than prevents eventual weight gain after smoking cessation.[18]

As noted previously, research has suggested that individuals who smoke for stimulation are most likely to experience residual withdrawal symptoms when using nicotine gum.[12] These individuals may be particularly responsive to the neuropharmacologic effects of nicotine boli and may have more withdrawal when using nicotine gum because the gum does not produce the high peaks in nicotine levels that occur during cigarette smoking.[10,11]

Enhancing Smoking Cessation

Controlled trials have demonstrated that nicotine gum is more effective than placebo in enhancing abstinence from smoking.[2,16,19,20] The increased benefit of active gum versus placebo is most marked when the gum is provided in the setting of formal smoking-cessation treatment program.[16,19,21] Lam and colleagues[19] published a meta-analysis of randomized controlled trials of nicotine gum in 1987. In seven trials, which were performed in specialized smoking-cessation clinics, the combined 12-month abstinence rates were significantly higher with nicotine gum (23%) than with placebo (13%).[19] Two more-recent studies also demonstrated the superiority of nicotine gum compared to placebo when used as an adjunct to group or behavioral treatment.[22,23] Moreover, two studies performed in a specialized smoking-clinic setting, which compared nicotine gum with a no-gum condition, found significantly better short-term abstinence rates with the addition of nicotine-gum treatment.[19]

Nicotine gum is less effective in enhancing smoking cessation in settings other than a specialized clinic-based treatment program.[16,19,21,24] Several placebo-controlled trials of nicotine gum conducted in physician office settings have found that, when evaluating long-term abstinence, nicotine gum is not significantly more effective than placebo.[16,19,21,24] However, when short-term outcomes are considered, nicotine gum appears to have some benefit over placebo.[16,21,24] The short-term, but not long-term, effectiveness of nicotine gum when compared to placebo in the medical setting is probably due to a number of interacting factors.

First, subjects in the medical setting are likely to have different characteristics than subjects attending smoking-cessation clinics. Only a small percentage of smokers will seek help by attending a formal treatment program.[25] Though Hughes and colleagues[24] found few demographic differences between subjects in a clinic-based trial and those in a trial in a general medicine practice setting, subjects in the general practice study scored lower on a scale of nicotine dependence and were less likely to have tried to quit smoking more than three times. This finding—and the fact that the subjects were not actively seeking treatment when they were enrolled in the study—suggests that the subjects in the general practice setting were less motivated to quit smoking at the time they received treatment than those seeking treatment the clinic setting.

Second, subjects in many of the trials in the medical setting were less likely to have received proper or complete instructions about effective chewing technique, as physicians providing the gum were not always adequately trained.[24] Even when adequate training about nicotine gum use is provided to physicians, the infrequent and brief contact received by smoking patients in the medical setting is not conducive to solving gum-use problems. Subjects in medical settings may also be less likely to use prescribed gum and may discontinue the gum too soon.[21]

Finally, and perhaps most importantly, little time and attention can be spent in the medical setting on the psychological and behavioral aspects of nicotine dependence.[17,21] Relapse-prevention training, an important component of most clinic-based treatment programs, can not be as easily addressed in the medical setting. The medical setting may also foster the development, or reinforcement, of the subject's reliance on extrinsic agents or forces to change behavior.[26] When the agent (i.e., nicotine gum) is discontinued, the absence of intrinsic or internal resources (e.g., self-efficacy) may increase susceptibility to relapse.[26]

Though placebo-controlled trials in the medical setting have found that nicotine gum is not significantly more effective than placebo in enhancing long-term abstinence, several studies performed in the medical and dental setting have found that nicotine gum is significantly more effective than no-gum treatment conditions.[16,19,27,28] These results indicate that the offer or provision of nicotine gum to medical patients may have significant placebo or nonspecific effects.[21,24] Another possible explanation is that the availability of gum in these studies served as a reminder to the physician or dentist to counsel patients about smoking.[27,28]

Nicotine gum has also been tested in combination with other minimal or low-contact treatment conditions. In two recent trials in which subjects also received self-help smoking-cessation modules, nicotine gum, when compared to placebo or no-gum conditions, produced significantly higher short-term (1–6 month), but not long-term (12 month) abstinence rates.[26,29] Sutton and Hallett[30] describe an effective brief individual treatment intervention using nicotine gum at the worksite. They found that workers randomly assigned to a 2 session, health-officer-delivered intervention, which included the provision of a prescription of nicotine gum, produced a 1-year abstinence rate of 12%, compared to a 2% rate in a no-intervention control group.[30] These results are consistent with the results found with brief intervention plus nicotine gum in the medical setting.

The preceding discussion raises the following important question regarding nicotine gum's efficacy: When prescribing nicotine gum, how much and what type of nonpharmacologic treatments are required to produce a successful long-term outcome? Though the answer to this question is unclear at this time, it appears that adequate instructions about nicotine-gum use, follow-up visits, and some form of relapse-prevention treatment are essential components of successful nicotine-gum treatment.[21]

Effect of Level of Nicotine Dependence on Nicotine-Gum Efficacy

When nonpharmacologic interventions are used, subjects who score high on measures of nicotine dependence, such as the Fagerstrom Tolerance Questionnaire, are generally less successful at quitting smoking than those with lower scores.[16] However, in most studies in which nicotine gum has been provided, highly dependent subjects have fared as well as subjects with low dependency.[16] This suggests that nicotine gum improves the chances that a highly dependent smoker will succeed in quitting smoking by directly addressing the pharmacologic aspect of nicotine dependence.[16]

Studies that have directly assessed the differential effectiveness of nicotine gum on the basis of the level of nicotine dependence have found that nicotine gum is consistently more effective than placebo gum in highly dependent subjects, while low-dependence subjects do not consistently fare better on nicotine gum compared to placebo.[2,16,31] Because almost all of these studies assessed the effect of level of nicotine dependence in a retrospective manner, this finding must be interpreted with caution. However, a recent study prospectively matched the smokers, on the basis of their level of nicotine dependence, either to a 4-mg or a 2-mg condition (for high-dependence subjects) or to a 2-mg or a placebo condition (for low-dependence subjects).[22] All subjects received weekly group counseling, led by a physician. Results indicated that (1) high-dependence subjects who received the 4-mg dose had significantly higher 2-year abstinence rates than those who received the 2-mg dose; and (2) low-dependence subjects who received the 2-mg dose had significantly higher 2-year abstinence rates than those who received placebo.[22]

Efficacy of Nicotine Gum—Other Considerations

Dose

As noted in the section on the pharmacology of nicotine gum use, use of the 4-mg dose produces blood nicotine levels that are closer to those obtained with regular smoking, especially in heavy smokers.[5] Though the 4-mg dosage form of nicotine gum is not available for general clinical use in the United States, it has been used and tested in Europe and Canada for several years. Two studies directly tested the differential effectiveness of 2-mg versus 4-mg nicotine gum and found no significant overall difference in smoking-cessation outcome between groups,[31,32] though one of these studies found that the 4-mg dose was significantly more effective than the 2-mg gum in high-dependence subjects.[32] Moreover, as noted previously, the results of another study that prospectively matched patients to treatments based on their level of nicotine dependence found that the 4-mg dose appears to be more effective for the heavily dependent smoker.[22] Thus, from the data presently available, it appears that the 4-mg dose may be especially useful for individuals with high levels of nicotine dependence. In the United States, simultaneous use of two pieces of 2-mg gum has been used in some studies. Fagerstrom and Tonnesen, two European investigators who have experience with the 4-mg preparation, have recommended that strengths even higher than the 4-mg variety be made available for the patient with very high nicotine dependence.[16,33]

SCHEDULE OF ADMINISTRATION

Most of the published studies that have tested the efficacy of nicotine gum have administered the gum on an ad lib, or as-needed, schedule. Patients are generally instructed to use the gum whenever they have an urge to smoke. However, a fixed schedule of tapering gum use has several theoretical advantages. First, a fixed schedule of nicotine gum use is likely to provide more stable blood nicotine levels than an ad lib schedule, and this, in turn, may improve control over withdrawal symptoms.[34,35] Second, a scheduled pattern of nicotine use may also help to break the conditioned link between craving and nicotine intake.[35] Third, use of a fixed schedule of gum, tapered over time, might also reduce the likelihood of developing dependence on the gum.[36] Thus, several lines of evidence suggest that a fixed schedule of administration may improve the effectiveness of nicotine-gum treatment.

However, the two studies that have tested fixed versus ad lib schedules of nicotine-gum administration have produced mixed results.[29,37] In a smoking-cessation clinic setting where weekly group treatment was provided, Goldstein and colleagues[37] found that schedule of nicotine gum administration had no overall effect on treatment outcome. However, the authors also reported that the fixed schedule was somewhat more effective than the ad lib schedule for subjects who were highly dependent on nicotine, as measured by the Fagerstrom Tolerance Questionnaire.

Killen and colleagues[29] compared a fixed schedule of nicotine administration with an ad lib schedule in a minimal contact, self-help treatment program. No-gum and placebo (ad lib) conditions were also included in the design. The overall results indicated that active gum was more effective than both placebo and no-gum conditions at 2- and 6-month follow-up and also suggest that the fixed condition accounted for much of the difference in abstinence rates.[29] However, the treatment effects were significant only for the men in the study. Additionally, men receiving nicotine gum had significantly higher abstinence rates 12 months after initiating treatment. The fixed schedule also accounted for most of the gum's benefit in men. Subjects in the fixed conditions chewed significantly more gum than those in the ad lib condition, suggesting that the increased benefit from the fixed condition was related to more complete nicotine replacement.[29] The findings of these two studies suggest that a fixed schedule may be more effective than an ad lib schedule in subgroups of smokers (e.g., men and high nicotine dependence), but also that further study is needed to determine the optimal schedule of nicotine gum administration.

COMBINED GUM AND BEHAVIORAL TREATMENT

To what extent does specific behavioral skills training enhance the effectiveness of nicotine gum when used in a clinic-based treatment program? Two studies have shown that the combination of nicotine gum and clinic-based behavioral treatment is more effective than either treatment component alone.[23,38] Killen and colleagues[38] compared extensive behavioral treatment plus nicotine gum with either treatment alone, but some behavioral skills training was provided for all subjects during a quitting phase prior to gum use, so this study cannot be considered a true assessment of the importance of adding behavioral skills treatment. Hall and colleagues[23] also compared extensive behavioral treatment plus nicotine gum with either treatment alone, but the gum-alone and the gum-plus-behavioral-treatment conditions were not equated for therapist contact time. A subsequent study performed by Hall et al., which used essentially the same nonpharmacologic interventions but included a placebo condition instead of the no-gum condition, found no advantage of intensive behavioral treatment over a low-contact condition.[39]

A recent study conducted by Goldstein and colleagues[37] is perhaps the best test of the effectiveness of adding specific behavioral skills training to clinic-based nicotine gum treatment program. This study compared a behavioral skills group treatment with a group providing nonspecific support and education. All subjects also received nicotine gum. At the 6-month follow-up, the subjects who received behavioral skills training had an abstinence rate that was twice that (36.7%) of the subjects in the education condition (17.5%).[37] The benefit of the behavioral skills treatment was associated with decreased relapse rates, rather than with increased initial quit rates, suggesting that the behavioral skills training was helpful in relapse prevention.[37] Another possible reason for the increased success of the addition of behavioral skills training to nicotine gum is the complementarity of these two interventions. Nicotine gum is not only a pharmacologic aid: it is also a coping strategy, which can be used by smokers along with other behavioral strategies that are taught in a behavioral skills treatment program. After other behavioral coping strategies are developed and practiced, they eventually can be substituted for nicotine gum as it is tapered to discontinuation. In contrast, if alternative behavioral coping strategies are not taught or developed during treatment with nicotine gum, patients may become overly reliant on the gum as a coping strategy and may fail to develop effective strategies to deal with cues and triggers. Once the nicotine replacement is discontinued, they may be more likely to relapse. Further study is needed to confirm the increased benefit of adding specific behavioral skills training to a clinic-based treatment program that includes nicotine gum.

Side Effects and Toxicity

Side effects of nicotine gum use occur in about 40–50% of patients.[40] However, only about 25% of patients in clinical trials discontinue use because of side effects.[40] Hiccups, nausea, decreased appetite, oral soreness or ulcers, jaw soreness, and gastrointestinal distress are the most frequent side effects, and headache, dizziness, light-headedness, and excessive salivation are not uncommon.[40] Most of these symptoms can be attributed to the act of chewing (e.g., jaw soreness, headache), the effects of excess nicotine in the mouth (e.g., oral soreness and ulcers), and the effects of swallowed nicotine (e.g., hiccups, nausea, gastrointestinal distress). Symptoms can be reduced by providing patients with instructions regarding proper use (see later section). Many patients also complain about the taste of the gum, which was best described by one of our patients as "stale peppermint."

Nicotine's toxic effects must be considered when making a decision about the use of nicotine gum in patients with smoking-related medical illnesses. The package insert for nicotine gum lists the following contraindications: recent myocardial infarction, life-threatening cardiac arrhythmia, severe or worsening angina, and active temporomandibular joint disease. Nicotine's effects on the vascular system promote and exacerbate cardiovascular, cerebrovascular, and peripheral vascular disease.[4,10] Regular use of nicotine gum will produce the same level of blood pressure elevation as cigarette smoking, but less heart rate acceleration.[4] Nicotine's effects on platelets, lipids, vascular muscle, and circulating catecholamines may promote atherosclerosis, thrombosis, ischemia, and arrhythmias.[4,10] Therefore, though the levels of nicotine achieved through the use of nicotine gum are generally lower than when smoking cigarettes, it is preferable to try alternative methods of smoking cessation when treating patients with known vascular disease. Because the use of nicotine gum is likely to lead to high concentrations of nicotine in the stomach and esophagus, nicotine gum use may also exacerbate peptic ulcer disease and esophageal reflux and should be avoided when these conditions are present.[4] Nicotine's toxic effects on the fetus, particularly during the third trimester of pregnancy, preclude its use in pregnant women. Use in nursing mothers is also contraindicated because nicotine also is secreted into breast milk.[4]

Nicotine gum has minimal adverse effects on oral health.[40] However, the mechanical forces of chewing can displace defective or loose restorations, and adequate dental repair is a prerequisite to nicotine gum use.[40] Though nicotine gum can stick to some dentures, most patients with dentures can chew the gum in an effective manner.[40,41]

Nicotine intoxication is characterized by nausea, vomiting, abdominal pain, weakness, dizziness, sweating, pallor, and headache.[4] Nicotine intoxication is theoretically possible from a nicotine gum overdose, but, unless a child chewed the gum, it is very unlikely to become a clinical problem unless multiple pieces are chewed actively at once.[4] Swallowing gum will not lead to significant toxicity because passive absorption from the gum is low.[4] In a study performed with volunteers, simultaneous ingestion of 10 pieces of 4-mg gum produced peak blood levels of nicotine that are well below the usual level achieved with one cigarette or one piece of nicotine gum, chewed as directed.[40]

Potential for Addiction

Individuals who use nicotine gum to stop smoking may become physically dependent on the gum and may experience withdrawal when they abstain from gum.[42–44] However, only 6–9% of subjects who receive nicotine gum in specialty clinics continue to use the gum 1 year after treatment.[44] Among the subset of subjects who successfully abstain from cigarettes, 34–54% use the gum for more than 6 months,[45] and about 25% continue to use gum after 1 year.[43] These individuals may require slow tapering of gum use over a longer period of time or the use of other pharmacologic treatments to treat withdrawal. To our knowledge, there have been no reports of nicotine gum misuse, abuse, or dependence among nonsmokers.

Cost

A box of 96 pieces of 2-mg gum presently (January, 1991) costs about $36 in the northeast United States. Data from clinical studies indicate that the average user consumes two to three boxes during the first month after quitting smoking.[33] Prescription plans available from third-party payers vary in their coverage of nicotine gum prescriptions.

Guidelines for Nicotine Gum Use

The general guidelines for nicotine gum use that follow are derived from the information summarized in preceding sections of this chapter. When considering nicotine gum treatment, the first step should be an assessment to ensure that the patient is an appropriate candidate for this form of treatment. Nicotine gum is best reserved for those patients who are (1) regular smokers, (2) motivated and ready to try to quit smoking, (3) moderately or highly nicotine dependent (as measured by the Fagerstrom Tolerance Questionnaire or an equivalent scale), (4) free of any contraindications (see the preceding section on toxicity) or known hypersensitivity to nicotine gum or gum products, and (5) willing to return for follow-up appointments to assess response to treatment and level of toxicity and side effects. Patients who have responded favorably to nicotine gum in the past or who have had significant withdrawal symptoms during prior cessation attempts are also good candidates for the gum.

Once a decision to use nicotine gum has been made, the choice of an appropriate dose and schedule of administration should be based on the patient's level of nicotine dependence and their previous experience, if any, with nicotine gum. Though 4-mg gum is not presently available in the United States, two 2-mg pieces may be used simultaneously in very dependent smokers. A fixed schedule may be more efficacious for the highly dependent subject. Adequate instructions about nicotine-gum use, follow-up visits, and some form of relapse-prevention treatment are essential components of successful nicotine-gum treatment. The efficacy of nicotine-gum treatment is most consistent when it is combined with a clinic-based treatment program, but minimum or low-contact conditions can also be enhanced by the provision of nicotine gum. There is some evidence to suggest that the combination of specific behavioral skills training and nicotine gum treatment is more effective than either treatment alone.

The pharmacologic properties of nicotine gum (see the foregoing section on pharmacology) require the provison of very specific instructions to the patient regarding proper use. These are outlined in Table 15.1. Patients should be told that nicotine gum should not be used to help them cut down the number of cigarettes they are smoking, as this defeats the purpose of replacement therapy and may actually lead to the attainment of higher nicotine levels than when smoking cigarettes without gum use.[33] It is helpful to share the rationale for using nicotine gum, to help patients to understand that the gum is most effective when enough gum is chewed to prevent the development of withdrawal symptoms.

TABLE 15.1. Instructions for patients using nicotine gum (seven S's).

1. Stop smoking cigarettes—do not smoke and chew.
2. Substitute gum for cigarettes—at each urge to smoke.
3. Several pieces per day—about 1 piece for every two cigarettes.
4. Slowly chew—only a few chews, then "park" the gum.
5. Stay on the gum for 2 to 3 months.
6. Staged reduction—decrease use over several weeks.
7. Stop using the gum.

Source. Adapted from the treatment protocol developed for the Waterloo Smoking Project, JA Best & D Wilson Principal Investigators, Waterloo University and McMaster University, National Cancer Institute, Smoking, Tobacco and Cancer Program, 1988.

When starting nicotine gum, we generally instruct patients to plan to chew one piece of nicotine gum for every two cigarettes they would otherwise smoke. They are also told to to titrate the amount of gum they chew to control withdrawal symptoms while minimizing side effects. We explain that it is best to chew gum at the first sign of withdrawal symptoms rather than waiting until they are intolerable because the slow rise in nicotine levels with gum use makes catching up with symptoms difficult. Instruction in proper chewing technique is crucial to effective use. We always ask the patient to chew a sample piece of gum in our presence, to correct improper techniques. Most individuals will start to chew the gum too rapidly, even when given instructions to chew slowly. We tell patients to think of nicotine gum as a lozenge that is occasionally chewed and "parked" in the mouth, rather than as a stick of chewing gum. We also recommend that patients plan to stay on the gum for 2–3 months. This recommendation is based on the findings of early British studies,[46] though we are not aware of any definitive evidence that suggests increased long-term benefit for patients who continue to chew nicotine gum for this period of time.[47] Establishing a target date for eventual discontinuation at the outset may decrease the risk of long-term dependence. Tapering of gum use before discontinuation is recommended, to prevent withdrawal symptoms upon cessation.[17]

References

1. Jarvik ME, Henningfield JE. Pharmacological treatment of tobacco dependence. Pharmacol Biochem Behav 1988; 30: 279–294.
2. U.S. Department of Health and Human Services. The health consequences of smoking: Nicotine addiction (a report of the Surgeon General). Rockville, MD: U.S. Department of Health and Human Services, Public Health Service, Office on Smoking and Health, 1988.
3. Jasinski DR, Henningfield JE. Conceptual basis of replacement therapies for chemical dependence. In: Pomerleau OF, Pomerleau CS, eds. Nicotine replacement: A critical evaluation. New York: Liss, 1988: 13–34.
4. Benowitz NL. Toxicity of nicotine: Implications with regard to nicotine replacement therapy. In: Pomerleau OF, Pomerleau CS. eds. Nicotine replacement: A critical evaluation. New York: Liss, 1988: 187–217.
5. Benowitz NL, Jacob P, Savanapridi C. Determinants of nicotine intake while chewing nicotine polacrilex gum. Clin Pharmacol Ther 1987; 41: 467–473.
6. McNabb ME, Ebert EV, McCusker K. Plasma nicotine levels produced by chewing nicotine gum. JAMA 1982; 248: 865–868.
7. Russell MAH, Sutton SR, Feyerabend C, Cole PV, Saloojee Y. Nicotine chewing gum as a substitute for smoking. Brit Med J 1977; 1: 1060–1063.
8. Henningfield JE, Jasinski DR. Pharmacologic basis for nicotine replacement. In: Pomerleau OF, Pomerleau CS, eds. Nicotine replacement: A critical evaluation. New York: Liss, 1988: 35–61.

9. Nemeth-Coslett R, Benowitz NL, Robinson N, Henningfield JE. Nicotine gum: Chew rate, subjective effects and plasma nicotine. Pharmacol Biochem Behav 1988; 29: 747–751.
10. Benowitz NL. Pharmacologic aspects of cigarette smoking and nicotine addiction. New Engl J of Med 1988; 319: 1318–1330.
11. Russell MAH. Nicotine replacement: The role of blood nicotine levels, their rate of change, and nicotine tolerance. In: Pomerleau OF, Pomerleau CS, eds. Nicotine replacement: A critical evaluation. New York; Liss, 1988: 63–94.
12. Niaura R, Goldstein MG, Ward KD, Abrams DB. Reasons for smoking and severity of residual nicotine withdrawal symptoms when using nicotine chewing gum. Brit J of Addict 1989: 84: 681–687.
13. Gross J, Stitzer ML. Nicotine replacement: Ten-week effects on tobacco withdrawal symptoms. Psychopharmacology 1989; 98: 334–341.
14. Hughes JR, Higgins ST, Hatsukami D. Effects of abstinence from tobacco: A critical review. In: Kozlowski LT, Annis HM, Cappell HD, Glaser FD, Goodstadt MS, Israel Y, Kalant H, Sellers EM, Vingilis ER, eds. Research advances in alcohol and drug problems. Vol. 10. New York: Plenum Press, 1990: 317–398.
15. Hughes JR, Gust SW, Skoog K, Keenan R, Fenwick JW. Symptoms of tobacco withdrawal: A replication and extension. Arch of Gen Psych 1991; 48: 52–59.
16. Fagerström K-O. Efficacy of nicotine chewing gum: A review. In: Pomerleau OF, Pomerleau CS, eds. Nicotine replacement: A critical evaluation. New York: Liss, 1988: 159–182.
17. West R. Nicotine: A dependence producing substance. In: Pomerleau OF, Pomerleau CS, eds. Nicotine replacement: A critical evaluation. New York: Liss, 1988: 237–259.
18. Gross J, Stitzer ML, Maldonado J. Nicotine replacement: Effects on postcessation weight gain. J of Consult Clin Psychol 1989; 57: 87–92.
19. Lam W, Sacks HS, Sze PC, Chalmers TC. Meta-analysis of randomized controlled trials of nicotine chewing-gum. Lancet 1987; 2: 27–30.
20. Schwartz JL. Review and evaluation of smoking cessation methods: The United States and Canada, 1978–1985. Bethesda, MD: National Institutes of Health, 1987.
21. Jarvis M. Nicotine replacement as sole therapy or as adjunct. In: Pomerleau OF, Pomerleau CS, eds. Nicotine replacement: A critical evaluation. New York: Liss, 1988: 145–162.
22. Tonnesen P, Fryd V, Hansen M, Helsted J, Gunnersen AB, Forchammer H, Stockner M. Effect of nicotine chewing gum in combination with group counseling on the cessation of smoking. New Engl J of Med 1988; 318: 15–18.
23. Hall SM, Tunstall C, Rugg D, Jones RT, Benowitz N. Nicotine gum and behavioral treatment in smoking cessation. J of Consult Clin Psychol 1985; 53: 256–258.
24. Hughes JR, Gust SW, Keenan RM, et al. Nicotine vs placebo gum in general medical practice. JAMA 1989; 261: 1300–1305.
25. Fiore MC, Novotny TE, Pierce JP, Giovino GA, Hatziandreu EJ, Newcomb PA, Surawicz TS, Davis RM. Methods used to quit smoking in the United States: Do cessation programs help? JAMA 1990; 263: 2760–2765.

26. Harackiewicz JM, Sansone C, Blair LW, Epstein JA, Manderlink G. Attributional processes in behavior change and maintenance: Smoking cessation and continued abstinence. J of Consult Clin Psychol 1987; 55: 372–378.
27. Cohen SJ, Stookey GK, Katz BP, Drook CA, Smith DM. Encouraging primary care physicians to help smokers quit: A randomized controlled trial. Ann of Internal Med 1989; 110: 648–652.
28. Cohen SJ, Stookey GK, Katz BP, Drook CA, Christen AG. Helping smokers quit: A randomized controlled trial with private practice dentists. J of the Am Dental Assoc 1989; 118: 41–45.
29. Killen JD, Fortmann SP, Newman B, Varady A. Evaluation of a treatment approach combining nicotine gum with self-guided behavioral treatments for smoking relapse prevention. J of Consult Clin Psychol 1990; 58: 85–92.
30. Sutton S, Hallett R. Randomized trial of brief individual treatment for smoking, using nicotine chewing gum in a workplace setting. Am J of Public Health 1987; 77: 1210–1211.
31. Tonnesen P, Fryd V, Hansen M, Helsted J, Gunnersen AB, Forchammer H, Stockner M. Two and four mg nicotine chewing gum in combination with group counseling in smoking cessation: An open, randomized, controlled trial with a 22 month follow-up. Addict Behav 1988; 13: 17–27.
32. Kornitzer M, Kittel F, Dramaix M, Bourdoux P. A double-blind study of 2 mg vs 4 mg nicotine chewing gum in an industrial setting. J of Psychosomatic Res 1987; 31: 171–176.
33. Tonnesen P. Dose and nicotine dependence as determinants of nicotine gum efficacy. In: Pomerleau OF, Pomerleau CS, eds. Nicotine replacement: A critical evaluation. New York: Liss, 1988: 129–144.
34. West RJ, Jarvis MJ, Russell MAH, et al. Effect of nicotine replacement on the cigarette withdrawal syndrome. Brit J of Addict 1984; 79: 215–219.
35. Hughes JR, Hatsukami D. Short term effects of nicotine gum. In: Grabowski J. Hall SM, eds. Pharmacologic adjuncts in smoking cessation. NIDA Research Monograph No. 53. Rockville, MD: National Institute on Drug Abuse, 1985: 68–82.
36. Hughes JR. Problems of nicotine gum. In: Ockene JK, ed. The pharmacologic treatment of tobacco dependence: Proceedings of the World Congress, November 4–5, 1985. Cambridge, MA: Institute for the Study of Smoking Behavior and Policy, 1986: 141–147.
37. Goldstein MG, Niaura, R, Abrams DB, Follick MJ. Effects of behavioral skills training and schedule of nicotine gum administration on smoking cessation. Am J of Psych 1989; 146: 56–60.
38. Killen JD, Maccoby N, Taylor CB. Nicotine gum and self-regulation training in smoking relapse prevention. Behav Ther 1984; 15: 234–248.
39. Hall SM, Tunstall CD, Ginsberg D, Benowitz NL, Jones RT. Nicotine gum and behavioral treatment: A placebo controlled trial. J of Consult Clin Psychol 1987; 55: 603–605.
40. Christen AG, McDonald JL, Jr. Safety of nicotine-containing gum. In: Pomerleau OF, Pomerleau CS, eds. Nicotine replacement: A critical evaluation. New York: Liss, 1988: 219–235.
41. Christen AG, Young JM, Beiswanger BB, Jackson RD, Potter R. Effects of nicotine gum on complete dentures and their soft-tissue-bearing areas. Intl J of Prosthodont 1989; 2: 155–62.

42. Hughes JR, Hatsukami DK, Skoog KP. Physical dependence on nicotine in gum: A placebo substitution trial. JAMA 1986; 255: 3277–3279.
43. Hughes JR. Dependence potential and abuse liability of nicotine replacement therapies. In: Pomerleau OF, Pomerleau CS, eds. Nicotine replacement: A critical evaluation. New York: Liss, 1988: 261–277.
44. West RJ, Russell MAH. Dependence on nicotine chewing gum. JAMA 1986; 256: 3214–3215.
45. Hughes JR, Hatsukami DK, Skoog KP. Dependence on nicotine chewing gum: Reply to a letter by R.J. West and M.A.H. Russell. JAMA 1986; 256: 3215.
46. Russell MAH, Jarvis MJ. Theoretical background and clinical use of nicotine chewing gum. In: Grabowski J, Hall SM, eds. Pharmacologic adjuncts in smoking cessation. NIDA Research Monograph No. 53. Rockville, MD: National Institute on Drug Abuse, 1985: 110–130.
47. Fagerstrom KO, Mellin B. Nicotine chewing gum in smoking cessation: Efficiency, nicotine dependence, therapy duration and clinical recommendations. In: Grabowski J, Hall SM, eds. Pharmacologic adjuncts in smoking cessation. NIDA Research Monograph No. 53. Rockville, MD: National Institute on Drug Abuse, 1985: 102–109.

16
Transdermal Nicotine and Nasal Nicotine Administration as Smoking-Cessation Treatments

JED E. ROSE

Nicotine replacement is currently the only approved pharmacologic treatment for smoking cessation, and for several years, the only formulation available has been nicotine chewing gum. While placebo controlled trials have shown that nicotine gum increases success rates when used as an adjunct to a behavioral treatment program, overall abstinence rates 6–12 months after initial cessation remain low. In a recent review of several clinical studies by Fagerstrom[1], abstinence rates averaged 26% with active gum treatment versus 16% with placebo gum. In an attempt to increase the magnitude of treatment effects, other routes of nicotine administration have been explored, including transdermal and intranasal routes. The hope is that an appropriate rate and dose of nicotine replacement can relieve smoking withdrawal symptoms and can greatly reduce the tendency of a smoker to relapse. However, one must be cautious to avoid a simplistic characterization of cigarette smoking. For example, while most people are aware that smoking is more than just a habit, it is also more complex than simply an addiction to nicotine, at least as that concept is often understood. In fact, both of these views are incomplete, and the development of effective treatments for smoking cessation may hinge on an understanding of the subtle interactions between conditioned cues and pharmacologic factors involved in the maintenance of smoking behavior. Before discussing the therapeutic application of both transdermal nicotine administration and nasal nicotine administration as adjuncts to smoking-cessation treatment, it will be helpful to review what we know about smoking and its relationship to nicotine dependence.

It has long been suspected that nicotine plays a major role in the maintenance of cigarette smoking[2] because nicotine is the most prevalent psychoactive constituent found in tobacco. Russell[3] has argued that every other plant substance smoked, such as marijuana and opium, is done so in order to obtain a psychoactive agent. Nicotine has profound effects on the

* This work was supported by Grant DA 02665 from the National Institute on Drug Abuse and by the Medical Research Service of the Veterans Administration.

nervous system, acting directly at nicotinic–cholinergic receptors and stimulating the release of several neurotransmitters, including dopamine and acetycholine.[4,5] Peripherally, nicotine has primarily sympathomimetic effects, elevating heart rate and blood pressure, and inducing vasoconstriction.[6] Nicotine can either stimulate or block autonomic ganglia. Nicotine can also release a variety of hormones.[7,8] In addition to direct peripheral effects and direct central nervous system (CNS) actions, nicotine evokes a number of reflexes, such as increasing heart rate by stimulating carotid chemoreceptors. Various subtypes of nicotinic receptors not only are found at autonomic ganglia and neuromuscular junctions but also have been mapped throughout the brain.[9] Behaviorally, nicotine has been shown to facilitate sustained vigilance performance,[10] enhance memory,[11] and decrease appetite[12] and aggression.[13] These are some of the key reasons people give for smoking cigarettes, and it is likely that nicotine is at least partially responsible for these reinforcing effects of smoking.

In spite of these findings, direct analysis of the role of nicotine in smoking behavior has been difficult. Initially, the main research strategy was to show that smokers regulate, or titrate their intake of nicotine to achieve a desired level. Thus, smokers take larger or more frequent puffs or inhale more deeply from low tar and nicotine cigarettes when switched from a higher nicotine brand. "Titrate" is perhaps an exaggeration, as smokers seem to exercise a very crude regulation of smoke intake in response to manipulations of nicotine delivery.[14] Instead of maintaining constant nicotine levels, most smokers seem to keep their nicotine levels within a broad range, somewhere between a high threshold of aversion and a low threshold of withdrawal.[15] This may be why even low doses of nicotine administered via gum or skin patches are effective at relieving some symptoms of smoking abstinence, such as irritability (see subsequent discussion). It also helps explain why administration of nicotine often has little effect on ongoing smoking behavior.[16,17] Even intravenous nicotine has less effect on the desire for cigarettes than does smoking itself.[18] Similarly, Fertig et al.[19] showed that nicotine rapidly absorbed from intranasal administration had no significant effect on craving for a cigarette, whereas smoking a nonnicotine cigarette did decrease craving.

Russell[3] has argued that brain nicotine concentrations equilibrate with high arterial blood nicotine levels following pulmonary absorption of nicotine from each puff of smoke—a *bolus* absorption effect that cannot be duplicated with slower routes of administration. To examine the effect of rapid nicotine absorption, we conducted a study in which the pulmonary absorption of nicotine from smoke was controlled while perception of the smoke was manipulated with local airway anesthesia.[20] Blockade of smoking-related sensations led to a decrease in satisfaction of the desire for a cigarette. It is likely that the cues accompanying smoking become potent conditioned reinforcers as a result of prior association with the effects of nicotine. Administration of nicotine without the behavioral and sensory characteristics of smoking may provide as little satisfaction to a smoker as does providing intravenous feeding instead of a meal to a hungry individual,[21] or giving caffeine capsules instead of a cup of coffee to a coffee drinker. Thus, the rationale for nicotine replacement in smoking-cessation treatment is mainly to relieve withdrawal symptoms rather than to replace all of the reinforcing effects of cigarette smoking.[22]

It is clear that nicotine replacement with gum, used in conjunction with behavioral treatment, has an effect in promoting smoking cessation.[1] Even though nicotine gum provides a lower dose and slower absorption of nicotine than does smoking, it seems to be effective in relieving withdrawal symptoms such as irritability. However, the gum does not substitute for the act of puffing and inhaling smoke, the unique taste and aroma of cigarette smoke, as well as the respiratory-tract sensations accompanying smoking. Also, many smokers find the taste of the gum aversive, and nicotine that is swallowed can upset the stomach. All of these factors may limit compliance and efficacy of the gum.[23] It was to overcome the problem of compliance that initially led Rose et al.[24,25,26] to explore transdermal nicotine administration.

The ability of nicotine to penetrate intact skin has been known for some time, and so it may seem rather surprising that this route has been exploited only relatively recently for therapeutic application to smokers. One reason for this may have been the psychological association between skin absorption and accidental poisoning from nicotine. Without any immediate feedback from the skin signalling that nicotine has been taken in, a lethal dose can easily be absorbed. More commonly, tobacco harvesters have fallen ill when handling wet tobacco leaves with the bare hands.[25] The occurrence of such "green tobacco sickness," together with the fact that nicotine is about as toxic as cyanide, encouraged the view that skin absorption of nicotine was something of which to be wary. Moreover, some researchers have attributed the low success rates obtained with nicotine gum to the absence of a rapid delivery of nicotine. Skin absorption, being even slower than buccal absorption, would not provide any obvious advantage over nicotine gum and may have been dismissed as being less likely to be effective. Finally, nicotine gum provides the user with some oral feedback, which may facilitate self-regulation of dose.

Each of these potential advantages of nicotine gum is a double-edged sword, and in fact is more likely to prove disadvantageous for many smokers. For example, the lack of sensory feedback from a nicotine patch also means that it does not have the bad taste or produce the stomach upset that limits many smokers' use of nicotine gum. The ability to self-regulate dose with nicotine gum, while advantageous in one respect, continues to reinforce the behavior of self-administration of nicotine on a frequent basis. This may increase the likelihood that a strong craving to engage in the behavior will develop. Once-a-day patch application minimizes the association between a smoker's behavior and immediate reinforcement.

A nicotine patch also creates the possibility, for the first time, of administering nicotine during sleep. This has the potential of preventing early morning withdrawal symptoms, but it could conceivably give rise to sleep difficulties. Weaning off of nicotine, ostensibly the ultimate goal of treatment, is difficult to control with nicotine gum, whereas with nicotine patches, it is possible to program practically any fading regimen desired.

Pharmacokinetics of Transdermal Nicotine Delivery

Nicotine is well absorbed through the skin, and care must be taken to limit the total dose or the rate of absorption to prevent toxic effects. In the first published study of nicotine patch pharmacokinetics, Rose et al.[25] reported saliva nicotine concentrations in a single nonsmoking subject following application of a patch containing 9 mg of nicotine in a 30% aqueous solution to the volar surface of the forearm. Concentrations peaked within 30 minutes and gradually declined over 4 hours. Using a patch containing 30 mg of nicotine in a gel matrix, Mulligan et al.,[27] in a study of 24 smokers, obtained relatively constant plasma nicotine concentrations over a 24-hour period. Approximately 8 hours were required to reach the peak level of nicotine (15.39 ± 5.05 ng/ml), although near maximal levels were obtained within 4 hours. Peak nicotine concentrations after 7 days of continuous application were similar to those of Day 1 (17.02 ± 6.89 ng/ml). Dubois et al.[28] also studied the pharmacokinetics of different doses of nicotine administered in patches applied to the scapula. Single doses of 10, 20, and 40 mg produced maximum levels of nicotine in plasma after 7–9 hours of 7.86 ± 3.48 mg/ml, 13.5 ± 6.1 ng/ml, and 24.6 ± 8.7 ng/ml, respectively. After repeated dosing for 10 days, there was little difference in the profile of nicotine concentrations across the day, indicating little long-term skin depot storage of nicotine.

Thus, nicotine patches can provide a relatively constant plasma nicotine level throughout the day. So far, most studies have used patches that reproduce the trough levels of nicotine typically occurring before smoking, rather than the peak levels occurring just after smoking a cigarette. It would be interesting to study the effects of maintaining peak levels of nicotine comparable to those reached after smoking, which could be done with larger patches or with concurrent application of more than one patch. Whether this would be beneficial, or whether toxic effects of nicotine would dominate, is not known.

Efficacy of Transdermal Nicotine in Smoking Cessation

There are a number of clinical trials in progress to evaluate the efficacy of nicotine skin patches in smoking-cessation treatment. While there are relatively few published studies to date, these studies uniformly suggest that nicotine replacement via the skin can relieve some smoking with-drawal symptoms and can enhance smoking-cessation rates. Generally, success rates have been approximately doubled or tripled. For example, Abelin et al.[29] found, in a study with 199 subjects, that success rates were 36% at 3 months in the nicotine group versus 22.5% in the placebo group. The nicotine group subjects received patches delivering either 21.2, 13.8, 7.7 mg/day, depending on their usual cigarette consumption and on whether they had relapsed. At 6 months, a nonsignificant trend of 22% abstinence in the nicotine-patch group versus 12.2% in the placebo group was re-ported. Similar results were obtained[30] in a study of 112 university students. In a short-term study, Mulligan et al.[27] found that a nicotine patch de-livering approximately 22.5 mg/day increased success rates at 6 weeks from 17.5% to 50%. Krumpe et al.[31] found an abstinence rate of 40% at 10 weeks in a group of heavily addicted smokers who received skin patches delivering 18 mg of nicotine/day versus 20% in a placebo group. It is im-portant to bear in mind that success rates often refer to abstinence at a given time; if a criterion of continuous abstinence at all previous times is imposed instead, success rates are often substantially lower. For example, Rose et al.[32] observed an abstinence rate at 22 days after smoking cessa-tion of 49% in a nicotine-patch group (receiving 18 mg/day), compared to 22% abstinence in a placebo-patch group. Continuous abstinence rates over the same period were 18% and 6%, respectively.

In a 12-month follow-up conducted by Buchkremer and Minneker,[33] success rates of 26% in a nicotine-patch group versus 18% in a placebo-patch group and 16% in a no-patch group were reported. All groups re-ceived behavioral treatment. In the same report, a comparison between doses of 10, 20 or 30 mg/day yielded no advantage for higher doses over a 9 week period.

Only one study has compared the efficacy of continuous nicotine delivery for 24 hours/day with that of 13 hours/day delivery in relieving withdrawal symptoms over 2 days.[34] Both nicotine schedules provided partial relief of withdrawal relative to a placebo control, but the two active conditions did not differ in efficacy. There was some suggestion of greater complaints of insomnia in the continuous 24-hour nicotine delivery condition. Hence, one of the unique potential advantages of transdermal nicotine, the ability to administer nicotine 24 hours/day, may not present any significant thera-peutic advantages and may in fact be disadvantageous. However, more research on this issue is clearly needed.

It is interesting that nicotine-patch treatment increased success rates even in the absence of behavioral treatment in the Abelin et al.[30] study, inasmuch as nicotine gum has generally been found to be effective only when combined with a behavioral program.

In contrast to smoking *cessation*, it is not clear that transdermal nicotine, at typical doses studied, is all that helpful in smoking *reduction*. Abelin et al.[30] reported that among nonabstinent smokers, carbon monoxide (CO) levels in the nicotine group receiving 21 mg/day from a patch averaged 18 ppm, versus 17 ppm in the placebo group. Thus, under these conditions, very little regulation of nicotine intake occurred. In contrast, Mulligan et al.[27] compared self-reports of the number of cigarettes smoked and detected a significant effect of nicotine replacement with a patch that delivered approximately 22.5 mg/day; number of cigarettes smoked per week averaged 53.99 (SD = 44.01) in the placebo group versus 35.80 (SD = 34.12) in the nicotine group. Converting to a daily average, this amounts to 7.7 cigarettes/day versus 5.1 cigarettes/day. Thus, at these low smoking levels, an amount of nicotine equivalent to over 20 cigarettes/day obtained from a patch reduced the number of cigarettes smoked by only 2.6/day. As mentioned, this is consistent with other data suggesting that regulation of nicotine intake is usually very imprecise, and one cannot assume that presenting nicotine from a patch will cause an equal decrement in nicotine obtained from smoking. Factors other than regulation of nicotine intake become very important in governing smoking when an individual is attempting to suppress smoking; perhaps the influence of environmental stress or the highly reinforcing aspects of certain cigarettes (e.g., right after a meal) become more important determinants of smoking in a nonabstinent smoker who is attempting to cut down or quit.

Relief of Withdrawal Symptoms

Tobacco withdrawal symptoms include craving, irritability, anxiety, concentration difficulties, daytime drowsiness, insomnia, hunger, restlessness, impatience, and physical symptoms, including headache, gastrointestinal disturbances, dizziness, and sweating.[35,36] Transdermal nicotine clearly provides some relief of some specific tobacco withdrawal symptoms. Most studies have examined nicotine effects on an aggregate measure of withdrawal. However, Rose et al.[32] conducted an analysis of individual withdrawal symptom clusters. While the nicotine patch was very effective at alleviating symptoms of negative affect (e.g., irritability) and hypoarousal (e.g., concentration difficulties), it had little or no effect on craving, hunger, and complaints about missing the act of smoking. This was generally consistent with data from Abelin et al.,[29] showing that the nicotine patch only reduced craving for cigarettes at 2 times out of 12, and at no time in the first 3 weeks, when craving was most intense. Based on the foregoing experiments, it is not surprising that nicotine replacement, in the absence of sensorimotor cues associated with the act of smoking, fails to completely eliminate the desire for cigarettes. Conceivably, a higher-dose patch or a faster route of administration would be more effective, but, as mentioned earlier, even rapid nicotine delivery has limited effects on craving. Transdermal nicotine treatment must therefore be viewed as a partial treatment for smoking withdrawal symptoms, but for those smokers who are especially disturbed by mood and arousal alterations after quitting, a nicotine patch can provide extremely effective relief in a substantial proportion of patients.

Side Effects of Transdermal Nicotine

The main side effect reported with the use of nicotine patches is skin irritation, including erythema, pruritis, and occasionally edema. These effects are due to the irritating properties of nicotine, above and beyond that produced by other patch components (e.g., adhesives). Abelin et al.[29] reported (1) intense erythema, occasionally associated with edema of the skin, in 7% of the nicotine group and 1% of the placebo group; (2) mild to moderate erythema in 25% of the nicotine group and 13% of the placebo group; and (3) pruritis in 29% of the nicotine group and 8% of the placebo group. In a related study with university students, intense skin reactions occurred in 8.6% of the nicotine group and 1.8% of the placebo group.[30] Mulligan et al.[27] reported a rate of 27.5% erythema or rash in the nicotine group and 12.5% in the placebo group. They also observed more complaints in the nicotine group that were not related to the skin, including gastrointestinal discomfort, sweating, dizziness, headache, tiredness, difficulty sleeping, nightmares, and a "pins and needles sensation." However, it is not clear whether subjects reporting these complaints were abstinent from smoking, and many of these symptoms are identical to tobacco withdrawal symptoms. Rose et al.,[32] using a patch with a higher flux rate (1.8 $mg/cm^2/24$ hours vs. $0.7 mg/cm^2/24$ hours in the Abelin et al. study[29] and vs. $0.75 mg/cm^2/24$ hours in the Mulligan et al. study[27]) reported that 97% of subjects had at least a mild skin reaction, 36% a moderate reaction, and 12% a severe reaction from the nicotine patches. Only 19% of subjects receiving placebo patches showed a mild skin reaction. Two subjects (6%) receiving nicotine patches developed a generalized rash. Interestingly, the most severe reactions occurred after wearing the nicotine patches 3–4 weeks. Eichelberg et al.[37] studied contact allergies induced by transdermal nicotine treatment, using patches delivering $0.72 mg/cm^2/24$ hours. They documented an allergic reaction to nicotine, beginning between the 16th and 28th day of patch application in 3.2% of subjects. They suggested that nicotine, being a hapten and protein bound, could act as a full antigen and could induce type IV sensitization. Interestingly, very few participants (3–7%) in any of the studies (except the Rose et al. study,[32] using a high-nicotine flux patch) dropped out because of skin-related side effects. Thus, skin irritation generally does not present a major problem for compliance and efficacy of transdermal nicotine treatment.

Weaning Schedules

Little is known about which weaning regimen would be optimal to implement with transdermal nicotine treatment. Abelin et al.[30] switched participants from patches delivering 21.2 mg/24 hours to those delivering 13.8 mg/24 hours and then 7.7 mg/24 hours, with each month of maintained abstinence. However, given that no experimental double-blind comparisons of different weaning regimens have been published, it is difficult to determine whether this reasonable strategy is indeed the best.

Nicotine Nasal Spray

Russell et al.[38] showed that nicotine absorbed through the nasal mucosa enters the bloodstream much more rapidly than through the buccal mucosa (e.g., when using nicotine gum) and almost as rapidly as from a cigarette. Hence, one might think that this could be a nearly ideal nicotine replacement strategy. In an uncontrolled clinical trial of nasal nicotine solution with 26 smokers, Jarvis et al.[39] reported that 65% of subjects stopped smoking in the short-term (11 days), and 35% were abstinent throughout 1 year of follow-up. In the absence of a control group, these results are difficult to evaluate. However, one is struck by the fact that success rates are not much, if at all, higher than those obtained with nicotine gum. If rate of absorption were the most critical consideration, one would expect to see more dramatic success with nasal nicotine administration. However, the small subject sample precludes an accurate estimate of the success rate, and further large-scale trials are currently underway to assess efficacy. The results of the Jarvis et al.[39] study may be compared with the foregoing findings with nasal snuff inhalation,[19] in which nicotine-containing snuff was not found to relieve smokers' craving for cigarettes. Both studies underscore the fact that smoking cannot easily be replaced by other forms of nicotine administration, even if a rapid boost in blood nicotine levels is achieved. However, subjects in the Jarvis et al. study did report that the nasal solution reduced their craving for cigarettes; they also reported a calming effect, light-headedness, and a euphoriant effect. Blood nicotine levels were only 7 ng/ml in the short-term, but subjects who became long-term users of the nasal solution had blood nicotine levels over 20 ng/ml, comparable to a smoker's trough levels. Side effects of nasal nicotine administration included nasal irritation, watering eyes, sneezing, and one instance of vomiting. Perhaps the local irritation and embarrassment of using the nasal solution in public prevented some subjects from using it more frequently and thereby maintaining higher nicotine levels. Conceivably, combining a nicotine patch with a nicotine spray would be helpful in providing a baseline nicotine level, and yet would allow a smoker the flexibility of obtaining a rapid intake of nicotine when desired.

Conclusions

Research to date has shown that nicotine skin patches are effective in combating some specific components of the tobacco withdrawal syndrome, especially negative affect and hypoarousal, and in promoting abstinence from cigarettes. Compliance is good, and many of the side effects of nicotine gum are avoided. Skin reactions appear to be well tolerated in general. Nicotine patches do not fully replace the pleasure derived from smoking, and many relapses occur even with nicotine patches that have been used thus far. As has been found in studies using other cessation techniques, withdrawal symptoms are only one trigger for relapse,[40,41] and alleviating these symptoms is but one, albeit important, technique for maintaining smoking abstinence.

Several key questions remain to be answered in order to facilitate the rational development of improved treatments for smoking cessation. First, it may be asked whether the limitations in success rates currently obtained with nicotine patches are due primarily to an inadequate dose or rate of administration of nicotine, which fail to mimic the peak bolus effect of cigarette smoking. If so, higher-dose patches, which maintain the peak, rather than trough, levels of nicotine in smokers may be more effective and may simultaneously yield an aversive effect if the individual smokes. However, the incidence of side effects would need to be evaluated, and there is the possibility that desensitization from a high-dose continuous administration may paradoxically reduce the level of nicotinic stimulation and may defeat the goal of relieving withdrawal symptoms. Alternatively, a nicotine patch may be useful in maintaining trough levels, and it could be supplemented by an inhaled spray that provides transient peak levels of nicotine when needed.

Another unanswered question is whether a key problem with the use of a skin patch in nicotine replacement therapy is the lack of sensorimotor aspects of smoking, which may be desired in their own right by many smokers. If so, behavioral substitutes for cigarettes, which can be combined with nicotine replacements, may be useful in relieving craving as well as other withdrawal symptoms.[42,43,44,45] One substitute that has been tested is a citric acid aerosol, which may reduce craving for cigarettes by producing sensations in the respiratory tract similar to those of smoking.[43,45] In addition, the use of nicotine antagonists[46] might be fruitfully combined with nicotine replacement. None of these combinations has yet been tested, and clearly, there are many promising strategies that will no doubt be evaluated in the near future.

References

1. Fagerstrom KO. Efficacy of nicotine chewing gum: A review. In: Pomerleau OF, Pomerleau CS, Nicotine replacement: A critical evaluation. New York: Liss, 1988: 109–128.
2. Armitage AK, Hall GH, Morrison CF. Pharmacological basis for the tobacco smoking habit. Nature 1968; 217: 331–334.
3. Russell MAH. Nicotine intake and its control over smoking. In: Wonnacott S, Russell MAH, Stolerman IP, eds. Nicotine psychopharmacology: Molecular,

cellular, and behavioral aspects. New York: Oxford University Press, 1990: 347–418.

4. Kellar KJ, Wonnacott S. Nicotinic cholinergic receptors in Alzheimer's disease. In: Wonnacott S, Russell MAH, Stolerman IP, eds. Nicotine psychopharmacology: Molecular, cellular, and behavioral aspects. New York Oxford University Press, 1990: 341–373.

5. Reavill C. Action of nicotine on dopamine pathways and implications for Parkinson's disease. In: Wonnacott S, Russell MAH, Stolerman IP, eds. Nicotine psychopharmacology: Molecular, cellular, and behavioral aspects. New York: Oxford University Press, 1990: 307–340.

6. Benowitz, NL, Porchet H, Jacob P. Pharmacokinetics, metabolism, and pharmacodynamics of nicotine. In: Wonnacott S, Russell MAH, Stolerman IP, eds. Nicotine psychopharmacology: Molecular, cellular, and behavioral aspects. New York: Oxford University Press, 1990: 112–157.

7. Fuxe K, Andersson K, Harfstrand A, Eneroth P, de la Mora MP, Agnati LF. Effects of nicotine on synaptic transmission in the brain. In: Wonnacott S, Russell MAH, Stolerman IP, eds. Nicotine psychopharmacology: Molecular, cellular, and behavioral aspects. New York: Oxford University Press, 1990: 194–225.

8. Pomerleau OF, Rosecrans J. Neuroregulatory effects of nicotine. *Psychoneuroendocrinology* 1989; 14: 1–17.

9. Wonnacott S. Characterization of nicotine receptor sites in the brain. In: Wonnacott S, Russell MAH, Stolerman IP, eds. Nicotine psychopharmacology: Molecular, cellular, and behavioral aspects. New York: Oxford University Press, 1990: 226–277.

10. Warburton DM. Psychopharmacological aspects of nicotine. In: Wonnacott S, Russell MAH, Stolerman IP, eds. Nicotine psychopharmacology: Molecular, cellular, and behavioral aspects. New York: Oxford University Press, 1990: 77–111.

11. Levin E, Lee C, Rose JE, Reyes A, Ellison G, Jarvik M, Gritz E. Chronic nicotine and withdrawal effects on radial-arm maze performance. Behav and Neural Biol 1990; 53: 269–276.

12. Grunberg NE. The effects of nicotine and cigarette smoking on food consumption and taste preferences. Addict Behav 1982; 7: 317–331.

13. Cherek DR. Effects of smoking different doses of nicotine on human aggressive behavior. Psychopharmacology 1981; 75: 339–345.

14. Jaffe JH. Tobacco smoking and nicotine dependence. In: Wonnacott S, Russell MAH, Stolerman IP, eds. Nicotine psychopharmacology: Molecular, cellular, and behavioral aspects. New York: Oxford University Press, 1990: 1–37.

15. Herman CP, Kozlowski LT. Indulgence, excess, and restraint: Perspectives on consummatory behavior in everyday life. J of Drug Issues 1979; 9: 185–196.

16. Kumar R, Cooke EC, Lader MH, Russell MAH. Is nicotine important in tobacco smoking? Clin Pharmacol Ther 1967; 21: 520–529.

17. Lucchesi BR, Schuster CR, Emley GS. The role of nicotine as a determinant of cigarette smoking frequency in man with observations of certain cardiovascular effects associated with the tobacco alkaloid. Clin Pharmacol Ther 1967; 89: 789–796.

18. Henningfield JE Woodson PP. Behavioral and physiologic aspects of nicotine dependence: the role of nicotine dose. In: Nordberg A, Fuxe K, Holmstedt B, Sundwall A. Progress in brain research. Vol. 79. Elsevier Science Publishers B. V., 1989: 303–312.
19. Fertig JB, Pomerleau OF, Sanders B. Nicotine-produced antinociception in minimally deprived smokers and ex-smokers. Addict Behav 1986; 11: 239–248.
20. Rose JE, Tashkin DP, Ertle A, Zinser MC, Lafer R. Sensory blockade of smoking satisfaction. Pharmacol Biochem Behav 1985; 23: 289–293.
21. Rose JE. The role of upper airway stimulation in smoking: In: Pomerleau OF, Pomerleau CS, eds. Nicotine replacement in the treatment of smoking: A critical evaluation. New York: Liss, 1988: 95–106.
22. Jasinski DR, Henningfield JE. Conceptual basis of replacement therapies for chemical dependence. In: Pomerleau OF, Pomerleau CS, eds. Nicotine replacement in the treatment of smoking: A critical evaluation. New York: Liss, 1988: 13–34.
23. Hughes JR. Problems of nicotine gum. In: Okene JK, ed. The pharmacologic treatment of tobacco dependence: Proceedings of the World Congress. November 4–5, 1985. Cambridge, MA: Institute for the Study of Smoking Behavior and Policy, 1986: 141–147.
24. Rose JE. Transdermal nicotine as a strategy for nicotine replacement. In: The pharmacologic treatment of tobacco dependence: Proceedings of the World Congress. November 4–5, 1985. Okene JK ed. Cambridge, MA: Institute for the Study of Smoking Behavior and Policy, 1986: 158–166.
25. Rose JE, Jarvik ME, Rose KD. Transdermal administration of nicotine. Drug and Alcohol Dependence 1984; 13: 209–213.
26. Rose JE, Herskovic JE, Trilling Y, Jarvik ME. Transdermal nicotine reduces cigarette craving and nicotine preference. Clin Pharmacol Ther 1985; 38: 450–456.
27. Mulligan SC, Masterson JG, Devane JG, Kelly JG. Clinical and pharmacokinetic properties of a transdermal nicotine patch. Clin Pharmacol Ther 1990; 47: 331–337.
28. Dubois JP, Siouf A, Muller P, Mauli D, Imhof PR. Pharmacokinetics and bioavailability of nicotine in healthy volunteers following single and repeated administration of different doses of transdermal nicotine systems. Meth and Findings in Exper and Clin Pharmacol 1989; 11: 187–195.
29. Abelin T, Buehler A, Muller P, Imhof PR. Controlled trial of transdermal nicotine patch in tobacco withdrawal. Lancet Vol. 1, 1989: 7–10.
30. Abelin T, Ehrsam R, Buhler-Reichert A, Imhof PR, Muller P, Thommen A, Vasanen K. Effectiveness of a transdermal nicotine system in smoking cessation studies. Meth and Findings in Exper and Clin Pharmacol 1989; 11: 205–214.
31. Krumpe P, Malani N, Adler J, Ramoorthy S, Asadi S, Corwin N, Dolan P, Geismar L. Efficacy of transdermal nicotine as an adjunct for smoking cessation in heavily nicotine addicted smokers. Amer Rev of Respir Disease 1989; 139: A337.
32. Rose JE, Levin ED, Behm FM, Adivi C, Schur C. Transdermal nicotine facilitates smoking cessation. Clin Pharmacol Ther 1990; 47: 323–330.
33. Buchkremer G, Minneker E. Efficiency of multimodal smoking cessation therapy combining transdermal nicotine substitution with behavioral therapy. Meth and Findings in Exper and Clin Pharmacol 1989; 11: 215–218.

34. Fagerström KO, Lunell E, Molander L, Forshell GP, Sawe U. Continuous and intermittent transdermal delivery of nicotine and blockade of withdrawal symptoms. Presented at the Seventh World Conference on Tobacco and Health. Perth, Australia, April, 1990.
35. Hughes JR, Hatsukami DK, Pickens RW, Krahn D, Malin S, Luknic A. Effect of nicotine on the tobacco withdrawal syndrome. Psychopharmacology 1984; 83: 82–87.
36. Shiffman SM, Jarvik ME. Smoking withdrawal symptoms in two weeks of abstinence. Psychopharmacology 1976; 50: 35–39.
37. Eichelberg E, Stolze P, Block M, Buchkremer G. Contact allergies induced by TTS-treatment. Meth and Findings in Exper and Clin Pharmacol 1989; 11: 223–225.
38. Russell MAH, Jarvis MJ, Feyerbend C, Ferno O. Nasal nicotine solution: A potential aid to giving up smoking? Brit Med J 1983; 286: 683–684.
39. Jarvis MJ, Hajek P, Russell MAH, West RJ Feyerabend C. Nasal nicotine solution as an aid to cigarette withdrawal: A pilot clinical trial. Brit J of Addict 1987; 83: 323–330.
40. Hughes JR, Gust SW, Keenan RM, Fenwick JW. Effect of dose on nicotine's reinforcing, withdrawal-suppression and self-reported effects. J of Pharmacol Exper Ther 1990; 252: 1175–1183.
41. Shiffman S. Relapse following smoking cessation: A situational analysis. J of Consult Clin Psychol 1982; 50; 71–86.
42. Behm FM, Levin ED, Lee YK, Rose JE. Low-nicotine smoke aerosol reduces desire for cigarettes. J Subst Abuse 1990; 2: 237–247.
43. Levin ED, Rose JE, Behm FB. Development of a citric acid aerosol as a smoking cessation aid. Drug and Alcohol Dependence 1990; 25: 273–279.
44. Rose JE, Behm FM. Refined cigarette smoke as a means to reduce nicotine intake. Pharmacol Biochem Behav 1987; 28: 305–310.
45. Rose JE, Hickman C. Citric acid aerosol as a potential smoking cessation aid. Chest 1988; 92: 1005–1008.
46. Rose, JE. Discussion. In: The biology of nicotine dependence. Chichester, England: Wiley, 1990: 82.

17
Clonidine in the Management of Nicotine Dependence

KAREN LEA SEES

For many years, physicians have been concerned about how to best facilitate patients in smoking cessation and, until recently, have had few tools other than advice. However, cigarette smoking and other forms of tobacco consumption are now acknowledged as causing nicotine dependence,[1,2] and with that recognition comes the acceptance of treating the use of tobacco products, not merely as a bad habit, or a nasty vice, but as the disease of nicotine addiction. This new recognition—that the use of tobacco products causes nicotine addiction—helps remove the long-accepted idea that it takes only willpower to stop smoking, and thereby brings all treatment modalities normally used in treating other chemical dependencies into the treatment arena for nicotine addiction.[3]

Medications to assist in detoxification from psychoactive drugs (e.g., benzodiazepines for alcohol, clonidine for opioids) have long been accepted as useful and often medically needed as part of the early treatment process of addiction. Medications are especially sanctioned for the treatment of withdrawal signs and symptoms. Likewise, the utility of medicinal adjuncts in the treatment of nicotine addiction is now more recognized and accepted.

Pharmacologic Adjuncts for Nicotine Withdrawal

Estimates indicate that more than 90% of cigarette smokers would like to stop smoking and that most cigarette smokers have tried unsuccessfully to quit several times.[4] It is thought that the majority of smokers who successfully quit are less dependent on nicotine.[5] Consequently, those who remain smokers today and in the future will be increasingly those who are physiologically addicted to nicotine.[6,7]

As smokers recognize the importance of the psychoactive effects of nicotine in their continuation of cigarette smoking, and the significance of the nicotine withdrawal symptoms in their relapse to smoking when attempting abstinence, their request for medical adjuncts to assist in nicotine withdrawal will increase as they attempt once again to abandon smoking. As a result, physiologic interventions should play a larger role in the effort to expedite smoking cessation. To maximize efficacy, these interventions need to be used in conjunction with a comprehensive treatment strategy.[3]

Pharmacologic adjuncts for nicotine withdrawal fall into four categories of medications: (1) replacement therapy, which provides nicotine maintenance via a less hazardous and more manageable form of the drug; (2) blockade therapy, which uses an antagonist medication that blocks the effects of nicotine; (3) deterrent therapy, which produces aversive effects when triggered by cigarette smoke; and (4) nonspecific supportive or symptomatic therapy, which diminishes or alleviates the craving and symptoms of nicotine withdrawal.[8,9] This chapter focuses on the medication clonidine, which falls into the symptomatic therapy (fourth) category.

Clonidine

Recently, a great deal of attention has focused on the use of the medication clonidine in nicotine withdrawal and smoking cessation. Clonidine, an alpha-2 adrenergic agonist, was developed and first used as a medication to treat hypertension. It has gained widespread recognition for its usefulness in treating many of the signs and symptoms of both opioid and alcohol withdrawal.[10-15] In the past several years, research studies have advocated clonidine's usefulness in diminishing cigarette craving and to a lesser degree the anxiety, tension, irritability, and restlessness that frequently occur during acute nicotine withdrawal.[16-20]

The first indication that clonidine seemed to have an effect in nicotine withdrawal was reported in *Science* in 1984.[16] In that study, Glassman et al. found that in heavy cigarette smokers, clonidine was useful in diminishing withdrawal symptoms and cigarette craving after 24 hours of abstinence. Those withdrawal symptoms decreased by the use of clonidine included anxiety, tension, irritability, and restlessness. The most exciting aspect of this original study was the noted decrease in cigarette craving perceived by their subjects.

Although clonidine appeared to reduce many of the symptoms of nicotine withdrawal and to decrease cigarette craving, that does not necessarily mean that it will facilitate smoking cessation: "Smokers may continue to smoke primarily because they derive positive effects from smoking and not because they experience withdrawal symptoms when they attempt to stop."[17] Several investigations have addressed, or are presently addressing, this aspect of clonidine's usefulness in smoking-cessation programs.

Subsequent to the publication of the first Glassman study in *Science*, Pearce described successful anecdotal results using 0.1 mg of oral clonidine twice a day in seven people, several of whom had been unsuccessful with smoking cessation in the past; all seven stopped smoking with reported ease.[21] Pearce and several colleagues at the University of Calgary are presently pursuing a randomized double-blind study to assess the efficacy of oral clonidine in smoking cessation. Three different dose regimes of oral clonidine with a placebo control group are being tested.[22] No results of this study are yet available.

Appel has conducted a study comparing transdermal clonidine (TTS #1) versus transdermal placebo in smoking cessation. His results are impressive, with 11 of the 18 subjects wearing the transdermal clonidine patch (Catapres-TTS) successfully quitting smoking, whereas only 2 of the 13 wearing the placebo patch were successful. Appel noted, as did Glassman, that craving was attenuated with the use of clonidine.[18]

Although, to date, only the abstract of the preceding study has been published, Appel presented the findings of his clonidine smoking-cessation research at the 83rd Annual Scientific Assembly.[23] Appel reported on 48 middle-aged subjects who were randomly assigned in a double-blind manner to either active or placebo transdermal clonidine (Catapres-TTS #1) for 6 weeks of a medication trial. Following the first 3 weeks of medication, those subjects who were still smoking were shifted to the other group, while those who had quit smoking continued in the same group. After 6 weeks total, all medication was stopped.

Previous to the study, all subjects were smoking at least one pack of cigarettes a day, had been smoking approximately 20 years, professed motivation to quit smoking, and had previous failures in smoking abstinence. By considering anyone smoking <4 cigarettes/day a quitter, Appel found that by the end of first 3 weeks, 15 of 24 (62.5%) subjects on the active medication had quit smoking, whereas only 3 of 24 subjects on the placebo medication had quit. Of those subjects who were transferred from placebo to active medication for the last 3 weeks of the medication phase of the study, 12 quit smoking. At a 9-month follow-up, 9 of the 15 who were on the active patch for all 6 weeks were still not smoking, compared to only 2 of the 12 who stopped smoking when switched to the active patch from the placebo after the first 3 weeks of the medication trial. Appel postulated that this decreased rate of abstinence noted in this second group may be related to a shorter course of treatment with the active medication (3 vs. 6 weeks).

In the most recent Glassman study,[17] a course of oral clonidine was evaluated for its usefulness in smoking cessataion; 4 weeks of oral medication with a maximum dose of 0.3 mg per day was followed by a medication taper, which averaged 12 days. Through this randomized clinical trial, Glassman et al. found that twice as many clonidine-treated patients succeeded in acutely quitting smoking, compared with the placebo-treated group.

An interesting observation in this study linked a history of major depression, which was unexpectedly high in the sample group, with a failure in attempts to quit smoking. Also significant was that clonidine treatment affected female smokers but did not influence the outcome in male smokers. Glassman et al. speculated that the gender difference of clonidine effectiveness on cigarette-smoking cessation might be due in part to small sample size or to inadequate doses used in males.[17] Their gender difference outcome is contrary to conventional observations that male smokers tend to respond more favorably to smoking-cessation programs.[24] An additional explanation for the gender differences has been speculated.[25] Shiffman reviewed and reanalyzed the data in several smoking-cessation studies, looking for gender differences.[24] This analysis found evidence suggesting that the abstinence syndrome is more severe in women, and women relapse more frequently due to anxiety and craving. Because clonidine, in addition to decreasing many nicotine withdrawal symptoms, is most noted for decreasing cigarette craving, Glassman et al.'s findings of gender differences may not be spurious.

Ornish and colleagues have completed a double-blind, randomized, placebo-controlled trial studying the effects of 1 week of transdermal clonidine (Catepres-TTS #2) on nicotine withdrawal symptoms.[19] Their results add further confirmation of clonidine's usefulness in smoking cessation. Significantly decreased cigarette craving was noted, and in addition, the irritability, anxiety, and restlessness usually experienced in nicotine withdrawal were also decreased. Side effects noted from transdermal clonidine were generally mild, but Ornish et al. concluded that side effects may be even fewer if a lower dose of transdermal clonidine were used initially. Unfortunately, Ornish and colleagues did not report their data separated by gender, and, therefore, they do not address the male–female differences noted by Glassman[17] and Shiffman.[24]

A study by Wei and Young[20] compared a 3-week medication trial of oral clonidine (0.075 mg/tablet three times/day) to diazepam (2.5 mg/tablet three times/day) to placebo (three times/day) when combined with a 3-week behavioral smoking-cessation program. The clonidine-treated group had significantly decreased withdrawal symptoms and significantly higher abstinence rates at the end of treatment, compared to the other two groups. Although the percentage of clonidine-treated individuals was still higher at 4.5 months after treatment, the differences in abstinence rates were no longer statistically significant. Wei and Young emphasized that the behavioral smoking-cessation treatment was an important part of this study. Perhaps if the behavioral treatment had been longer and in greater depth, the positive effects of medication-assisted nicotine withdrawal would have persisted.

The first study to dispute clonidine's effectiveness as an adjunct in stopping smoking was recently published.[26] Franks and colleagues found that oral clonidine, 0.2 mg twice per day, had no effect on nicotine withdrawal and smoking abstinence when used in what they called "a primary care setting." This study involved merely prescribing the medication, advising patients to stop smoking, recommending that patients read smoking-cessation literature, and weekly assessments to ensure that the patients were medically stable. Just as Nicorette has questionable effectiveness when used without being a part of a comprehensive stop-smoking program, so may clonidine. Just as simple detoxification from alcohol rarely helps an alcoholic stay sober, and simple detoxification from opioids rarely helps an opioid addict stay clean, simple nicotine detoxification will probably not assist many smokers in maintaining smoking abstinence.

Boehringer Ingelheim Pharmaceuticals, Inc., the manufacturers and distributors of Catapres-TTS (the transdermal clonidine patch), have conducted a multicenter study of 213 smokers; apparently, data on file with the company from that study detected no statistically significant advantage for smokers treated in a 7-week protocol with transdermal clonidine, compared with transdermal placebo in smoking abstinence attempts.[23]

Oral Versus Transdermal Clonidine

It is commonly accepted that the less frequently a medication needs to be taken, the more likely it will be taken as prescribed. The dosing regimen for the oral tablet of clonidine is usually twice a day for treating hypertension, but it may be given four to six times per day or more, when used for treating opioid and/or alcohol withdrawal. In those studies using oral clonidine for smoking cessation and nicotine withdrawal, the dose has been given twice per day and occasionally three times per day. In contrast, the transderemal patch (Catapres-TSS) needs to be replaced only once every 7 days.,

Blood levels from oral medication normally fluctuate. The level peaks shortly after ingestion, then gradually declines, with the lowest level occurring immediately prior to the next dose. In this type of dosing regime, the peak level of a medication may be excessive and is often associated with undesired medication side effects. In contrast, immediately prior to the next dose, the level may be inadequate and, therefore, not fully therapeutic. The transdermal patch, however, offers the advantage of steady-state blood levels. Once a patch is placed on the skin, the medication begins slowly diffusing through its semipermeable membrane, through the skin, and into the bloodstream. This diffusion continues at a constant rate for at least 7 days and thereby maintains a constant blood level. Therefore, the problems associated with the peaks and troughs of fluctuating blood levels are not present.

When considering using oral clonidine as an adjunct in smoking-cessation programs, the implications of the fluctuating blood levels are quite clear. If relapses occur, a thorough medication history would need to be taken to ascertain not only that the medication was taken as often as it was prescribed but also that the dosing interval was properly maintained. If an oral medication is postponed or forgotten, as frequently happens when a drug is supposed to be taken several times per day, the blood level and therapeutic effect drop even lower. Because the transdermal patch needs to be changed only weekly, forgetting to take the medication should be a minor problem, if a problem at all. With the transdermal clonidine, there is no need to rely on a patient's memory to take the medication several times a day, and there is no need to worry about a patient undermedicating or overmedicating.[25]

In addition to eliminating much of the potential difficulty from patient compliance and fluctuating blood levels, transdermal clonidine offers other advantages. Many of the side effects with oral clonidine are not experienced with transdermal therapy. Dry mouth, drowsiness, and sexual dysfunction all tend to decrease in severity and frequency, and often resolve completely when patients are switched from oral to transdermal clonidine.[27-30]

Rebound hypertension is a concern when blood pressure medications that have been used on a long-term basis are abruptly discontinued. For this reason, Glassman et al.[17] tapered the oral clonidine dose slowly over approximately 12 days at the end of the medication part of their study; tapering was done even though the medication had been taken for only 4 weeks. When a transdermal clonidine patch is removed, a reservoir of medication remains in the skin. The dermal store of clonidine continues to be absorbed, and the drug blood level falls slowly over several days. The transdermal clonidine patch is therefore essentially a self-tapering medication once it has been removed, and this feature may help to prevent rebound hypertension.[30,31] Although transdermal clonidine has been reported to cause rebound hypertension when stopped abruptly in elderly patients who were using the medication for long-term hypertensive therapy,[32] it is doubtful that this should be a problem when used in normotensive patients on a short-term basis, such as 2–4 weeks, in treating nicotine withdrawal. However, in part because of this concern, but mainly because of not wanting to abruptly discontinue a medication that may be relieving nicotine withdrawal symptoms and thereby assisting smoking abstinence, when transdermal clonidine is used in smoking cessation the medication dose (patch size) is frequently decreased from a TTS #2 to a TTS #1 for the week prior to total discontinuation of the medication. In addition, the final patch is frequently left on the patient's skin for a total of 10, not 7, days. Steady-state clonidine blood levels begin to drop after 7 days of patch placement, but some medication is still present in the transdermal patch, and leaving it on the skin the extra days slows the tapering of the medication even more. Despite this, monitoring blood pressure and heart rate is recommended at 24 and 48 hours after the final patch is removed.

Because clonidine is an antihypertensive medication, there may be reluctance to use it in patients for nicotine withdrawal, especially if the patient has low normal blood pressure.

The onset of action of transdermal clonidine is gradual, because it is slowly absorbed through the skin into the bloodstream. The effect peaks and reaches equilibrium in 2–3 days after the patch is applied to the skin.

With this slow onset of action, blood pressure is lowered less precipitously than with oral clonidine, where the serum level peaks shortly after each dose ingested. Also, the amount of the medication absorbed from the transdermal system depends on where it is placed on the body: the thicker the skin, the less medication absorbed. The plasma concentration of clonidine from a transdermal patch placed on the thigh equals 70% of the plasma concentration when it is placed on the arm or chest.[28] In patients with low normal blood pressure, transdermal therapy may be the only option if clonidine use is desired.

In 1986, Clark and Longmuir[11] suggested that transdermal clonidine should, when possible, be used for opioid detoxification instead of the oral form. They concluded that the patch was less disruptive in terms of recovery-oriented treatment program participation, and it offered the advantage of maintaining a therapeutic steady-state drug level without frequent dosing. Their impression was "that patients treated with oral clonidine have more withdrawal symptoms than those treated with the transdermal patches. (p. 2)"[11] This impression and rationale for the use of clonidine should also hold true in a comprehensive recovery-oriented smoking-cessation program. Transdermal clonidine should offer a practical solution to many of the limitations of oral clonidine.

Side Effects and Exclusion Criteria

All of this is not to suggest that there are no unpleasant side effects associated with transdermal clonidine, but to suggest that it is a very feasible alternative to oral clonidine and offers several advantages. There are arguments against using transdermal clonidine. The most significant is that the medication cannot be abruptly discontinued. Because it is stored in the skin, it may take several days for its effects to completely subside once the patch is removed. For this reason, many practitioners, before using the transdermal systems for nicotine withdrawal, give an oral challenge dose of 0.1 mg of clonidine. Blood pressure is measured 30 and 60 minutes after the oral clonidine test dose. If there is no precipitous decrease in blood pressure, and/or the patient does not become uncomfortably symptomatic from the side effects of the clonidine, it is then deemed safe to proceed with using transdermal medication. Special attention is paid to the development of light-headedness, dizziness, and postural hypotension.

Even though blood pressure is lowered much less in normotensive patients exposed to clonidine, blood pressure should be monitored throughout its use for nicotine withdrawal. Evaluating blood pressure and heart rate at 24 and 48 hours after the first patch is placed, and then at weekly intervals when the patch is changed is suggested.

When the transdermal form of clonidine is used for nicotine withdrawal, the day on which the patient quits smoking is generally not the day the patch is placed; because the onset of action for the transdermal form of the medication is gradual, the day on which the patient quits smoking is scheduled for when the medication peaks in the bloodstream, usually the morning of the second day (about 36–48 hours) after the transdermal patch is placed. An alternative method is to place the transdermal clonidine patch and to supplement with oral clonidine for the first day or day and a half, until the transdermal medication peaks; in this case, the day the patient quits smoking would be the day the patch was placed and the oral medication started. This is the standard method for detoxification when transdermal clonidine is used for opioid withdrawal. A word of caution, however: This method does increase the incidence of immediate side effects from the oral clonidine. These side effects may unfortunately limit the patient's interest in continued use of the medication.

There may be a reluctance to employ clonidine as an adjunct in the primary intervention for nicotine withdrawal. This reluctance could stem in part from the fact that clonidine is a potent antihypertensive medication. Naturally, then, there are inclusion and exclusion criteria that must be considered in treatment, and side effects that should be recognized and dealt with.

Clonidine is a medication with potentially serious side effects, and therefore several exclusion criteria must be observed. Most of the recommended exclusion criteria for using clonidine for nicotine withdrawal are self-explanatory. Clonidine should not be used in someone with surgery planned during the medication trial because of potential problems this medication could cause with blood pressure maintenance during surgery. It seems prudent also to have the medication out of the patient's system for several weeks before elective surgery is planned. Other exclusion criteria include hypotension, hypersensitivity to tape (if the transdermal medication is used), hypersensitivity to clonidine, concurrent amitriptyline medications, history of auditory hallucinations, history of delirium, significant liver disease, pregnancy, lactation, concurrent heavy alcohol consumption, Sjögren-Larsson syndrome, cerebrovascular disease, severe coronary insufficiency, recent myocardial infarction, chronic renal failure, and age of less than 12 years.[25] Finally, using clonidine for nicotine withdrawal in patient's who are taking antihypertensive medications other than diuretics is probably not reasonable.

In addition to exclusion criteria, there are side effects of the medication that may limit its usefulness; those most frequently noted include postural hypotension, causing light-headedness and dizziness; dry mouth; tiredness, fatigue, sedation, drowsiness, and lethargy; and headaches. Rarely, sexual dysfunction occurs. These side effects decrease or may not occur when the transdermal patch form of the medication is used in place of oral medication.[28–31] These side effects also tend to diminish with continued therapy.

On the other hand, transdermal clonidine is frequently associated with local skin irritation. Up to 50% of patients using the transdermal patch experience itching under the patch, and 25% experience some erythema under the patch.[33] Although these numbers are relatively large, patients may tolerate these side effects fairly well; the skin reactions are usually mild and self-limiting, but occasionally, the patch must be removed.[29] Moreover, only 5% experience a more serious skin reaction of allergic contact sensitization.[33]

Furthermore, if a patient is taking ongoing medications prescribed from another physician, it is a good idea to consult that physician about the appropriateness of combining clonidine with the other medications. This type of consultation is met with widespread appreciation from the other physician and also provides another source of support for the patient to stop smoking.

A final word of caution about clonidine is needed. Because it is a power-ful medication, patients must be warned about keeping it out of the reach of children. Although this applies most obviously to the oral medication, because a supply will probably be taken home by the patient, the caution applies also to the transdermal patch, even while the patient is wearing it. Inadvertent exposure of others to the medication must be avoided. Several cases of children coming in contact with the patches and suffering adverse consequences have been reported.[34,35] It is therefore judicious to advise patients who are receiving the transdermal patch that care must be taken to avoid transfer of the patch to another person during close contact; patients are advised to have the patch covered with clothing whenever they are handling babies and small children. This is one of the reasons the transdermal patch is frequently placed on the upper back or the scapular area. Care must be exercised also in the disposal of the used patches be-cause some medication is still present after the 7-day wearing time; when used in smoking-cessation programs, the old patch is frequently removed and the new weekly patch placed by the treating physician or investigator. Thereby, patient compliance is not a problem, and safe disposal of the used patch is ensured. Patch changing can easily be arranged at the time of the weekly behavioral smoking-cessation group meeting or at a medication follow-up appointment.

Nicotine Polacrilex and Catapres-TTS

Both nicotine-replacement therapies and clonidine are proving useful in smoking-cessation programs. A unique and perhaps more thorough physiologic intervention for nicotine dependence has been developed at the Haight-Ashbury Free Medical Clinic's Drug Detoxification, Rehabili-tation & Aftercare Project[36]; this approach combines both a rapidly de-creasing dose of a nicotine-replacement therapy (nicotine polacrilex) and a medication for symptomatic treatment of nicotine withdrawal (clonidine). The rate of nicotine withdrawal can be controlled by the amount of the nicotine polacrilex used in 24 hours, and the withdrawal symptoms can be controlled with the dose (number and/or strength) of the Catapres-TTS. Both of these medications can be adjusted. Nicotine detoxification is thereby accomplished effectively and comfortably.

As with any prescription medicine, this intervention for nicotine detoxification first requires an evaluation by a physician, including a history and physical examination, to determine a patients eligibility for the use of both of these medications. After a thorough explanation of the approach is given, and if the patient is interested, one Catapres-TTS #2 (clonidine patch) is placed on the skin of the upper back and the patient is given a prescription for Nicorette® (nicotine polacrilex). Both verbal and written detailed instructions on the use of nicotine polacrilex are provided to the patient.

Instruction on the proper use of nicotine polacrilex is reviewed elsewhere in this textbook and must be detailed by the physician prescribing the polacrilex. Patients should not simply be told to read the package insert on how to chew the polacrilex; most patients assume that they know how to chew polacrilex and therefore do not read it.

The day after patch placement is the day that the patient quits smoking. The patient is instructed that when awakening in the morning, she or he is not to smoke cigarettes, but instead to chew the nicotine polacrilex, as much as necessary for comfort (usually 10–15 pieces in a day for a one-pack-a-day smoker). This also continues on the day after quitting: As much nicotine polacrilex as is necessary to relieve nicotine withdrawal symptoms is to be chewed. This covers nicotine withdrawal symptoms until the clonidine from the transdermal patch reaches its peak effect (36–48 hours). Gradual reduction by 1–2 pieces per day of the nicotine polacrilex is begun on the third day. The nicotine polacrilex is not to be increased to an amount higher than the previous day, but if the previous day was difficult for the patient due to some minor withdrawal symptoms or due to craving cigarettes, the same amount should be used for 1–2 days and then the taper begun again. If withdrawal symptoms persist after stabilizing the daily nicotine polacrilex consumption for a day or 2, additional transdermal clonidine (usually a Catapres-TTS #1) may be started. The clonidine patch(es) is (are) replaced every 7 days. This routine is continued for as long as necessary, planning for a clonidine patch to remain in place for at least 3–4 days after the last nicotine polacrilex has been chewed. Occasionally, it may be necessary to use an additional patch after the nicotine polacrilex is discontinued; for this purpose, a smaller-sized patch is used, a Catapres-TTS #1 when the patient had been on a #2 patch, or a #2 patch when the patient had been on a higher transdermal amount of clonidine (this patch size may then be decreased from a #2 to a #1 prior to discontinuing the clonidine). Most of the patients who have used this method of nicotine detoxification are successfully off cigarettes and off the nicotine polacrilex in less than 1 month (nicotine polacrilex dependence is thus avoided), and off the clonidine in less than 6 weeks.

By combining a nicotine polacrilex taper with clonidine, the physician can control the rate of nicotine withdrawal (via nicotine polacrilex) and the extent to which withdrawal symptoms are treated (via clonidine). This appears to be an effective, comfortable method for detoxification off cigarettes and nicotine, not unlike using clonidine as an adjunct at the end of a methadone detoxification for heroin addiction. This may prove especially useful in chemical dependency units that have chosen to go smoke free and find nicotine withdrawal a significant problem.

Although a scientific study is not underway to investigate the efficacy of this approach to nicotine detoxification, it is the observation at the Haight-Ashbury Free Medical Clinic's Drug Detoxification, Rehabilitation & Aftercare Project that approximately 80% of patients using this approach stop smoking successfully, at least on a short-term basis. Of those who return for a second nicotine detoxification with this method, they frequently admit that this method was the most comfortable nicotine detoxification they have ever been through, and they usually identify what needs to be done differently (usually behavioral) to be successful in smoking cessation on their next attempt.

Clonidine and Buspirone

Some practitioners and some researchers are combining clonidine with buspirone, a nonbenzodiazepine antianxiety medication, as medication adjuncts for smoking cessation. This is done in an attempt to increase the efficacy of relieving nicotine withdrawal and prolonging smoking abstinence. Both medications are started simultaneously. Clonidine is used for acute nicotine withdrawal for a 2- to 3-week period of time. Buspirone, with a delayed onset of action of several weeks, is continued on a longer-term basis. As an antianxiety agent, it is postulated and hoped that buspirone will decrease the stress intolerance, restlessness, nervousness, depression, irritability, impatience, anxiety, tension, and fatigue frequently experienced in nicotine withdrawal and during early smoking cessation. No clinical trials of this medication combination to date have been completed.

Conclusion

In the past 6 years, much research has been done searching for a cure or a "quick fix" for smokers who want to quit. The correlation between the success rate of simply assisting nicotine withdrawal and maintenance of long-term cigarette abstinence is not known. However, speculation based on other chemical dependencies can be made. Detoxification is easy; maintaining abstinence is difficult. Just as alcoholism and other chemical dependencies are relapsing diseases, so is nicotine dependence. Quitting smoking is rarely a one-time proposition. It is estimated that more than 80% of smokers fail to quit on the first attempt, and even after seven attempts, more than half return to smoking.[37] In other words, multiple attempts are usually made before long-term success is achieved.

Therefore, it is ideal for physicians to have additional resources to support smoking abstinence and/or to know what community services/ programs are available for patients who would like to stop smoking.

Stop-smoking programs have traditionally dealt with the psychological and overlearned behavioral aspects of cigarette smoking. Behavioral, cognitive, psychodynamic, and peer-support treatments of nicotine addiction will continue to play a primary role in smoking-abstinence successes. Physiological interventions now play an important part in efforts to facilitate smoking cessation, but medications that assist with nicotine withdrawal are usually not enough; it is important to remember that they are only adjuncts in a comprehensive smoking-abstinence program.

References

1. American Psychiatric Association. Diagnostic and statistical manual of mental disorders. 3rd ed, rev. Washington, DC: Author, 1987.
2. U.S. Department of Health and Human Services. The health consequences of smoking: Nicotine addiction (a report of the Surgeon General). Washington, DC: U.S. Government Printing Office, 1988.
3. Sees KL. Cigarette smoking, nicotine dependence and treatment. West J of Med 1990; 152(5): 578–584.
4. Fielding JE. Smoking: Health effects and control. Pt 2. New Engl J of Med 1985; 313: 555–561.
5. Pechacek TF. Modification of smoking behavior. In: Smoking and health (a report of the Surgeon General). Washington, DC: U.S. Department of Health, Education, and Welfare, U.S. Government Printing Office, 1979.
6. Hughes JR. Clonidine, depression, and smoking cessation. JAMA 1988; 259: 2901–2902.
7. Hughes JR, Gust SW, Pechacek TF. Prevalence of tobacco dependence and withdrawal. Am J of Psychi 1987; 144: 205–208.
8. Prignot J. Pharmacologic approach to smoking cessation. Eur Respir J 1989; 2: 550–560.
9. Jarvik ME, Henningfield JE. Pharmacological treatment of tobacco dependence. Pharmacol Biochem & Behav 1988; 30: 279–294.
10. Baumgartner GR, Rowen RC. Clonidine vs. chlordiazepoxide in the management of acute alcohol withdrawal syndrome. Arch of Internal Med 1987; 147: 1223–1226.
11. Clark HW, Longmuir N. Clonidine transdermal patches: A recovery oriented treatment of opiate withdrawal. Cal Soc for the Treatment of Alcoholism and Other Drug Dependencies News 1986; 13: 1–2.
12. Mahem P, Nilsson LH, Moberg A, Wadstein J, Hokfelt B. Alcohol withdrawal: Effects of clonidine treatment on sympathetic activity, the renin–

aldosterone system, and clinical symptoms. Alcoholism: Clin and Exper Res 1985; 9: 238–243.

13. Walinder J, Balldin J, Bokstrom K, Karlsson L, Lundstrom B. Clonidine suppression of the alcohol withdrawal syndrome. Drug and Alcohol Dependence 1981; 8: 345–348.

14. Gold MS, Pottash AC, Sweeney DR, Kleber HD. Opiate withdrawal using clonidine. JAMA 1980; 243: 343–346.

15. Gold MS, Redmond DE, Kleber HD. Clonidine in opiate withdrawal. Lancet 1978; 1: 929–930.

16. Glassman AH, Jackson WK, Walsh BT, Roose SP. Cigarette craving, smoking withdrawal, and clonidine. Science 1984; 226: 864–866.

17. Glassman AH, Stetner F, Walsh T, Raizman PS, Fleiss JL, Cooper TB, Covey LS. Heavy smokers, smoking cessation, and clonidine. JAMA 1988; 259: 2863–2866.

18. Appel D. Clonidine helps smokers stop smoking. Am Rev of Respir Disease (Suppl) 1987; 135: A354.

19. Ornish SA, Zisook S, McAdams LA. Effects of transdermal clonidine treatment on withdrawal symptoms associated with smoking cessation. Arch of Internal Med 1988; 148: 2027–2031.

20. Wei H, Young D. Effect of clonidine on cigarette cessation and in the alleviation of withdrawal symptoms. Brit J of Addict 1988; 83: 1221–1226.

21. Pearce KI. Clonidine and smoking. Lancet 1986; 2: 810.

22. Pearce KI. Personal communication; April 1988.

23. Drug therapy for the withdrawal syndrome—Another study confirms benefits of clonidine. Peer to Peer, A Clinical Digest of the 83rd Annual Scientific Assembly 1990, Washington, DC: 9–10.

24. Shiffman SM. The tobacco withdrawal syndrome. In: Cigarette smoking as a dependence process. NIDA Research Monograph Series No. 23. Washington, DC: U.S. Department of Health, Education, and Welfare, U.S. Government Printing Office, 1979.

25. Sees KL, Clark HW. Clonidine use in nicotine withdrawal. J of Psychoactive Drugs 1988; 20: 263–268.

26. Franks R, Harp J, Bell B. Randomized, controlled trial of clonidine for smoking cessation in a primary care setting. JAMA 1989; 262: 3011–3013.

27. Hollifield J. Clinical acceptability of transdermal clonidine: A large-scale evaluation by practitioners. Am Heart J 1986; 112: 900–906.

28. Weber MA. Clinical experience with transdermal antihypertensive therapy. Practical Cardiol 1986; 12: 104–120.

29. Burris JF, Mroczek WJ. Transdermal administration of clonidine: A new approach to antihypertensive therapy. Pharmacotherapy 1986; 6: 30–34.

30. Josse S, Danays T, Lafferre M, Fillastre JP. Substitution of oral clonidine with transdermal clonidine in hypertensive patients. Current Therapeutic Res 1987; 42: 579–584.

31. Lowenthal DT, Saris S, Paran E, Cristal N, Sharif K, Bies C, Fagan T. Efficacy of clonidine as transdermal therapeutic system: The international clinical trial experience. Am Heart J 1985; 112: 893–900.

32. Metz S, Klein C, Morton N. Rebound hypertension after discontinuation of transdermal clonidine therapy. Am J of Med 1987; 82: 17–19.

33. Physicians' desk reference. 44th ed. Oradell, NJ: Medical Economics. 1990.

34. Hamblin JE. Transdermal patch poisoning. Pediatrics 1987; 79: 161.
35. Reed MT, Hamburg EL. Person-to-person transfer of transdermal drug-delivery systems: A case report. New Engl J of Med 1986; 314: 1120–1121.
36. Sees KL, Stalcup SA. Combining clonidine and Nicorette® for treatment of nicotine withdrawal. J of Psychoactive Drugs 1989; 21: 355–359.
37. U.S. Department of Health and Human Services. The health consequences of smoking: Chronic obstructive lung disease (a report of the Surgeon General). Washington, DC: U.S. Government Printing Officer, 1984.

18
Anticholinergics and Other Medicines

ROBERT P. CLIMKO

Over 350,000 Americans die each year from the effects of nicotine dependence, and yet few physicians are involved in treating patients for this devastating disease. Perhaps the critical issue is that until recently, many physicians, as well as the general public, considered cigarette smoking not an addictive illness, but simply a bad habit. Indeed, many of our friends and relatives are dying each year, from an extremely bad habit. Everett Koop (the former U.S. Surgeon General) has certainly heightened both lay and physician awareness about the true nature of smoking (i.e., an addiction to nicotine, which drives continued use). Even though I have been involved in the treatment of chemical dependency for 5 years, it is only in the past 3 years that I have been concerned with nicotine addiction. Like others, I told many patients that they could take care of the smoking habit later and that for the moment, we had to address the alcohol, cocaine, marijuana, or drug other dependence. Unfortunately, later never comes for the majority of patients. It would seem to be a collective denial that those of us in the chemical dependency field have used, probably because 80% of us are smokers. Most of our patients describe having much greater fears about giving up the cigarettes than about giving up cocaine, heroin, or alcohol. Although this chapter is concerned with the medical management and early intervention in the treatment of nicotine dependence, it must be noted that medication must only be used as an adjunct and that multimodal treatment of nicotine dependence is the rule. Other chapters in this book outline various other intervention strategies. Many initial treatment efforts are at least partially unsuccessful, but this should not be viewed as failure, only that a more intense, individualized or expanded approach is necessary.

Physicians have contact with approximately 70% of all smokers each year and with 61% of smokers who consider themselves to be in "excellent health".[1] Given this high frequency of contact, it is imperative that physicians become more involved in the effort to treat this devastating disease before multisystem failure begins, such as chronic obstructive lung disease, cardiovascular disease, or lung cancer. (The majority of patients who

TABLE 18.1 Actions of nicotine in humans.

Cardiovascular
   Increased heart rate
   Increased contractility
   Increased blood pressure
   Cutaneous vasoconstriction
Metabolic
   Increased free fatty acids
   Increased glycerol and lactate
Central nervous system
   Arousal of relaxation
   EEG changes
   Tremor
Endocrine
   Increased growth hormone
   Increased adrenocorticotropic hormone and cortisol
   Increased vasopressin
   Catecholamine release
   Increased beta-endorphins

Source. Adapted with permission from Benowitz[7]

smoke would like to quit; however, they share the pessimism that nothing can be done.) As our ability to help patients overcome nicotine dependence improves, and physician pessimism decreases, we may begin to see a more enthusiastic approach in addressing the patient who has yet to experience secondary illness from cigarette smoking.

I discuss the basic pharmacology of nicotine, the active ingredient in cigarettes, and I review literature on pharmacologic interventions as aids to nicotine cessation. These studies are reviewed in detail, as the results are somewhat unclear.

Physiologic Dependence

Traditionally, nicotine is viewed as a ganglionic stimulant. It is an alkaloid that has both stimulant and depressant actions. As noted in Table 18, the metabolic effects of nicotine are protean. Pomerleau and Rosecrans[2] suggest that by altering the bioavailability of various neuroregulators, nicotine serves as a pharmacologic coping response that alters affective performance in response to various environmental demands.

Pharmacologic intervention in early nicotine-cessation programs are most useful for those who have a higher degree of physical dependence. The Fagerstrom Tolerance Questionnaire was developed by Fagerstrom, in order to assess probable physical dependence on nicotine.[3] We currently use this questionnaire in order to assess whether pharmacologic management of early nicotine withdrawal would be beneficial to the patient.

The Fagerstrom Tolerance Questionnaire

1. How many cigarettes a day do you smoke? (High frequency of use probably means more physical dependence.)
2. What brand do you smoke? (Brands that hold a higher dose of nicotine point to possible greater physical dependence.)
3. Do you inhale? _____ Always _____ Sometimes _____ Never (Making the nicotine more effective by inhalation points to probable greater physical dependence.)
4. Do you smoke more during the morning than during the rest of the day? (Smoking more in the morning, when the level of nicotine in the body is low indicates greater physical dependence.)
5. How soon after you wake up do you smoke your first cigarette? (Smoking immediately after getting up in the morning is taken as a sign of stronger physical dependence.)
6. Which cigarette would you hate to give up? (Rating the first cigarette in the morning as the most precious one points to greater physical dependence.)
7. Do you find it difficult to refrain from smoking in places where it is forbidden (e.g., in church, at the library, cinema)? (Little external and relatively more internal stimulus control manifested as frequent urges in forbidden places points to greater physical dependence.)
8. Do you smoke if you are so ill that you are in bed most of the day? (Smoking while ill is taken as a sign of greater physical dependence.)

Those patients scoring higher on the Fagerstrom Tolerance Questionnaire have a higher degree of physical dependence on nicotine and many benefit from pharmacologic management of early nicotine cessation. (For scoring the Fagerstrom Tolerance Questionnaire, please see Fagerstrom[3]).

Pharmacologic Interventions

Jarvik and Henningfeld[4] discussed four pharmacologic approaches for treatment of nicotine detoxification:

1. Nicotine replacement therapy
2. Deterrent therapy
3. Blockade therapy
4. Nonspecific pharmacotherapy

Nicotine Replacement and Deterrent Therapies

The use of nicotine replacement for detoxification is discussed in Chapters 15 and 16 of this book. The search for an effective pharmacologic deterrent continues. Silver acetate in gum or lozenge form has been used as such an agent because it combines with cigarette smoke to produce an extremely noxious taste. The efficacy of silver acetate has been studied[5,6] and is reviewed in Chapter 12.

BLOCKADE THERAPY

Blocking agents or antagonists for the opioids are well known and frequently used in the treatment of narcotic dependence. Naloxone is a short-acting narcotic antagonist used in acute overdose situations. Naltrexone is much longer-acting and useful for blocking and euphoric effects of opiates as an adjunct to longer-term recovery. These drugs are quite specific in their action on the opioid receptors. It is important to note that the various biogenic amine systems have numerous interconnections. Nicotine may stimulate a specific receptor,[7] but activation or stimulation of a certain neuron may be the outcome (serotonin, 5-HT; norepinephrine, NE; or dopamine, DA).[2] Although a specific and complete antagonist would be difficult to find, given the complicated effects of nicotine an various neurohormonal pathways, there are some medications that show some efficacy.

Mecamylamine

Mecamylamine, a secondary amine, is a ganglionic blocking agent that has been in use since the mid-1950s as an antihypertensive drug. Stolerman[8] notes that pharmacologic studies identified acetylcholine as an important neurotransmitter in the ganglia, and these receptors were characterized as *nicotinic*: That is; the effect of acetylcholine could be mimicked by administration of nicotine.

Tenant et al.[9] studied the effectiveness of mecamylamine in the treatment of nicotine dependence. Fourteen subjects were included with the following selection criteria: smoked at least one pack of cigarettes per day; had not been abstinent from nicotine more that 1 day for at least 1 year; and had no history of hypertension, pregnancy, cardiovascular disease, prostate enlargement, glaucoma, or other chemical dependency. Subjects attended a clinic daily for 5 consecutive days and every other day for 2 weeks. Mecamylamine, in doses of 2.5 mg, was administered, to reach a total of 5.0–7.5 mg over the first 24 hours. On Day 2, doses were raised by 2.5–5.0 mg per day until the subject experienced nicotine blockade or significant secondary effects. At this point, dosage was either reduced or held constant. The subject continued on mecamylamine for up to a maximum of 21 days. Results indicated that 93% reported at least partial blockade of the effects of nicotine and reduced nicotine craving. Fifty percent of the subjects completely discontinued smoking. The mean dose of mecamylamine on the day that each stopped smoking was 26.7 mg. Side effects were common and caused 36% to drop out. Urinary retention, constipation, abdominal cramps, and weakness were the most distressing side effects. The authors note that mecamylamine should be reserved for those who are refractory to other treatment methods. Clinical experience with this protocol remains limited.

Anticholinergic Medication Strategies

Nicotine withdrawal may be mediated by an excessive acetylcholine-rebound phenomenon after chronic blockade of certain cholinergic synapses by nicotine.[10] Bachynsky[11] reports significant efficacy of anticholinergic medications in order to block this possible rebound stimulation. This pilot study included 500 smokers who had a desire to stop smoking and who did not have any medical contraindication for the use of anticholinergic medications, such as glaucoma, prostate enlargement, or cardiac arrhythmias. The screening protocol included assessment of medical history, chest x-ray, urinalysis, electrocardiogram, laboratory analysis of blood, and history regarding and hypersensitivity to anticholinergic drugs. The treatment protocol (synopsis) included the following:

1. An initial intramuscular injection of a 2-ml saline solution with 0.2 mg of scopolamine and 0.2 mg of atropine.
2. Monitoring of the patient for 5 minutes, followed by an assessment of normal pupillary contriction and mild xerostomia.
3. Two additional injections are administered over each mastoid area. The total regimen is 0.2 mg of atropine, 0.2 mg of scopolamine, and 10 mg of chlorpromazine.
4. On Day 2 through Day 14, the patient takes an oral anticholinergic medication or uses a scopolamine patch.

Results indicated 87% of the subjects were abstinent at 2 months; 40% remained nonsmokers at the end of 1 year. This is an uncontrolled study, and the investigator gives no information regarding untoward effects.

Another uncontrolled study using anticholinergic medicine was conducted using transdermal patches of scopolamine. This is a less costly and less physician-intensive protocol than reported in the previous study. Cocores et al.[12] treated 31 nicotine-dependent employees of a single corporation. Each was assessed for nicotine dependence, caffeinism, nutrition and exercise habits, alcohol and other drug abuse, and psychiatric history. Excluded were those with a history of glaucoma, psychosis, or current pregnancy. Two 1-hour educational groups were conducted, reviewing nicotine dependence and emphasizing the use of medication. Each subject was instructed to apply the scopolamine patch (1.5 mg) in the right mastoid area at 10 P.M. and to remain abstinent from smoking. The patch was worn for 3 consecutive days then replaced with another patch for 3 days, placed in the left mastoid area. The patients returned for a second session, at which time they were instructed to take 10 mg of imipramine in the morning and 10 mg at noon for 1 week. Imipramine was prescribed because of its anticholinergic properties. Use of the scopolamine patch is not recommended beyond 6 days. Also during that session, relapse-prevention techniques were discussed. Four additional support groups were held on a weekly basis. Also, a self-help group was established at the company. Follow-up showed that 87% of 31 subjects remained abstinent at 6 months. This study incorporated multiple treatment strategies, which complicates interpretation of the data. Although side effects were reported, such as dry mouth, fatigue, and blurred vision, no one discontinued treatment on that basis. The relatively high success rate may be attributable to the effective use of the support network available to the employees.

An important consideration is the use of medication in the person already in recovery from other drug dependencies Cocores et al.[13] treated 16 subjects (eight control and eight recovering drug addicts) with anticholinergic medication. The recovering addicts had a minimum of 3 years of abstinence from drugs other than nicotine. All subjects attended two groups regarding nicotine dependence and use of medication and a third group dealing with stress management and self-help techniques. A transcutaneous patch of scopolamine (1.5 mg) was applied to the right mastoid area at bedtime 1 hour after the last cigarette. This patch was removed and replaced with another patch to the corresponding left side for another 3 days. Then 2.5 mg of clidinium bromide was dispensed, to be used on an as-needed basis four times daily for cigarette craving for the next 5 days. The subjects also had two other group meetings on Days 7 and 14 of the study. Results indicated that 75% of the control group and 38% of the recovering addict group had remained abstinent from nicotine for 90 days. Although all patients reported dry mouth and visual disturbances, the recovering drug-addict group reported significantly more side effects, such as fatigue, depression, and impaired memory. The majority of the recovering group complained of mood-altering effects of the scopolamine. The authors concluded that scopolamine should be avoided in those recovering from other drug dependencies but it is useful for other nicotine-dependent persons.

NONSPECIFIC PHARMACOTHERAPY

Discontinuation of chronic nicotine use is usually followed by a well-described withdrawal syndrome,[14] which can include irritability, anxiety, insomnia, impaired concentration, decreased heart rate hyperphagia and weight gain, craving, headache, gastrointestinal disturbances, dysphoria, and impaired cognitive functioning. It is impossible to attribute all of these signs and symptoms to a specific neuroregulatory mechanism, nicotine may modulate the activity of acetylcholine, serotonin, dopamine, beta-endorphin, and norepinephrine.[2] Many pharmacologic agents have been used in order to treat withdrawal phenomena.

Bromocriptine

The rewarding properties of nicotine may be linked to stimulation of dopamine neurotransmission in the limbic area of the brain.[15] Cessation of smoking could lead to acute nicotine craving secondary to dopamine depletion. A dopamine agonist like bromocriptine may reduce this craving by stimulating postsynaptic dopamine receptors.[16] One investigator suggests prescribing an initial dose of 0.625 mg every 4 hours while awake and titrating upward on a weekly basis to 2.5 mg three times per day. There are no controlled studies confirming the efficacy of this protocol, however, studies are ongoing. Relatively few side effects are reported with this dosage schedule.

Doxepin

Doxepin hydrochloride is a dibenzoxepin tricyclic compound used most commonly as an antidepressant medication. One double-blind study compared doxepin hydrochloride to placebo.[17] Nineteen subjects were studied with the following eligibility criteria: age of at least 18 years, a previous smoking-cessation failure that was accompanied by withdrawal symptoms, no history of psychiatric complaints, and no contraindications for use of doxepin (e.g., pregnancy, use of monoamine oxidase inhibitors, or excessive alcohol use). The subjects were randomized to two groups. The active medication group initially received 50 mg of doxepin at bedtime, which was increased to 150 mg per day over the first week. Weekly appointments were held, to monitor the subjects and to reinforce cessation efforts. Abstinence was to begin on Day 22. Subjects who failed to stop smoking by the sixth week were discontinued from the study. At 12 weeks, abstinence was 78% in the doxepin subjects versus 10% in the placebo group. Given the small sample size and other complexities of this study, these findings need to be corroborated by further research. It cannot be established by what mechanism doxepin may be effective as an adjunct to smoking cessation. It may help secondary to its anticholinergic potential or through its noradrenergic, serotonergic, or histaminic effects. The subjects in this study did report various side effects, such as dry mouth and sedation.

Buspirone

Buspirone hydrochloride is an antianxiety agent unrelated to the other sedative or anxiolytic medications, such as the barbiturates and benzodiazepines. It is less sedating than other anxiolytics and reportedly has no abuse potential.

As uncontrolled 6-week trial using buspirone without any psychological interventions showed some promise as a pharmacologic adjunct in early smoking-cessation efforts.[18] The researchers selected buspirone because of its nonsedating anxiolytic properties. They opined that it might antagonize the characteristic withdrawal symptoms of nicotine discontinuation. Eight subjects were treated, all of whom smoked more than 1.5 packs of cigarettes per day for more than 5 years. The subjects were given buspirone in divided doses, beginning at 15–30 mg per day and titrated in 10-mg increments to 60 mg per day. The subjects reported the effects of buspirone in the second to fourth weeks, and all reported reduction of the urge to smoke. All subjects reported reduction to seven cigarettes per day or less for at least 1 week. Dizziness was reported as a side effect.

As suggested by the authors, the mechanism through which buspirone is effective may be clinically, by way of decreasing anxiety, or neurochemically through its effect on dopaminergic functioning. Again, further investigation is warranted.

Fluoxetine

Fluoxetine hydrochloride is an antidepressant medication that is unrelated pharmacologically to the tricyclics, the tetracyclics, or the monoamine oxidase inhibitors. Its antidepressant effects are thought to be secondary to inhibition of neuronal reuptake of serotonin in the central nervous system. Anecdotal evidence by me and other colleagues suggests a role for use of this compound for selected patients, to alleviate nicotine withdrawal symptoms. My own experience is with patients who were being treated for unipolar depression, who had suspended cigarette use after their mood disorders had improved. They all expressed amazement at the absence of significant withdrawal symptoms while taking fluoxetine hydrochloride. Fluoxetine may also show promise in alleviating the weight gain experienced by many patients during the initial phase of abstinence. Clearly, a controlled, double-blind study is needed to corroborate these findings. Also, because antidepressant medications have significant contraindications, this should probably not be used as a first-line medication.

Conclusion

The effective treatment of nicotine dependence is clearly in the development stage. Many approaches are discussed in this comprehensive volume. Pharmacologic intervention is only one part of a necessarily holistic approach to this potentially devastating addiction. Physicians need to become more involved in treatment efforts for cigarette smokers prior to the occurrence of the legion secondary diseases. All smoking patients should be informed of the various treatment options. Physician assessment and management of smoking-cessation efforts can greatly enhance abstinence rate. Smoking-intervention strategies employing more than one modality and involving physicians as well as nonphysicians have a more significant cessation rate.[19] Pharmacologic intervention is most beneficial for those patients exhibiting a higher degree of physiologic tolerance. Judicious use of appropriate medications allows may patients to engage successfully in longer-term treatment modalities.

Acknowledgment. I wish to thank Patricia Rue for her superb aid in the preparation of this manuscript.

References

1. Ockene JK. Physician's delivered interventions for smoking cessation: Strategies for increasing effectiveness. Prev Med 1987; 16: 723–737.
2. Pomerleau OF, Rosecrans J. Neuroregulatory effects of nicotine. Psychoneuroendocrinology 1989; 6: 407–423.
3. Fagerstrom KO. Measuring degree of physical dependence to tobacco smoking with reference to individualization of treatment. Addict Behav 1978; 3: 235–241.
4. Jarvik ME., Henningfield JE. Pharmacologic treatment of tobacco dependence. Pharmacol Biochem Behav 1988; 30: 279–294.
5. Malcolm R, Currey B, Mitchell M, et al. Silver acetate chewing gum as a deterrent to smoking. Chest 1986; 10: 107–111.
6. Rosenberg A. An investigation into the effect on cigarette smoking of a new antismoking chewing gum. J of Internal Med Res 1977; 5: 68–70.
7. Benowitz NL. Toxicity of nicotine: Implications with regard to nicotine replacement therapy. In: Nicotine replacement: A critical evaluation, New York: Liss, 1988: 187–217.
8. Stolerman IP. Could nicotine antagonists be used in smoking cessation. Brit J of Addict 1986; 81: 47–53.
9. Tennant FS, Tarver AL, Rawson RA. Clinical evaluation of mecamylamine for withdrawal from nicotine dependence. In: Problems of drug dependence. NIDA Research Monograph Series No. 49. Rockville, Maryland U.S. Department of Health, Education and Welfare 1984.
10. Dahlstrom A, et al. The effect of chronic nicotine use and withdrawal on intraneuronal dynamics of acetylcholine and related enzymes in preganglionic neuron system of the rate. Acta Phys Scand 1980; 110: 13–20.
11. Bachynsky N. The use of anticholinergic drugs for smoking cessation: A pilot study. Intl J of Addict 1986; 21(7): 789–805.
12. Cocores JA, Goias PR, Gold MS. The medical management of nicotine dependence in the workplace. Ann of Clin Psychiatry 1989; 1: 237–240.
13. Cocores JA, Gold MS. Transcutaneous scopolamine for nicotine dependence: Use in non-addicts versus recovering addicts. 20th Annual Conference of the American Society of Addiction Medicine, in Atlanta April 1989.
14. Henningfield JE. How tobacco produces drug dependence: Pharmacologic treatment of tobacco dependence. In: proceedings of the World Congress, 1985. CAMBRIDGE, Massachusetts Institute for the Study of Smoking Behavior, 1986.
15. Imperato A, Mulas A, DiChiara G. Nicotine preferentiality stimulates dopamine release in the limbic system of freely moving rats. Eur J of Pharmacol 1986; 132: 337–338.
16. Mueller PS. Method of controlling tobacco use: Application for U.S. Patent No. 4800204, 1989.
17. Edwards NE, Murphy JK, Downs AD, et al. Doxepin as an adjunct to smoking cessation: A double blind pilot study. Am J of Psychi 1989; 146(3): 373–376.

18. Gawin F, Compton M, Byck R. Buspirone reduces smoking. Arch of Gen Psych. 1989; 46: 288–289.
19. Kôttke TE, Battista RN, DeFriese GH, et al. Attributes of successful smoking cessation interventions in medical practice: A meta-analysis of 39 controlled trials. JAMA 1988; 259(1a): 2883–2889.

19
Clinical Laboratory Testing of Nicotine

WALLACE B. PICKWORTH, EDWARD B. BUNKER, and
JACK E. HENNINGFIELD

A large subject sample is typically employed in studies designed to test the efficacy of drug treatments or behavioral therapies for smoking cessation. Large sample sizes are also required for an estimation of the risk of cigarette smoking to the health of the smoker or the smoker's nonsmoking associates. In contrast, the laboratory evaluations described in this chapter utilize small numbers of research subjects (generally $N < 10$). The validity and significance of such studies is maintained by other characteristics of the protocols, such as rigorous subject-selection criteria, objective measures of nicotine consumption, quantitative evaluation of nicotine-withdrawal symptoms, the systematic manipulation of the medication dose, and the use of closely monitored residential subjects. These issues determine the validity and reliability of the research and are reviewed in the present chapter.

Subject Selection

While the subjects of clinical research experiments are typically referred to as "smokers" or "nonsmokers," it is clear that neither group is homogeneous. *Nonsmokers* have been variously categorized as persons who have never smoked, who have not smoked in the past 2 years, or who have not smoked or used other tobacco or nicotine-containing products during a particular period of time. Smokers differ in their smoking history, daily consumption, puff topography, reasons for smoking, and smoking response to external factors such as concomitant drug ingestion or stress. The amount of nicotine intake is an important determinant of dependence level, severity of withdrawal symptoms, difficulty of quitting, and medication efficacy.[1,2] A variety of means of its quantification are employed in clinical experiments.

The most basic estimate of nicotine intake in smokers is the number of cigarettes smoked per day; a cutoff of 16 is typical to define modestly dependent smokers. Additional reliability may be achieved using the

1. How many cigarettes a day do you smoke? (Scoring − 15 cigarettes = 0 points, 16 to 25 = 1 point, and 26 = 2 points)

2. What brand do you smoke? (Scoring − .9 mg of nicotine or less = 0 points, 1.0 to 1.2 mg = 1 point. and 1.3 mg or more = 2 points)

3. Do you inhale? (Scoring − Never = 0 points, Sometimes = 1 point, and Always = 2 points)

4. Do you smoke more during the first two hours of the day than during the rest of the day? (Scoring − No = 0 points, Yes = 1 point)

5. How soon after you wake up do you smoke your first cigarette? (Scoring − More than 30 mins after waking = 0 points, 30 mins or less = 1 point)

6. Which cigarette would you hate to give up? (Scoring − First cigarette in the morning = 1 point, Any other = 0 points)

7. Do you find it difficult to refrain from smoking in places where it is forbidden, e.g., in church, at the library, cinema etc.? (Scoring − No = 0 points, Yes = 1 point)

8. Do you smoke if you are so ill that you are in bed most of the day? (Scoring − No = 0 points, Yes = 1 point)

FIGURE 19.1. Fagerstrom Tolerance Questionnaire. Updated version with specified cutoffs and revised wording (8). Used with permission.

Fagerstrom Tolerance Questionnaire (FTQ), which is frequently used to assess the degree of nicotine dependence of smokers.[3] The test is useful because it correlates with other measures of nicotine dependence, such as expired carbon monoxide (CO),[4] plasma cotinine,[5] and nicotine levels.[6] The FTQ is an eight-item, self-report instrument that estimates the quantity of nicotine consumed, the temporal patterns of use, and the situational factors in an individual's smoking pattern.[3] The relationship between the FTQ score and withdrawal symptoms is moderate, and the FTQ does not predict treatment success in all conditions.[7] In general, a score of 7 or higher indicates a substantial degree of nicotine tolerance and predicts the appearance of withdrawal discomfort. Because the maximum score on the FTQ is 11, small scoring errors can influence subject selection and the determination of individual treatment.[7,8] A commonly used version of the FTQ and its scoring is illustrated in Figure 19.1.

Motivation for smoking (and motivation to quit smoking) is not identical for all subjects, nor are the problems that lead to relapse following smoking cessation. For example, some smokers seek stimulation from cigarettes, whereas others smoke to relax.[9] Fear of withdrawal symptoms, including weight gain, contributes to some smokers maintaining their addictions. Tiffany[10] recently suggested that the process of smoking is partially a purposive behavior and partially an automatic behavior. These psychological factors involved in the smoking process[2,9] may be important to document in laboratory studies of etiological factors. The diverse factors may account for an undefined and important confounding variable in the results of these small-sample studies. Additionally, there is a high incidence of smoking among alcoholics[11,12] and persons with other drug-dependency disorders.[13] The prevalence of smokers (overall 50%) among psychiatric patients is significantly higher than national population-based samples[14] (30%) and was especially high in patients with schizophrenia (80%) and mania (70%). Smoking prevalence is also elevated among nonhospitalized persons with drug-abuse diagnoses.[15] The presence of comorbidity with tobacco use is important to ascertain because it can exacerbate difficulty in quitting smoking and may impair the efficacy of medications to treat nicotine dependence.[16] The identification of psychiatric illness using a standard diagnostic assessment such as the *Diagnostic and Statistical Manual of Mental Disorders* (3rd ed., rev.) (*DSM-III-R*)[17] is an important part of the subject-selection criteria of small-sample studies.

Thus, it can be seen that subject-selection criteria are important considerations in the laboratory study of nicotine. Smokers are not a homogeneous group. They differ in smoking history, reasons to smoke, smoking topography, and typology. These individual differences may affect the validity and variability of results. Such considerations are especially important in designing and interpreting the data from small-sample studies.

Biochemical Indexes of Smoking Behavior

Biochemical markers correlate with smoking and are sensitive and quantitative measures of smoking behavior. They are typically used in clinical studies to verify the smoking behavior of the subjects, to ensure abstinence and to quantify the effects of smoking-cessation treatments. Benowitz and Jacob[18] studied the biochemical correlates of cigarette smoking in 22 subjects. They correlated several biochemical markers of smoking with daily intake of nicotine. They found that afternoon blood-nicotine samples correlated most strongly ($r = .81$) with nicotine intake. Carboxyhemoglobin (COHb), urinary cotinine, and saliva thiocyanate levels are other frequently used biochemical indexes of nicotine intake.[19]

Blood Nicotine

Nicotine is rapidly metabolized in the liver of humans so that blood levels of nicotine depend on the time elapsed since the last cigarette. In the morning, smokers have blood nicotine levels of less than 10 ng/ml, but afternoon levels average around 30 ng/ml (range 10–50 ng/ml). The half-life of nicotine in blood is approximately 2 hours.[20] This half-life value results in well-documented patterns of plasma nicotine, whereby the nicotine level increases over the first 6–8 hours of the day and persists for several hours until bedtime. Nicotine plasma levels gradually decline overnight.

Carboxyhemoglobin

The inhaled CO generated from the burning tobacco combines with hemoglobin to form COHb. Its concentration is ordinarily expressed as a percentage of the total hemoglobin. This percentage varies with the time of day but plateaus in the afternoon at levels around 8%.[20] The CO levels in expired air can also be used to quantify smoking behavior. These are commonly measured in parts per million (ppm) of CO in expired air. Expired air CO levels are highly correlated with COHb, with a ratio of 5 to 1. Most smokers have late afternoon levels of approximately 25 ppm or greater.[19] After overnight abstinence, exhaled CO levels typically average 10 ppm or lower. Recent data suggest that genetically determined factors (e.g., lactase enzyme) can influence the utility of CO measures in the determination of the smoking status of the subject.[21,22]

Cotinine

Only about 10% of nicotine is excreted unchanged. A major liver metabolite of nicotine is cotinine.[2] Unlike nicotine and COHb, cotinine has a half-life that averages 18–20 hours (range: 11–37 hours). Therefore, cotinine levels are subject to less fluctuation than those of nicotine. A recent study indicates that racial differences in cotinine levels may exist.[23] In smokers, cotinine levels average between 250 and 300 ng/ml.

Thiocyanate

Hydrogen cyanide (30–200 μg) is delivered to the smoker with each cigarette. It is metabolized in the liver into thiocyanate, which is slowly excreted by the kidney. The half-life of thiocyanate is 14 days. Thiocyanate can be measured in saliva or serum samples, but it is seldom used in laboratory studies because of its prolonged half-life.[19]

Utility of Biochemical Markers

The definition of a smoker by means of biochemical markers enhances the objectivity of the description. Biochemical markers should be used to verify treatment success and to ensure compliance with the study protocol. The exact cutoff for each marker is determined by the prevalence of deception.[24] The calculated optimal cutoff levels for smokers are as follows: expired CO, ≥16 ppm; COHb, ≥2.8%; plasma cotinine, ≥14 ng/ml; plasma nicotine, ≥7.8 ng/ml. These biochemical indexes can be used to verify the smoking behavior in subjects involved in small clinical laboratory studies. They are used to determine whether subjects are truly abstinent or to determine whether medications have actually diminished smoking.[25] They are also used to estimate the success of attempts to regulate nicotine dosage, as described in the following section.

Laboratory Studies of Smoking Behavior

Tobacco smoke is a complex mixture of gases and particles, (Figure 19.2) and smoking behavior is a major determinant of the intake of these constituents. Among the methodologic considerations in smoking research is puff behavior, sometimes referred to as "smoking topography." Of major interest is the understanding of the complex relationship between the ingestion behavior of smoking, the availability and dose level of nicotine in the cigarette, and the eventual change in blood nicotine content.

Administration and Regulation of Nicotine Intake

It has been observed in many studies that smokers regulate their puffing behavior in response to the availability of cigarette nicotine.[26] In a sum-

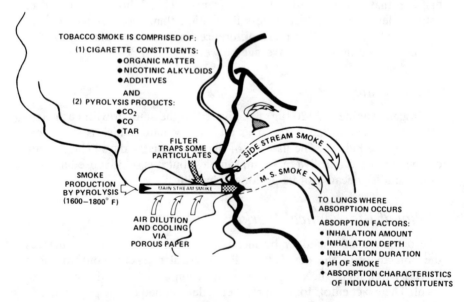

FIGURE 19.2. Tobacco smoking is a complex process involving the inhalation of cigarette constituents and pyrolysis products through the cigarette and from side stream smoke (25). Used with permission.

TABLE 19.1. Average puff topography values from Surgeon General report.[2]

Measurement	Puffs/ cigarette	Interpuff interval (sec)	Cigarette duration (sec)	Puff duration (sec)	Puff volume (ml)	Peak flow (ml/sec)	Inhalation volume (ml)
Mean	11	34	346	1.8	43	36	591
Median	11	28	351	1.9	42.5	35.5	560
Range	8–16	18–64	232–414	1.0–2.4	21–66	28–48	413–918

Note. Values are the mean, median, and range of puff topography data from 36 studies.

mary of more than 30 studies,[2] the puffing characteristics of smokers were measured. Despite wide methodological variations among the studies, the findings summarized in Table 19.1 are remarkably consistent.

A typical example of a study of smoking topography is that of Woodman et al.[27] They gave 10 smokers three cigarettes of varying nicotine content to smoke. By means of a tracer gas, they were able to quantify the puff-by-puff activity of the subjects. Generally, high-nicotine cigarettes decreased puff volume and total number of puffs, compared to the low-nicotine cigarette.

Guyatt et al.[28] found that the puff volume, puff duration, and interpuff interval increased during the smoking of a single cigarette. There was a large between-subject variation, but the within-subject measures were consistent over the six-cigarette test. There was a correlation between the tar content of the cigarette and the decrease in puff volume and an increase in interpuff interval. These data suggest that the tar content, as well as the nicotine content, of cigarettes influence smoking topography.

Nemeth-Coslett et al.[29] studied the effects of *mecamylamine*, a centrally acting nicotine antagonist, on smoking in eight volunteers. It was found that increases in mecamylamine dosage were associated with increases in puffs per session, cigarettes per session, puffs per cigarette, interpuff interval, and intercigarette interval. Greater overall smoking activity was confirmed with increases in expired CO.

DOSAGE CONTROL

Knowing that individuals can alter their smoking behavior in response to both dose manipulations and nicotine antagonists creates a methodologic problem. If one attempts to study the effects of nicotine ingestion by smoking, there must be a way to control dosing. Self-regulation of nicotine intake thus becomes a confounding factor, not a stabilizing one. One attempt to control dosing is the paced puffing paradigm. *Paced puffing* is a method by which an experimenter rigidly regulates variables such as depth of inhalation, number of puffs, interpuff interval, puff volume, and puff duration. Pomerleau et al.[30] proposed to validate this procedure by measuring pre and post blood-nicotine levels. They compared blood-nicotine changes in five subjects before and after highly controlled smoking sessions with those of five subjects who were not subjected to the pacing procedures. All subjects were tested on 2 different days. Their findings indicated that paced puffing did not lead to consistent increases in plasma-nicotine boosts across sessions. These observations suggest that fixed-dosing methods can benefit from validation using plasma nicotine and other biochemical measures.

AN INTERACTIVE MODEL OF NICOTINE DOSING

Puffing behavior and intake of nicotine seem to be closely related. Herning et al.[31] suggested a model whereby both puffing behavior and nicotine content of cigarettes need to be considered when estimating nicotine delivery. They measured the number, duration, and volume of puffs, as well as interpuff interval and volume and duration of inhalation, in 11 overnight-deprived smokers. Blood nicotine levels were collected before and after smoking. The machine-measured Federal Trade Commission (FTC) nicotine yields of the cigarettes only modestly correlated ($r = .52$) with the increases in blood-nicotine levels. However, when the factors of individual puffing behavior where considered together with the nicotine yields of the cigarettes, the correlations reached values between $r = .84$ and $.93$.

From the studies reviewed in this section, it is apparent that the regulation of nicotine dosage from smoked tobacco is a complex issue. Overall, it seems that no single factor accounts for the actual changes in blood nicotine levels. It is the interaction of cigarette yield and individual smoking characteristics (smoking topography) that is most predictive of nicotine delivery. An implication of this research is that simple manipulation of the number of cigarettes smoked or the nicotine delivery of the cigarette may not produce the intended effect on nicotine intake.

Quantification of Nicotine Administration and Deprivation

Among methods used to assess drug effects in humans, the electroencephalogram (EEG) provides objective and quantitative data. Psychoactive drugs are also known to affect performance. In this section, the effects of nicotine and nicotine deprivation on the EEG and performance is reviewed.

EFFECTS OF NICOTINE ON EEG

The spontaneous EEG recorded from the scalp of the subject is a convenient and noninvasive measure of the effects of drugs in the brain. Ulett and Itil[32] reported that overnight cigarette deprivation in heavy smokers decreased alpha frequency and increased power in the lower-frequency bands. This observation was confirmed and extended by Herning et al.,[33] who reported that overnight cigarette deprivation caused increases in alpha and theta power and a slowing of the dominant alpha frequency. Further, they observed that increases in theta power occurred as early as 30 minutes after the last cigarette. Pickworth et al.[34] recorded the spontaneous EEG before, during, and after 10 days of smoking deprivation in heavy smokers. They found the decrease in alpha frequency persisted for at least 7 days and the increase in theta power was elevated significantly above baseline ad lib smoking levels for the entire 10-day deprivation (Figure 19.3).

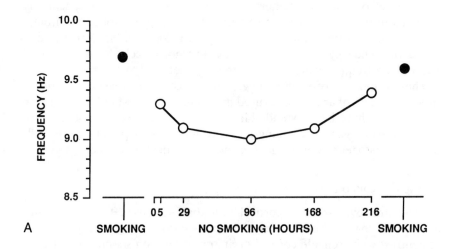

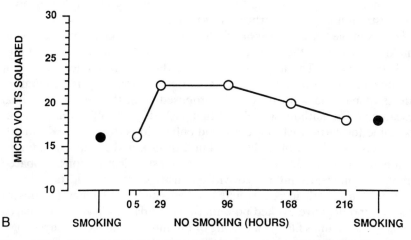

FIGURE 19.3. Decreases in (A) alpha frequency and increases in (B) theta power during a ten-day nicotine abstinence (open circles) compared to *ad lib* smoking (closed circles) (34). Used with permission.

Knott[35] used quantitative EEG analyses on a puff-by-puff basis of cigarette smoking. By the fourth puff, a characteristic psychostimulant profile was present, which consisted of decreased delta and theta power and increased alpha power and frequency. These data indicate that cortical arousal occurs during cigarette smoking in nondeprived volunteers. This conclusion was supported by data from Surwillo,[36-38] who postulated that the speed of information processing in the brain is related to the alpha frequency.

Knott and Venerables[39] used a sham smoking control procedure to indicate that the EEG effects were specific for the nicotine ingestion and not the act of smoking. Others have found that nicotine is specifically involved in the EEG effects of smoking.[40] These observations apparently extend to other forms of nicotine delivery. For example, Pickworth et al.[41] found that chewing nicotine polacrilex, but not placebo gum, increased EEG alpha frequency and reduced theta power.

Thus, a number of studies suggest that nicotine increases electrophysiologic indexes of arousal measured by spontaneous (resting) EEG. These observations have been extended in evoked-potential experiments, where the effects of cigarette smoking and nicotine or its deprivation are evaluated on endogenous or exogenous evoked cortical potentials.

CORTICAL EVOKED POTENTIAL STUDIES

Evoked and event-related cortical potentials are used to quantify the neurophysiologic effects of treatment conditions on cognitive processes. In contrast to its reliable cortical excitatory effects on spontaneous EEG, nicotine has variable and equivocal effects on cortical evoked potentials. The general conclusion of the few studies available has been that nicotine administration improves cortical information processing.

For example, Knott[42] reported that tobacco smoking, but not sham smoking, increased the amplitude of wave V of the brain stem auditory evoked response. The authors interpreted this as a facilitatory action of nicotine on subcortical (thalamic, midbrain) neural centers. Excitatory effects of nicotine were previously proposed from the results of animal research.[43] The authors speculated that such subcortical actions were responsible for cortical EEG arousal and enhanced performance. Knott[44,45] compared the effects of auditory stimuli in task and nontask conditions in female smokers during smoking and nonsmoking sessions. Tobacco smoking significantly interacted with intensity of stimuli and task conditions to cause both increases and decreases in short-latency (100 msec) positive and negative evoked potentials. These data indicate that tobacco can act as a stimulus filter, enhancing or diminishing the electrophysiologic consequences of external stimuli to the smoker. Woodson et al.[46] similarly found that high-nicotine-containing, but not low-nicotine-containing, cigarettes increased cortical potentials evoked by visual stimuli. Edwards et al.[47] found that cigarette smoking tended to enhance the speed of information processing of visually presented stimuli. Among the measures they studied was the P300 latency, an electrophysiologic marker of the time to update working memory. Nicotine decreased the P300 latency, results that support the common self-report by smokers that smoking aids concentration. However, Michel et al.[48] found that 4-mg nicotine gum changed the cortical spontaneous EEG but had no effect on performance task accuracy or response times. Further, the gum did not change the amplitude or latencies of evoked potentials. It seems that the speed of nicotine delivery affects the cortical electrical activity; rapid nicotine delivery (from smoking) causes changes in evoked potentials and spontaneous EEG, whereas slower delivery (from nicotine gum) changes only the resting EEG.

Performance Effects of Nicotine and Nicotine Deprivation

Smokers claim that smoking enhances concentration. This is among the most commonly cited reasons for smoking[2,49], and inability to concentrate is also a frequently mentioned symptom of withdrawal[50]. The impairment on performance of tasks requiring concentration is a formally recognized symptom of tobacco abstinence by the American Psychiatric Association's *DSM-III-R*.[17] Laboratory studies of the effects of smoking deprivation and nicotine administration tend to substantiate the anecdotal reports of smokers.

Snyder et al.[51] studied the performance on a battery of five computer-delivered cognitive tests of smokers after 12 hours of tobacco deprivation. They found that when subjects were given placebo, the response time was lengthened. On the other hand, when subjects chewed nicotine polacrilex before the tests, the speed of responding increased to rates not different than those during the freely smoking training period (Figure 19.4). Hughes et al.[50] investigated tobacco withdrawal on a sustained attention task. They found that 24-hour nicotine abstinence impaired the ability to respond and increased both the variability of responding and the ability to inhibit responding. The authors interpreted these results to indicate that abstinence decreased concentration and enhanced impatience. *Fatigue* (operationally defined as a decrement in performance) was not changed by abstinence. Revell[52] studied rapid visual-information processing while tobacco-deprived subjects smoked at a rate of one puff per minute. His results indicated that speed and accuracy of performance increased as soon as the second nicotine puff. Not all cognitive tests are enhanced by nicotine administration to tobacco-deprived subjects. For example, Dunne et al.[53] found that nicotine administration not only failed to enhance speed or

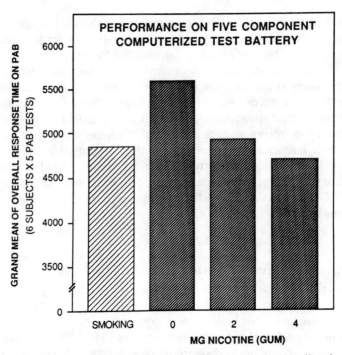

FIGURE 19.4. Nicotine polacrilex (2 and 4 mg) but not placebo (0 mg) prevents the increase in response time on performance tasks after overnight cigarette deprivation (51). Used with permission.

accuracy of word and number tasks, but it also impaired both delayed and immediate recall and recognition. Snyder et al.[54] reported that nicotine deprivation increased response time on several cognitive tasks, whereas accuracy was decreased on only two of the tasks—namely, digit recall and serial addition/subtraction. These tasks were distinguished from the unaffected tasks by their reliance on short-term or working memory, which was evidently affected by nicotine abstinence. There were no significant changes in episodic memory of subjects who exhibited profound changes in the resting EEG during nicotine deprivation.[34]

Snyder et al.[54] followed the time course of the cognitive effects of tobacco abstinence (Figure 19.5). They found that the speed of response was slowed within 4 hours of deprivation, was maximal at 24–28 hours, and began to return to ad lib smoking values over the next 8 days. Accuracy in some tests (e.g., serial addition/subtraction) on resumption of smoking performance measures was partially reversed within 1 hour, and all values returned to control level within 24 hours of resumption of smoking.

Performance decrements that occur as a consequence of nicotine deprivation have practical implications for the aviation industry. A 1978 NIH

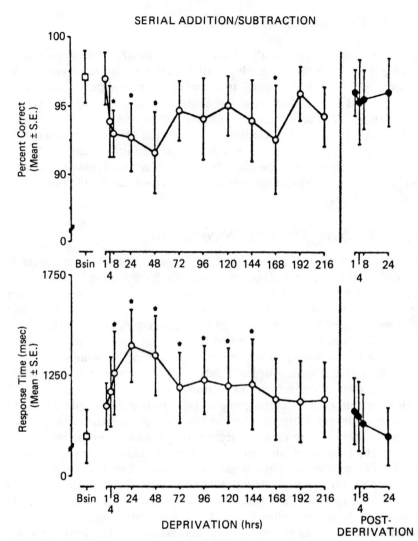

FIGURE 19.5. Nicotine deprivation decreases accuracy and increases response time on a rapid arithmetic test over a ten-day period of abstinence. Upon the resumption of smoking, performance rapidly returns to baseline levels (54). Used with permission.

study indicated that smoking per se did not affect flight performance, but nicotine withdrawal had adverse effects. The study conclusion was that the adverse effects of withdrawal in a chronic smoker were significant and may have a net adverse effect on overall flight safety.[55] With this report in mind, federal regulators exempted smoking in the cockpit from the overall ban on smoking during domestic airline flights.[56]

Clinical Psychopharmacologic Studies

Addictive drugs or drugs with a liability for abuse are of concern in part because the availability of such drugs will lead to their abuse by susceptible individuals. The ability of drugs to act as reinforcers appears to be complexly related to their potential for abuse and ability to cause physical dependence.[57] The abuse liability of drugs can be estimated in laboratory studies. The 1988 Surgeon General report on the "Health Consequences of Smoking"[2] came to the conclusion that the physical characteristics of nicotine delivery systems can affect their toxicity and addictiveness. Therefore, new nicotine delivery systems should be evaluated for their toxic and addictive effects.

Abuse Liability Studies of Nicotine

Studies that purport to assess the abuse liability of drugs were generally adapted from the extensive literature on the effects of morphine and morphinelike compounds in humans.[58-60] Such studies typically ascertain whether the drug in question is (1) psychoactive, (2) a euphoriant, and (3) a reinforcer. Psychoactivity and euphoriant properties of drugs are measured by means of subject self-reports of drug effects. The reinforcing properties of drugs in humans are estimated from the drug's ability to maintain and strengthen orderly patterns of self-administration when subjects are given free access to the drug.[61]

Henningfield et al.[62] administered nicotine or placebo in a double-blind study to volunteer subjects. The nicotine was given intravenously or in tobacco smoke from research cigarettes using standardized puffing procedures. They found that intravenous and smoked nicotine caused the same profile of subjective and physiological responses, whereas placebo had no effect. The subjects reliably discriminated nicotine from placebo, indicating that nicotine is psychoactive. The self-reported and physiologic effects of nicotine occurred within 1 minute of administration and dissipated within 5 minutes after either route of administration. The peak response and duration of action was directly related to the dose of nicotine.

The two indicators of drug-induced euphoria used in the study were the drug-liking scale of the Single Dose Questionnaire (SDQ)[59] and the Morphine–Benzedrine Group (MBG) scale of the Addiction Research Center Inventory (ARCI).[63] On the five-point drug-liking scale of the SDQ, nicotine by both routes of administration was rated as highly as other subjects rated their liking for morphine and amphetamine (Figure 19.6). When the subjects were instructed to identify the drug condition from a list of commonly used and abused substances, they frequently identified the intravenous nicotine as cocaine. Similar physiologic effects, including increases in pupil diameter, heart rate, and blood pressure, occurred after intravenous nicotine or inhaled tobacco smoke. The similarity in response

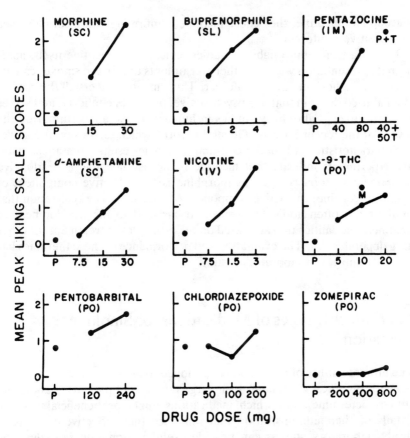

FIGURE 19.6. Drug liking scores after a variety of psychoactive drugs. Intravenous nicotine increased scores to the same extent as other abused drugs (P + T = pentazocine 40 mg = tripelennamine 50 mg, M = marijuana smoked, P = placebo) (59). Used with permission.

between intravenous nicotine and inhaled tobacco smoke indicated that nicotine was the responsible constituent in the smoke.

Another type of abuse liability study involves the characterization of the conditions under which an animal or human subject will self-administer a drug. Variations of this paradigm in animals provides a means of generalizing the administration of a drug while controlling for uniquely human characteristics such as personality, social, and cultural variables. A high degree of concordance over a wide range of drugs exists between animal self-administration and human abuse potential.[64] Nicotine has been shown to be an effective reinforcer, as judged by its self-administration in several animal species.[65] Smokers deprived of nicotine for 1 hour reliably self-administered intravenous nicotine, but not saline placebo injections.[66] Another study showed that when subjects had simultaneous access to both placebo and nicotine, they chose nicotine, confirming that nicotine served as a positive reinforcer.[67]

The data from abuse liability studies indicate that nicotine itself, apart from its presentation with the other constituents of tobacco smoke, can act as both a euphoriant and a reinforcer. Thus, nicotine meets all the criteria of an abused drug, in that it is psychoactive, produces euphoria, and serves as a reinforcer. Laboratory studies in humans and animals supported the results of the recent Surgeon General report,[2] which focuses on the addictive characteristics of tobacco consumption. The results from abuse liability experiments indicate that nicotine is the psychoactive and addictive component of tobacco, just as morphine is the addictive component of opium or cocaine, the active component of coca leaf. The realization that smokers are often addicted to nicotine has lead to the development of treatment modalities that are based on the principles of treatment for other drug dependencies. The evaluation and performance of these therapies has been the subject of laboratory testing.

Laboratory Studies of Medications for Smoking Cessation

The ultimate utility of medications developed to assist in smoking cessation depends on efficacy estimates from large numbers of patients. Laboratory studies determine both which medications might be beneficial and the details of their administration that influence their effectiveness. Specifically, laboratory studies can provide useful information regarding the efficiency of drug treatment on signs and symptoms of withdrawal (e.g., performance deficits, EEG effects), as well as possible liabilities of use (e.g., abuse liability, cardiovascular toxicity).

The most thoroughly evaluated medication for use in the treatment of nicotine dependence and its withdrawal symptoms is nicotine polacrilex. Nicotine polacrilex was developed as a substitution or replacement therapy to aid in smoking cessation. The preparation consists of nicotine, combined with an ion-exchange resin. Upon slowly chewing the gum, between 1 and 2 mg of nicotine is released over 20–30 minutes.[68] These doses are similar to the amount of nicotine from a single cigarette. Laboratory studies have provided data regarding the effectiveness of nicotine polacrilex in the treatment of acute withdrawal signs and symptoms, as well as the evaluation of parameters, such as dose and determinants of bioavailability.

Benowitz et al.[69] analyzed nicotine plasma levels in subjects chewing the polacrilex. The kinetic characteristics of 12 pieces of 2- and 4-mg nicotine polacrilex (chewed for 20 minutes every hour) were compared with ad lib smoking. They found that extraction of nicotine from the polacrilex was incomplete (53% of 2 mg; 72% of 4 mg) and variable. Furthermore, the

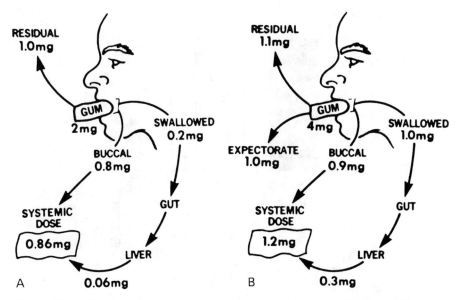

FIGURE 19.7. Metabolic fate and systemic dose of nicotine polacrilex 2 mg (A) and 4 mg (B); (69). Used with permission.

systemic dose of nicotine was less than expected, and there was evidence that some of the nicotine was swallowed and metabolized before reaching the bloodstream (Figure 19.7).

Pickworth et al.[41] tested whether nicotine polacrilex could reverse or prevent the EEG effects of nicotine deprivation. They found that overnight cessation of smoking increased theta power and decreased alpha frequency effects, which were reversed by paced chewing of nicotine polacrilex in doses of 2 and 4 mg. These findings were replicated and extended in a subsequent study,[34] in which subjects chewed 12 pieces of polacrilex or placebo at 2-hour intervals for 3 days (Figure 19.8).

The EEG effects of nicotine abstinence reliably occurred as early as 5 hours in the placebo condition, but they were prevented in the active-dose polacrilex condition. These results indicate that it is the nicotine component of tobacco smoke responsible for the EEG effects of deprivation. Furthermore, EEG signs of tobacco withdrawal are in the direction of decreased cortical arousal. These may account for the inability to concentrate, an effect of tobacco deprivation frequently mentioned by abstinent smokers. Similarly, Snyder et al.[54] reported that nicotine polacrilex, but not placebo gum, prevented performance decrements on a computerized performance assessment battery.

Nemeth-Coslett et al.[70] studied the effects of variations in the chewing rate of nicotine polacrilex on plasma levels of nicotine and subjective effects. While there was an overall trend for more nicotine to be extracted at

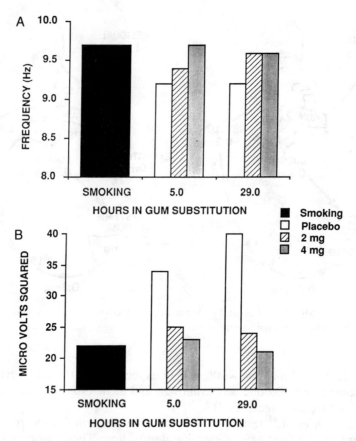

FIGURE 19.8. Nicotine polacrilex but not placebo gum prevents the decrease in (A) alpha frequency and increase in (B) theta power, EEG effects of nicotine deprivation (34). Used with permission.

higher chew rates (1 chew/second), than at lower rates (1 chew/8 seconds), the relationship was weak and not correlated with changes in blood-nicotine levels. The authors concluded that, despite instructional charges, subjects regulated the chew rate to obtain optimal nicotine absorption, much like smokers autoregulate their puffing to control nicotine absorption from cigarettes of various strengths.[26] Thus, the rate of chewing makes a difference in the amount of nicotine extracted from the polacrilex, but variations in gum chewing is probably not an effective way to regulate consistently the dose of nicotine.

Nemeth-Coslett and Henningfield[71] investigated the effects of eight pieces of placebo, 2-, or 4-mg nicotine polacrilex (given at 2-hour intervals) on ad lib smoking. The 4-mg nicotine polacrilex decreased the number of cigarettes smoked and the number of puffs taken, but the 2-mg polacrilex had no effect. The expired CO was not changed. The subjective effects of gum chewing were assessed with the SDQ, a tobacco questionnaire[71] and the ARCI. Generally, there were no subjective effects, although the authors found that higher doses of the nicotine polacrilex were reliably perceived and rated as objectionable. There was a tendency for coughing, hiccuping, and heartburn to be more evident after the higher dose. In this study, nicotine gum produced a low level of euphoria. The authors speculated that the route of administration and the rate of absorption are primary determinants of the abuse liability of nicotine.

Laboratory experiments on the effects of concomitant ingestion of beverages on nicotine blood levels following administration of nicotine polacrilex were reported by Henningfield et al.[72] In smoke-deprived volunteers, mouth rinses with acidic beverages (coffee and cola) decreased oral pH and diminished nicotine absorption and subjective effects of nicotine polacrilex. Other food products decreased saliva pH and were presumed to diminish nicotine absorption. In a subsequent study,[73] concomitant chewing of nicotine polacrilex and sugar-containing chewing gum (e.g., Juicyfruit®) decreased saliva pH and diminished nicotine absorption. However, simultaneous chewing of sugarless gum did not change the absorption of nicotine or salivary pH.

Mecamylamine is a centrally acting nicotine antagonist that has intermittently been proposed as a therapeutic aid in smoking cessation.[74–76] Several clinical laboratory studies have investigated the effects of mecamylamine in cigarette-smoking volunteers. Henningfield et al.[76] found that mecamylamine pretreatment (2.5, 5, and 10 mg) attenuated behavioral and physiologic effects of intravenous nicotine. Specifically, mecamylamine pretreatment prevented nicotine-induced decreases in skin temperature and eliminated the biphasic (initial mydriasis, subsequent miosis) pupillary response. Mecamylamine also decreased drug-liking scores, drug identification as amphetamine, and the weak nicotine-dose-related decrease in desire to smoke. The effects of mecamylamine on smoking were further investigated by Nemeth-Coslett et al.[29] They found that mecamylamine pretreatment increased the number of cigarettes smoked, the number of puffs per cigarette, and the expired CO level. However, after the high dose of mecamylamine (20 mg), subjects occasionally complained of dizziness, weakness in their legs, and blurred vision.

Reductions in functional nicotine doses by a variety of means are associated with increased smoking behavior.[26] For example, Pomerleau et al.[77] reported that plasma nicotine levels increased more after smoking two research cigarettes in subjects who were pretreated with mecamylamine than in those pretreated with placebo. Their findings indicated that subjects evoke compensatory behaviors to overcome mecamylamine blocking effects. Pickworth et al.[78] showed that mecamylamine pretreatment prevented the EEG effects of nicotine gum in subjects that were deprived of tobacco for 12 hours. They also showed that mecamylamine (10 mg) alone had EEG effects on the deprived smokers. These effects included slowing of the alpha frequency and increased theta power—two consistently observed EEG effects of nicotine withdrawal.

In another clinical laboratory study, Rose et al.[79] reported that mecamylamine produced dose-related decreases in ratings of puff strength and harshness and reduced desire for a cigarette. However, mecamylamine pretreatment increased the subject-selected self-administered dose of nicotine. In this study, mecamylamine was administered over a range of doses, enabling the authors to distinguish those aspects of cigarette smoking that are not nicotine dependent, such as ratings of harshness, from nicotine-dependent processes, such as desire for a cigarette.

Summary

In this chapter, the data from selected clinical laboratory studies of nicotine have been reviewed. The advantages of the clinical laboratory study include both the careful monitoring of subjects and their smoking topography and the quantitative evaluation of experimental manipulations. Such studies are useful for an understanding of the role of nicotine in smoking behavior and in the development of treatment strategies for tobacco dependence. Data from clinical laboratory studies have practical and theoretical importance. For example, low-yield cigarettes do not reliably decrease the frequency of certain smoking behaviors or blood levels of nicotine, findings that belie the claim that low-yield cigarettes are safer. The finding that nicotine absorption from the gum is affected by salivary pH or by the concomitant ingestion of certain foods has led to new instructions on the use of the nicotine polacrilex. The low absorption of nicotine from the polacrilex dictates that heavily dependent smokers need up to 20 pieces of nicotine polacrilex per day. Furthermore, the limited nicotine absorption from the commercially available 2-mg nicotine polacrilex supports the need for a 4-mg preparation in the United States. Finally, data from psychopharmacology studies indicate that nicotine is an addictive substance. Smokers and clinicians need not be intimidated by this realization. Rather, advances in the treatment of opiate and alcohol addiction (e.g., substitution and replacement therapy, relapse prevention, 12-step programs) may ultimately benefit smokers seeking abstinence.

References

1. Henningfield JE. Improving the diagnosis and treatment of nicotine dependence. JAMA 1988; 260: 1613–1614.
2. U.S. Department of Health and Human Services. The health consequences of smoking: Nicotine addiction (a report of the Surgeon General). Washington, DC: U.S. Government Printing Office, 1988.
3. Fagerstrom KO. Measuring degree of physical dependence to tobacco smoking with reference to individualization of treatment. Addict Behav 1978; 3: 235–241.

4. Fagerstrom KO. Effects of a nicotine-enriched cigarette on nicotine titration, daily cigarette consumption, and levels of carbon monoxide, cotinine and nicotine. Psychopharmacology 1982; 77: 164–167.
5. Hall SM, Killen JD. Psychological and pharmacological approaches to smoking relapse prevention. In: Grabowski J, Hall SM, eds. Pharmacological adjuncts in smoking cessation. NIDA Research Monograph No. 53. Washington, DC: U.S. Government Printing Office, 1985: 131–143.
6. Tonnesen P, Fryd, V, Hansen M, et al. Effect of nicotine chewing gum in combination with group counselling on the cessation of smoking. New Engl J of Med 1988; 318: 15–18.
7. Fagerstrom KO, Schneider NG. Measuring nicotine dependence: A review of the Fagerstrom Tolerance Questionnaire. J of Behav Med 1989; 12: 159–182.
8. Moore BL, Schneider JA, Ryan JJ. Fagerstrom's Tolerance Questionnaire: Clarification of item and scoring ambiguities. Addict Behav 1987; 12: 67–68.
9. Russell MAH, Peto J, Patel UA. The classification of smoking by factoral structure of motives. J of Roy Stat Soc 1974; 137: 313–364.
10. Tiffany ST. A cognitive model of drug urges and drug-use behavior: A role of automatic and non-automatic processes. Psychol Rev 1990; 97: 147–168.
11. DiFranza JR, Guerrera MP. Hard-core smokers. JAMA 1989; 261: 2634.
12. DiFranza JR, Guerrera MP. Alcoholism and smoking. J of Stud Alcohol, 1990; 51: 130–135.
13. Henningfield JE, Clayton R, Pollin, W. Involvement of tobacco in alcoholism and illicit drug use. Brit J of Addict 1990; 85: 279–292.
14. Hughes JR, Hatsukami DK, Mitchell JE, Dahlgren LA. Prevalence of smoking among psychiatric outpatients. Am J of Psychiat 1986; 143: 993–997.
15. Breslau N, Kilbey M. Co-dependency of nicotine, alcohol and drugs in an urban population of young adults. Problems of drug dependence 1990. NIDA Research Monograph. Washington, DC: U.S. Government Printing Office, in press.
16. Glassman AH, Stetner F, Walsh BT, et al. Heavy smokers, smoking cessation and clonidine: Results of a double-blind, randomized trial. JAMA 1988; 259: 2863–2866.
17. American Psychiatric Association. Diagnostic and statistical manual of mental disorders 3rd ed, rev. (DSM-III-R). Washington DC: Author, 1987.
18. Benowitz NL, Jacob P. Daily intake of nicotine during cigarette smoking. Clin Pharmacol Ther 1984; 35: 499–504.
19. Benowitz NL. The use of biological fluid samples in assessing tobacco smoke consumption. Grabowski J, Bell CS, eds. In: Measurement in the analysis and treatment of smoking behavior. NIDA Research Monograph No. 48. Washington, DC: U.S. Government Printing Office, 1983: 6–26.
20. Benowitz NL, Kuyt F, Jacob P. Circadian blood nicotine concentrations during cigarette smoking. Clin Pharmacol Ther 1982; 32: 75.
21. McNeill AD, Owen LA, Belcher M, Sutherland G, Fleming S. Abstinence from smoking and expired-air carbon monoxide levels: Lactose intolerance as a possible source of error. Am J of Public Health 1990; 80: 1114–1115.
22. Henningfield JE, Cohen C, Giovino GA. Can genetic constitution affect the "objective" diagnosis of nicotine dependence? Am J of Public Health 1990; 80: 1040–1041.

23. Wagenknecht LE, Cutter GR, Haley NJ, et al. Racial differences in serum cotinine levels among smokers in the CARDIA study. Am J of Public Health 1990; 80: 1053–1056.

24. Cummings SR, Richard RJ. Optimum cutoff points for biochemical validation of smoking status. Am J of Public Health 1988; 78: 574–575.

25. Henningfield JE. Behavioral pharmacology of cigarette smoking. In: Thompson T, Dews PB, Barrett JE, eds. Advances in behavioral pharmacology. New York: Academic Press, 1984: 131–210.

26. Gritz ER. Smoking behavior and tobacco abuse. In: Mello NK, ed. Advances in substance abuse: Behavioral and biological research. Greenwich, CT: JAI Press, 1980: 91–158.

27. Woodman G, Newman SP, Pavia D, Clarke SW. Inhaled smoke volume and puff indices with cigarettes of different tar and nicotine levels. Eur J of Respir Disease 1987; 70: 187–192.

28. Guyatt AR, Kirkham AJT, Baldry AG, Dixon M, Cumming G. How does puffing behavior alter during the smoking of a single cigarette? Pharmacol Biochem Beh 1989; 33: 189–195.

29. Nemeth-Coslett R, Henningfield JE, O'Keeffe MK, Griffiths RR. Effects of mecamylamine on human cigarette smoking and subjective ratings. Psychopharmacology 1986; 88: 420–425.

30. Pomerleau CS, Majchrzak MJ, Pomerleau OF. Paced puffing as a method for administering fixed doses of nicotine. Addict Behav 1989; 14: 571–575.

31. Herning RI, Jones RT, Benowitz NL, Mines AH. How a cigarette is smoked determines blood nicotine levels. Clin Pharmacol Ther 1983; 33: 84–90.

32. Ulett JA, Itil TM. Quantitative electroencephalogram in smoking and smoking deprivation. Science 1969; 154: 969–970.

33. Herning RI, Jones RT, Bachman J. EEG changes during tobacco withdrawal. Psychophysiology 1983; 20: 507–512.

34. Pickworth WB, Herning RI, Henningfield JE. Spontaneous EEG changes during tobacco abstinence and nicotine substitution in human volunteers. J of Pharmacol Exper Ther 1989; 251: 976–982.

35. Knott VJ. Dynamic EEG changes during cigarette smoking. Neuropsychobiology 1988; 19: 54–60.

36. Surwillo W. Frequency of the "alpha" rhythm, reaction time and age. Nature 1961; 191: 823–824.

37. Surwillo W. The relation of simple response time to brain wave frequency and the effects of age. EEG Clin Neurophysiol 1963; 15: 105–114.

38. Surwillo W. Some observations on the relation of response speed to frequency of photic stimulation under conditions of EEG synchronization. EEG Clin Neurophysiol 1964; 17: 194–198.

39. Knott VJ, Venables PH. EEG alpha correlates of non-smokers, smokers, smoking, and smoking deprivation. Psychophysiology 1977; 14: 150–156.

40. Edwards JA, Warburton DM. Smoking, nicotine and electrocortical activity. Pharmacol Ther 1983; 19: 147–164.

41. Pickworth WB, Herning RI, Henningfield JE. Electroencephalographic effects of nicotine chewing gum in humans. Pharmacol Biochem Beh 1986; 25: 879–882.

42. Knott VJ. Effects of tobacco on human brainstem evoked potentials. Addict Behav 1987; 12: 375–379.

43. Domino E. Electroencephalographic and behavioral arousal effects of small doses of nicotine: A neuropsychopharmacological study. Ann of the NY Acad of Sci 1967; 142: 216–244.
44. Knott VJ. Tobacco effects on cortical evoked potentials to distracting stimuli. Neuropsychobiology 1985; 13: 74–80.
45. Knott VJ. Effects of tobacco and distraction on sensory and slow cortical evoked potentials during task performance. Neuropsychobiology 1985; 13: 136–140.
46. Woodson PP, Battig K, Etkin MW, et al. Effects of nicotine on the visual evoked response. Pharmacol Biochem Behav 1982; 17: 915–920.
47. Edwards JA, Wesnes K, Warburton DM, Gale A. Evidence of more rapid stimulus evaluation following cigarette smoking. Addict Behav 1985; 10: 113–126.
48. Michel C, Hasenfratz M, Nil R, Battig K. Cardiovascular, electrocortical, and behavioral effects of nicotine chewing gum. Klinische Wochenschrift 1988; 66: 72–79.
49. Wesnes K, Warburton DM. Effects of smoking on rapid information processing performance. Neuropsychobiology 1983; 9: 223–229.
50. Hughes JR, Keenan RM, Yellin A. Effect of tobacco withdrawal on sustained attention. Addict Behav 1989; 14: 577–580.
51. Snyder FR, Henningfield JE. Effects of nicotine administration following 12 h of tobacco deprivation: Assessment on computerized performance tasks. Psychopharmacology 1989; 97: 17–22.
52. Revell AD. Smoking and performance—A puff-by-puff analysis. Psychopharmacology 1988; 96: 563–565.
53. Dunne MP, MacDonald D, Hartley LR. The effects of nicotine upon memory and problem solving performance. Physiol Behav 1986; 37: 849–854.
54. Snyder FR, Davis FC, Henningfield JE. The tobacco withdrawal syndrome: Performance decrements assessed on a computerized test battery. Drug Alcohol Dependencies 1989; 23: 259–266.
55. National Institutes of Health. Cigarette smoking and airline pilots: Effects of smoking and smoking withdrawal on flight performance. Bethesda, MD: Author, 1978.
56. Booth W. Smoking lamp still lit in most airline cockpits. Washington Post, March 3, 1990: A3.
57. Henningfield JE, London ED, Jaffe JH. Nicotine reward: Studies of abuse liability and physical dependence potential. In: Engel J, Oreland L, eds. Brain reward systems and abuse. New York: Raven Press, 1987: 149–164.
58. Jasinski DR. Assessment of the abuse potential of morphinelike drugs (methods used in man). In: Martin WR, ed. Handbook of experimental pharmacology. Heidelberg, Germany: Springer-Verlag, 1977: 197–258.
59. Jasinski DR, Johnson RE, Henningfield JE. Abuse liability assessment in human subjects. Trends Pharmacol Sci 1984; 5: 196–200.
60. Brady JV, Lukas SE. In: Testing drugs for physical dependence potential and abuse liability. NIDA Research Monograph No. 52. Washington, DC: U.S. Government Printing Office, 1984.
61. Henningfield JE, Goldberg SR. Stimulus properties of nicotine in animals and human volunteers: A review. In: Behavioral pharmacology: The current status. New York: Liss, 1984: 433–449.

62. Henningfield, JE, Miyasato K, Jasinski DR. Abuse liability and pharmacodynamic characteristics of intravenous and inhaled nicotine. J of Pharmacol Exper Ther 1985; 234: 1–12.
63. Haertzen CA. An overview of the Addiction Research Center Inventory scales (ARCI): An appendix and manual of scales. Washington, DC: U.S. Government Printing Office, 1974.
64. Griffiths RR, Bigelow GE, Henningfield JE. Similarities in animal and human drug taking behavior. In: Mello NK, ed. Advances in substance abuse: Behavioral and biological research. Greenwich, CT: JAI Press, 1980: 1–90.
65. Goldberg SR, Henningfield JE. Reinforcing effects of nicotine in humans and experimental animals responding under intermittent schedules of IV drug injection. Pharmacol Biochem Behav 1988; 30: 227–234.
66. Henningfield JE, Miyasato K, Jasinski DR. Cigarette smokers self-administer intravenous nicotine. Pharmacol Biochem Behav 1983; 19: 887–890.
67. Henningfield JE, Goldberg SR. Progress in understanding the relationship between the pharmacological effects of nicotine and human tobacco dependence. Pharmacol Biochem Behav 1988; 30: 217–220.
68. McNabb ME, Ebert RV, McCusker K. Plasma nicotine levels produced by chewing nicotine gum. JAMA 1982; 258: 865–868.
69. Benowitz NL, Jacob III P, Savanapridi C. Determinants of nicotine intake while chewing nicotine polacrilex gum. Clin Pharmacol Ther 1987; 41: 467–473.
70. Nemeth-Coslett R, Benowitz NL, Robinson N, Henningfield JE. Nicotine gum: Chew rate, subjective effects and plasma nicotine. Pharmacol Biochem Behav 1988; 29: 747–751.
71. Nemeth-Coslett R, Henningfield JE. Effects of nicotine chewing gum on cigarette smoking and subjective and physiologic effects. Clin Pharmacol Ther 1986; 39: 625–630.
72. Henningfield JE, Radzius A, Cooper TM. Drinking coffee and carbonated beverages blocks absorption of nicotine from nicotine polacrilex gum. JAMA 1990; 264: 1560–1564.
73. Henningfield JE, Radzius A, Cooper TM. Oral pH: A factor in the treatment of nicotine addiction. J Am Dental Association, in press.
74. Tennant FS, Tarver AL, Rawson RA. Clinical evaluation of mecamylamine for withdrawal from nicotine dependence. In: Harris LS, ed. Problems of drug dependence. NIDA Research Monograph No. 49 Washington, DC: U.S. Government Printing Office, 1984: 239–246.
75. Stolerman IP. Could nicotine antagonist be used in smoking cessation? Brit J of Addict 1986; 81: 47–53.
76. Henningfield JE, Miyasato K, Johnson RE, Jasinski, DR. Rapid physiologic effects of nicotine in humans and selective blockade of behavioral effects by mecamylamine. In: Harris LS, ed. Problems of drug dependence. NIDA Research Monograph No. 43. Washington, DC: U.S. Government Printing Office, 1983: 259–265.
77. Pomerleau CS, Pomerleau OF, Majchrzak MJ. Mecamylamine pretreatment increases subsequent nicotine self-administration as indicated by changes in plasma nicotine level. Psychopharmacology 1987; 91: 391–393.
78. Pickworth WB, Herning RI, Henningfield JE. Mecamylamine reduces some EEG effects of nicotine chewing gum in humans. Pharmacol Biochem Behav 1988; 30: 149–153.

79. Rose JE, Sampson A, Levin ED, Henningfield JE. Mecamylamine increases nicotine preference and attenuates nicotine discrimination. Pharmacol Biochem Behav 1989; 32: 933–938.

20
Outpatient Management of Nicotine Dependence

JAMES A. COCORES and A. CARTER POTTASH

Physicians in all specialties, dentists, pharmacists, chiropractors, psychologists, social workers, nurses, and other health-care professionals need continuing education regarding the treatment of nicotine dependence. Education is prevention, and education fosters intervention. Clinicians should be able to educate their patients, aid in the prevention of nicotine dependence, and familiarize themselves with both phases of recovery (primary treatment and aftercare or relapse prevention).

Health professionals are progressing with regard to their active participation in the management of nicotine dependence. Although the number of nurses that smoke is still above the national average,[1] the general trend among other groups of health professionals is improving. The number of physician smokers is down to 9%.[2] This is a marked improvement from the 1950s, when physicians smoked as much as most other groups. Physicians were portrayed in cigarette advertisements: "Rosalind Russell says, L&M Filters are Just What the Doctor Ordered!" "More Doctors Smoke Camels Than Any Other Cigarette!" and "20,679 Physicians say Luckies are less irritating."[3] The number of dentists who smoke is also declining, but up to a third do not advise patients about smoking cessation.[4] Clearly, an increasing number of health professionals are beginning to learn that nicotine dependence in any form or amount is hazardous to their health. However, what remains unclear is why clinicians are not as aggressive as they could be in educating, diagnosing, treating, or referring their patients, and being more a part of the national movement toward the prevention, and treatment of nicotine dependence.

Why would health-care workers ignore nicotine dependence? Is it because nicotine use is not viewed as a part of their patients mental or physical health? Why are blood pressure and cholesterol problems swiftly followed up with education and intervention, but too often, essentially nothing is said or done about nicotine dependence? Clinicians are justifiably concerned about AIDS and its psychological and physical consequences; but more people died last year from complications of nicotine dependence than have ever died of AIDS. Why do psychiatrists say and do nothing about their patients' nicotine dependence? Why do dentists concern themselves with caries and cleanings, and ignore tar-stained teeth? Why do gynecologists focus on Pap smears and routine pelvic examinations and say nothing about nicotine dependence? Why does the psychotherapist probe insight and self-esteem, and ignore nicotine dependence? Perhaps health specialists living in an age of specialization assume that enough nicotine-dependence specialists exist to service all their patients who use nicotine, or simply "it is not my job!"

Before a clinician can consider becoming part of the solution, he or she must first stop any personal use of nicotine delivery systems of any kind and in any amount. Next, the clinician should consider engaging relatives or friends into nicotine recovery. The American Cancer Society keeps it simple: "Adopt a Smoker." After the clinician has had experience engaging and treating nicotine-dependent persons at home or in the workplace, he or she is better able to begin the practice of nicotine-dependence treatment with patients. In addition, clinicians who have not piloted smoking-cessation techniques at home and in the workplace are more likely to encounter frustration when attempting to recruit patients into recovery. Nicotine-naïve clinicians are also likely to convey their own denial, rationalization, intellectualization, and minimization about nicotine use to their patients. A nicotine-dependence fellowship, consisting of experience in using various techniques outlined in this book, is a prerequisite to effective intervention with patients. It is easier to sell nicotine-dependence recovery to patients after the clinician develops confidence and the necessary skills.

All health-related clinicians are needed and are in the position to engage nicotine users into treatment. Smokers are six times more likely to quit for good if their doctors help them.[2]

Resistant Recruiters

There are several reasons why clinicians resist recruiting nicotine users into recovery. One of the most common reasons is lack of the facts, in part due to a rapidly changing and expanding literature on the topic of substance-use disorders in general and of nicotine dependence in particular. Many clinicians are fixed in an archaic belief that nicotine users stop when they are ready and that "nothing I say or do will change that."

Clinicians may convey the willpower philosophy to their patients. The *willpower view* usually conveys a sense of failure, weakness, stupidity, and ignorance to the patient who is unable to stop independently. Frustration and a sense of failure is perceived by both the patient and the clinician. A clinician's experiences may have been uncomfortable because of confrontations and unnecessary verbal battles with patients. Because of this discomfort, a clinician may have elected to stop trying to engage nicotine users.

The nicotine-dependent person may be viewed by the clinician as lacking willpower and being weak or ignorant. Understanding the disease concept, as described by Miller in chapter 6 not only helps the addict recover by taking the blame out of treatment but also helps clinicians view patients in a manner that they are accustomed to—as a victim. The disease concept is not intended to make excuses for addictive behavior, nor does it foster irresponsibility. The disease concept is conveyed as follows: "You are not responsible for your disease. . . . You are responsible for your recovery."

Clinicians may overlook a patient's need for nicotine-dependence treatment or for minimal guidance out of habit. They may have initially attempted some intervention by using scare tactics or by threatening patients with health consequences. This method often leads to aggression and defensiveness on the user's part. Scare tactics are not effective methods of engaging patients into recovery.

Other clinicians may be accustomed to immediate gratification in their clinical practice. For example, an abdominal surgeon may be accustomed to the immediate success or failure accompanying treatments such as surgical intervention in appendicitis. These clinicians avoid counselling nicotine-dependent patients because of the perceived chronicity, hopelessness, and frustration associated with the treatment of a chronic, relapsing disorder.

Some clinicians may view a smoker's relapse as a shared personal failure instead of an expected part of a broad-based, lifelong, recovery process. The clinician may want to avoid these "losers." As Glidden states in chapter 22: "Failure should be seen as temporary, an interlude between successes."

Clinicians who are uncomfortable discussing treatment options with drug addicts often avoid doing so because of fear. Many clinicians prefer to avoid drug addicts of any variety for fear of their frequent ability to manipulate, intimidate, and outtalk inexperienced clinicians. Many clinicians are not trained, experienced, skilled, or confident in communicating with users who are defensive and in a state of denial. Most clinicians do not want to aggravate their patients. Inexperienced clinicians often fear losing a patient if they discuss nicotine-dependence treatment options.

Still others do not treat nicotine dependence because most patients are not reimbursed by insurance companies for their treatment. Although some smokers present with significant primary depression (which, as Taylor discusses in chapter 24, must be addressed first), the majority of patients will not have coverage for the treatment of nicotine dependence. In our clinic, patients who pay for their own treatment without insurance appear to be more motivated and have a better prognosis than patients who are reimbursed. In any case, we are hopeful that insurance companies will pay for nicotine-dependence treatment in the near future. Blue Cross of Washington, for example, has adopted this policy, and others are expected to follow.

Most nicotine-dependent patients welcome support and guidance toward recovery from nicotine dependence. The clinician should not attempt to make just one intervention. Instead, the clinician should begin the process toward recovery through multiple, small, nonthreatening interventions. This may be initiated simply by adding a nicotine section to the history and physical or psychosocial evaluation. If nicotine use is identified, it should be tracked with each visit. The clinician should inquire briefly about signs of progress. Reading material can be assigned and discussed briefly at the next appointment. Many clinicians assume that someone else will help their patient or that a simple "you know you ought to stop" is sufficient. Many are waiting for multiple double-blind studies of a particular treatment before they are willing to take action. Many believe that enough is being done.

Utopia

It would be ideal if we knew the precise phenomenology of nicotine dependence. It would be wonderful if there was a magic cure. However, there is no magic bullet for nicotine dependence, and there probably never will be one, because the development of nicotine dependence is multifactorial, involving genetics, neuroendocrinology, the environment, and personality. Because its origins are multifaceted, recovery must address each aspect of the disease. Medicine (for drug craving and withdrawal symptoms) represents only a very small portion of the larger recovery picture. Many clinicians do not understand the difference between abstinence and recovery.[5]

Even if we were to believe in the medicine-only approach, as clinicians, we do not have the luxury to wait idly for someone to discover the ideal medication to cure nicotine dependence. The most realistic solution to the current pandemic problem of nicotine dependence is to know which medical and nonmedical approaches have been tried and which can serve as aids. Knowing both the resources and the research challenges that these approaches have undergone is where science ends. Deciding which smoking-cessation techniques to employ with a given patient is an art. The clinician must be aware of patient variables, which include motivational factors, effective cessation skills, social supports, psychosocial assets, and smoking-habit factors.[6]

It would be ideal if each community had a nicotine-dependence education and treatment center staffed by experienced nicotine-dependence treatment specialists. The center would furnish nicotine-dependence educators to local elementary schools to teach children to say "no" to nicotine in all its forms. Educators would also visit local junior high schools to educate students about the insidious evolution from controlled nicotine use to nicotine dependence and the loss of choice. The center would educate high school students about the gateway drug of nicotine[7] and how this drug regularly progresses to alcohol and other drug experimentation and

TABLE 20.1. Nicotine dependence treatment menu.

Level (number of cigarettes)	Intervention
1 (0–5/wk)	Education
	Bibliotherapy
	Willpower
2 (5/wk–10/day)	Minimal guidance
	Set target date
	Change brands
	Log use
	Fade by 20% every 4 days
	Silver acetate
3 (10–20/day)	Review Levels 1 and 2 attempts/relapses
	Behavioral and cognitive therapy
	Counterconditioning program
	Smokenders®
	Live for Life®
	Nicotine Anonymous
4 (over 20/day)	Review Levels 1–3 attempts/relapses
	Rule out mental disorders
	Rule out other addictions
	Hypnosis
	Acupuncture
5—Severe withdrawal	Review Levels 1–4 attempts/relapses
	Nicotine replacement
	Clonidine
6—Over 3 prior treatments	Review Levels 1–5 attempts/relapses
	Anticholinergic and other experimental medicines
7—Difficult-to-treat patients	Review Levels 1–6 attempts/relapses
	A new combination or inpatient treatment

Source. Adapted with permission from Cocores.[8]

addiction progression. The center would teach nicotine abusers about the disease concept of addiction and how it relates to nicotine.

The center would have an assessment center that would diagnose in a specific way the level of nicotine dependence and the presence of other mental, social, and physical problems. The center might offer a menu similar to Table 20.1.[8] A specific treatment plan would be generated for each of the addicts and their support persons. The treatment plan would draw from all the considerations in this book and would apply the most appropriate methods to the person and his or her history. Young nicotine users would be educated by attending early intervention programs, which would provide bibliotherapy, individual education, brief behavioral and cognitive therapy, and implementation of nicotine-fading techniques without medication or nicotine replacement. Nicotine-dependent persons who have been unable to abstain without the support and guidance of a structured program would be educated about the numerous treatment modalities available. They would then formulate their own treatment plan in conjunction with their treatment team, consisting of a physician, a therapist, and a family member or friend. Severely dependent patients would attend group and individual sessions five times during the first week, four times during the second week, three times during the third week, two times during the fourth week, and once each week for an additional 8 weeks. Ideally, the 3-month outpatient treatment program would be covered by most insurance companies.

The ideal outpatient nicotine-dependence education, resource, and treatment center probably does not exist in your community. It probably does not exist, as such, anywhere. However, most of the components do exist independently in your community. What is almost always missing is a community coordinator. Clinicians should, therefore, familiarize themselves with all the resources available to them. They should carefully review Goldsmith's chapter 7 on engaging the nicotine-dependent person into treatment. Regardless of clinical specialty or degree, clinicians are in the best position to identify nicotine dependence and to make treatment recommendations and interventions.

Prevention

Education is the best preventive measure we have. Education can help children to "just say no" to nicotine. Education has helped people stop using nicotine on their own, and nicotine-dependent persons are most attracted to minimal-intervention self-help approaches that can be learned through a number of mediums. As Fey and his associates point out in chapter 13, mass education may help as few as 4% of the smokers it reaches, while structured programs servicing 200 people per year may help as many as 80% or 160 smokers. However, if the mass-media approach reaches 10,000 people, then 400 smokers are helped. Both approaches are necessary because they target addicts in different stages of physical dependence, psychological dependence, and disease progression.

Nicotine-dependence education in particular and drug-dependence education in general is becoming more commonplace in schools and businesses. Some clinicians experienced in the diagnosis and treatment of substance-use disorders elect to volunteer their time a few times each year to address school assemblies and businesses. This is usually done in conjunction with employee assistance personnel or student assistance programs to educate and recruit users into trying willpower, bibliotherapy, other self-help aids, or one of many structured treatment programs available in their area.

Know Your Resources

Clinicians must first familiarize themselves with the educational material available to smokers and then facilitate its distribution. Table 20.2[9] lists a

TABLE 20.2. Selected smoking-cessation material and programs for clinicians and the general public.

Kits for clinicians
  Available from local divisions of the American Cancer Society
    Patient self-administered risk-assessment test
    Program package for health professionals
    Program package for pregnant women
    Kit for health professionals
  Available from the National Cancer Institute, Bethesda, MD
    Kit for pharmacists
    Kit for health professionals
  Available from the National Heart, Lung, and Blood Institute, Bethesda, MD
    A physician's guide to intervention
    Clinician's role for school-based intervention
    Risk of "Chronic Obstructive Pulmonary Disease" (COPD) using spirometer
  Available from the American Academy of Family Physicians, Kansas City, MO
    Stop smoking kit for physicians and patients
    Audiotape: "How to Stop Smoking"
  Available from the National Audio Visual Center, Capital Heights, MD
    A slide presentation
  Available from local offices of the American Lung Association
    Smoking and pregnancy kit for clinicians (patient materials available in Spanish)
    Program for parents and the physician of the newborn child

Videotape smoking-cessation programs
  Available from local offices of the American Lung Association
    "In Control; A Video Freedom from Smoking program"
  Available from Lorimar Home Video (1-800-323-5275)
    "Larry Hagman's Stop Smoking for Life"
  Available from local divisions of the American Cancer Society
    "Breaking Free"
  Available from the National Audio Visual Center, Capitol Heights, MD
    "We Can't Go On Like This"
  Available from the American Academy of Family Physicians, Kansas City, MO
    "The Family Physician's Guide to Smoking Cessation"

Self-help materials
  Available from local divisions of the American Cancer Society
    Quitter's Guide—Seven-Day Plan to Help You Stop Smoking
    How to Quit Cigarettes (made for blue-collar workers)
    Breaking Free Comic Book
  Available from local offices of the American Lung Association
    A Lifetime of Freedom from Smoking
    Freedom from Smoking for You and Your Baby
    Freedom from Smoking for You and Your Family
    Freedom from Smoking Clinic—A seven-session group program
  Available from local offices or the national office of the American Heart Association
    Smoking and Heart Disease
    Children and Smoking: A Message to Parents
    Calling It Quits
  Available from the Office on Smoking and Health, Rockville, MD
    Smoking Tobacco and Health: A Fact Book
    Pregnant? That's Two Good Reasons to Quit Smoking (Spanish version available)

Available from the National Cancer Institute, Bethesda, MD
  Clearing the Air
Available from Health Promotion Group, Inc., Homewood, AL
  A Pregnant Women's Self-Help Guide to Quit Smoking
Nicotine Anonymous (415) 922–8575

Group smoking-cessation programs sponsored by the American Cancer Society and the
American Lung Association
  Fresh Start
  Breaking Free
  Freedom from Smoking

Source. Adapted from Gritz,[9] with permission.

wealth of resources available to clinicians and their patients. There are
many easy-to-read books on the topic of smoking cessation.[10] There are
many easy-to-read books on the topics of relapse prevention and of recovery in general.[5] In addition, clinicians should familiarize themselves
with all the nicotine-dependence treatment programs in their locale. Each
provider is usually contacted, and specific methods of treatment, as well
as cost, are discussed. Each providers' flexibility and willingness to work
with you is assessed.

Clinical Symbiosis

Only after clinicians familiarize themselves with the educational materials
available to smokers and the treatment providers in their area are they best
able to manage nicotine dependence. What is researched simultaneously
are the treatments that are not available to nicotine users in a particular
geographic area. Most clinicians can find room to expand their practice to
include a specialized nicotine-dependence treatment and simultaneously
fill a void in their community.

  For example, suppose that a gynecologist discovers that no one in her
community prescribes clonidine or other medication-oriented treatments.
The gynecologist speaks to a local psychologist who conducts group and
individual therapy using behavioral and cognitive techniques for smoking
cessation. The psychologist prefers to treat patients without medications
but agrees to refer multiple relapsers or difficult-to-treat patients to the
gynecologist. The gynecologist prescribes and monitors nicotine replacement or another medication to help reduce withdrawal symptoms. The
psychologist conducts parallel treatment by simultaneously reviewing
relapse-prevention techniques and stress management, establishing a
support system, and referring the patient to a local nutritionist for exercise
and nutrition guidance.

  There are many creative instances of clinical symbiosis like this one.
For example, a psychiatrist researches local smoking-cessation programs

and discovers that most providers have great difficulty treating nicotine-dependent persons who also have major psychiatric disorders. The psychiatrist may have several high-functioning individual psychotherapy patients who smoke but does not want to dilute the psychotherapy process by treating their nicotine dependence. The psychiatrist chooses to refer these high-functioning psychotherapy patients to the local behavior-modification smoking-cessation program, while the program refers psychiatric patients who smoke to the psychiatrist for stabilization of the mental condition with medication before repeating the nicotine-dependence recovery program. As Taylor indicates in chapter 24, it is close to impossible to treat nicotine dependence if the coexisting untreated major psychiatric condition is not first stabilized.

In another example, a certified alcoholism counselor decides to advise her patients who smoke to set a nicotine-cessation target date to coincide with their 6-month anniversary of alcohol recovery. The counselor advises her patients to apply the knowledge and skills they developed for alcohol recovery to nicotine recovery. If the recovering alcoholic finds it difficult to stop smoking using this plan, then the counselor refers the smoker to a physician who prescribes nicotine replacement or a medicine considered safe for recovering alcoholics, such as clonidine.[11]

Conclusion

Nicotine-use treatment is optimal when tailored to the individual's level of motivation, level of dependence, social supports, and psychosocial assets, and when the treatment plan is negotiated between the clinician and the patient.[8] A particular treatment plan or method may be useful for some patients but not for others. To the best of our knowledge, there are no treatment centers that offer all possible combinations on an outpatient basis. Therefore, regardless of their specialty, health-care clinicians who are interested in helping their nicotine-dependent patients can do so by acting as community coordinators. At the same time, with a minimal amount of research, clinicians can also create their own specialized contributions toward the establishment of the ideal nicotine-dependence education and treatment program that should exist in every community.

References

1. Cinelli B, Glover ED. Nurses' smoking in the workplace: Causes and solutions. J of Commun Health Nursing, 1988; 5(4): 255–261.
2. Greene HL, Goldberg RJ, Ockene JK. Cigarette smoking: The physician's role in cessation and maintenance. J of Gen Internal Med 1988; 3: 75–87.
3. Carrell S. When more doctors smoked Camels. Am Med News 1989; 6(23): 35–36.

4. Geboy MJ. Dentists' involvement in smoking cessation counseling: A review and analysis. J of the Am Dental Assoc 1989; 118: 79–83.
5. Cocores JA. The 800-COCAINE book of drug and alcohol recovery. New York: Villard Books, 1990.
6. Orleans CT. Understanding and promoting smoking cessation: Overview and guidelines for physician intervention. Annu Rev of Med 1985; 36: 51–61.
7. Henningfield JE, Clayton R, Pollin W. Involvement of tobacco in alcoholism and illicit drug use. Brit J of Addiction 1990; 85: 279–292.
8. Cocores JA. The clinical management of nicotine addiction. In: Miller NS, ed. A handbook of drug and alcohol addiction. New York: Marcel-Dekker, 1990.
9. Gritz ER. Cigarette smoking: The need for action by health professionals. CA–A Cancer J for Clinicians 1988; 38(4): 194–212.
10. Schneider N. How to use nicotine gum & other strategies to quit smoking. New York: Pocket Books, 1988.
11. Cocores JA, Gold MS. Trancutaneous scopolamine for nicotine dependence: Use in non-addicts versus recovering addicts. Am Soc of Addiction Med 1989; 8: 23.

21
Residential Treatment

JOHN P. DOCHERTY

The apathy of our society in regard to the treatment of its most serious health hazard has been widespread. This apathy persists despite the numerous well-documented hazards for the individual smoker, the effects of passive smoking, and other tangible effects, such as the fact that cigarette smoking is responsible for more than 65,000 fires, causing more than $300 million in property damage per year. Local, state, and national fire data all list cigarette-caused fires as the leading cause of fire fatalities.[1]

Minimization has followed denial. We have offered treatments that are too brief, too restricted, and too simple. We have offered too little and often too late. Stop for a moment and consider the reaction that would occur if we were to purport to treat heroin addiction with seven group sessions of 20–50 participants, providing some education regarding the nature of heroin abuse and some take-home behavioral techniques to aid the addict on her or his way. Yet this is the way we have approached much of our effort to help the addicted smoker overcome his or her disease. It is no wonder then that the statistics with regard to the success of smoking-cessation efforts have been so dismal. Relapse rate within a year of quitting smoking is approximately 75%.[2]

We clearly have not addressed the treatment of cigarette smoking and nicotine addiction with sufficient seriousness. We have partaken of our culture's nonchalance with regard to this fatal and devastating illness. It is clear that we need to address this illness with at least as much seriousness as we address any other serious illness. This means that we employ research in the design of clinical practice, that we achieve an appropriate individual diagnosis prior to beginning treatment, and that we subsequently employ the panoply of appropriate therapeutic procedures referenced to the individual patient's diagnosis. This basic skeleton structure of medical treatment has not been applied to cigarette smoking. In addition, we should make available for the treatment of this problem the full range of resources that we know provide us with appropriate and necessary therapeutic leverage. One such resource that has demonstrated itself to be critical for many illnesses, including serious substance abuse problems, is the use of hospital residential care. Residential or inpatient care is an essential component of a continuum of services for the treatment of nicotine addiction. There are several important advantages that can be claimed for a residential setting.

Benefits of a Residential Setting

Control of the Availability of the Addictive Substance

We know well that the most important risk factor for the development and maintenance of any addiction is the availability and ease of access to the substance of abuse. This risk factor accounts for the higher rates of addiction of medical personnel. It is one of the rationales preventing legalization of substances of abuse, and ultimately it underlies every interdiction effort. On the immediate clinical level, we know that many addicts cannot begin to be successfully treated unless they are removed from a setting in which access to substances of abuse, such as nicotine, can be well-controlled. The outpatient setting, particularly in our contemporary society, does not afford this protection for the previously addicted individual.

Control of Social Influence

We also know that a second critical factor predicting substance abuse is the prevailing social influence to which a person is exposed. Many individuals who have difficulty with their problems of addiction do so because they are in a social environment that continues to facilitate the abuse. Such encouragement for continued substance abuse occurs in both overt and covert forms. A residential setting provides a method for removing individuals from such negative influence. Reciprocally, it provides an opportunity for formulating and delivering a social influence force strongly directed toward overcoming the addiction and maintaining abstinence. Such control of social influence is not possible in an open system such as outpatient or even partial hospital care.

Intensity of Treatment Intervention

A residential setting provides the framework and opportunity for an extremely intense treatment intervention. In essence, all of the patient's day can be turned toward therapeutic use. Kottke's[3] observation that treatment efficacy is related to the intensity of intervention, the amount of face-to-face contact, argues strongly for the availability of such a treatment option.

Coordination of Clinical Services

It is notably difficult in an outpatient setting, given the pragmatics of therapists' schedules, patients' schedules, travel time, and so on, to effectively and efficiently organize diagnostic and therapeutic services in a comprehensive and synergistic manner. The closed residential inpatient setting provides the opportunity to accomplish such a coordination and integration in an expeditious and effective manner.

There are various forms that a residential or inpatient treatment program may take. Variation may occur with regard to specific indications for admission to a particular program, such as age, gender, comorbid illnesses, program duration, spectrum of services provided and program intensity. The determination of the relative value of the different designs of such programs will ultimately benefit from empirical assessment. We present here the outline of a specific program that our preliminary work has indicated has greater than expected efficacy. We present it as one example of the form such a program may take. This chapter's presentation reviews the following:

1. Indications for admission to residential care
2. Major program elements and program structure
3. Program implementation issues

Indications for Hospitalization

We have identified three major indications for hospitalization and residential treatment:

1. Repeated failures at previous smoking-cessation attempts
2. Serious medical disorders exacerbated by smoking
3. Psychiatric disorders that may be exacerbated by smoking cessation

Repeated Failed Efforts to Stop Smoking

There are many patients who have tried to quit smoking but have failed repeatedly to stop or to remain smoke-free. These patients are often the ones who are the most highly dependent on nicotine, are the heaviest smokers, and experience the most severe withdrawal symptoms. For such patients who have shown failure in previous efforts that were assisted by treatment, residential treatment is indicated.

Medical Disorders

Hospitalization and residential treatment is also indicated for those patients who are suffering from a medical condition (e.g., disorders of the cardiovascular system, pulmonary disorders, or failure to control smoking during pregnancy made worse) by continued cigarette smoking. Most physicians are familiar with a number of tracheostomized patients who continue to try to smoke even through their tracheostomy holes. Similarly, there is the awful condition of persons with Buerger's disease, whose fingers and toes are falling off but who are unable to refrain from smoking because of the depth of their addictions. Less dramatic but still consequential indications for hospitalization are those patients suffering from numerous other serious medical conditions that are either complicated by or complications of cigarette smoking, such as coronary artery disease, chronic obstructive pulmonary disease, and lung cancer. Such patients cannot afford trials of the various treatments of less-restrictive environments.

Psychiatric Disorders

Treatment in a residential facility may also be indicated when the smoker has a psychiatric disorder or history of a psychiatric disorder that may be exacerbated by smoking cessation. The most common examples of these are anxiety disorders and depression. Previous reports have indicated, and our own data reflect, the development of full-blown depressive syndromes in the aftermath of smoking cessation.[4,5] Other data have revealed that serious smokers with comorbid psychiatric disorders, particularly depression, in outpatient treatment show an extremely high recidivism rate.[6] In such settings, it is likely that the psychiatric disorder will be inadequately recognized, evaluated, and treated during the smoking-cessation effort.

The Main Program Components

The program consists of two major components:

I. Evaluation component
   A. Comprehensive nicotine-addiction evaluation
   B. Physical assessment, including pulmonary function test, and carbon monoxide monitoring
II. Treatment component
   A. Group treatment module
      1. Psychoeducational groups
      2. Psychotherapy groups
   B. Individual behavioral treatment module
      1. Behavioral assessment and goal setting
      2. Relaxation training
      3. Relapse-prevention planning
      4. Planning for generalization of learned skills

    C. Family module
      1. Nature of nicotine addiction
      2. Reasons for quitting
      3. Relapse prevention
      4. Importance of family support
    D. Self-help module
      1. Invited speakers twice per month
      2. Nicotine Anonymous meetings
      3. Introduction to an aftercare outpatient group
    E. Biomedical module
      1. Nicorette
      2. Clonidine
      3. Antidepressant
    F. Health and nutrition module

The program is structured to cover a period of 2 weeks. We have experimented with various time frames and feel that 2 weeks is adequate time to contain most of the acute withdrawal period, to allow each individual to identify major issues related to the smoking problem, and to provide, for most people, adequate plans for aftercare. There usually are patients who will require further care in relationship to an emergent psychiatric syndrome. However, for the most part, 2 weeks seems to be an adequate time frame. Each aspect of this program is discussed next.

Evaluation Component

See Table 21.1. The nicotine evaluation that we use is based on a specialized set of instruments for the assessment of cigarette use and nicotine addiction. This set of instruments is proprietary and available through Health Enhancement Services, Inc.[7] It consists of a series of semistructured interviews providing detailed information about the most relevant aspects of the smoking problem. This set of instruments was developed based on review of the literature and was pilot-tested and refined for ease of use and reliability of scoring. It yields responses by the patients, which can be coded and quantified. In addition, through a computerized scoring method, a narrative report is generated, summarizing the main findings of the interview series. This body of information, in conjunction with several other instruments, forms the basis for specific treatment planning for the individual patient. The components of the nicotine assessment are the following:

1. Smoking history evaluation
2. Cessation history evaluation
3. Family smoking analysis

TABLE 21.1. Comprehensive nicotine addiction assessment.[7]

Smoking history evaluation	Cessation history evaluation	Family smoking analysis
Length of substance use	Previous cessation attempts (timeline)	Smoking behavior in family of origin
Environmental effects on use	Motivation for these attempts (e.g., children)	Smoking behavior in current family and/or living situation
Comorbidity with other substance use	Methods used in previous attempts	Cessation attempts used by family members who smoke
Patterns of use over time	Reasons for failure in previous attempts	Smoking-related illnesses suffered by family members
	Motivation for present cessation attempt	Level of familial support

SMOKING HISTORY EVALUATION

The following is a brief clinical example of some of the information that will be gleaned from the use of this instrument:

Mr. G. is a 55-year-old, white, married, father of six, who lists his occupation as truck driver but considers himself semiretired. Mr. G. has been smoking regularly since the age of 22, when he entered the armed services and tried his first cigarette. For the past 5 years, he has smoked a low-tar and low-nicotine cigarette. He reports that during the week, he smokes an average of 2 packs of cigarettes a day, but not while on the job, where it is prohibited. He says he smokes more on weekends and when he drinks coffee (he averages 15–20 cups per day) or alcohol. He feels that he is quite addicted to cigarettes and that quitting would be difficult, even if he really wanted to quit, which he is not sure he does.

CESSATION HISTORY EVALUATION

The following clinical example illustrates the type of information gleaned herein:

Mr. A.'s wife was a social smoker in the past (occasionally lighting up a cigarette at a party), she has been a strong force in his history of cessation attempts, pushing him from program to program. He feels that for the first time, this attempt will be different because he wants to quit as much as his wife wants him to quit. Therefore, he believes the environment at home will be highly supportive. In the past 2 years, he has thought about smoking almost all of the time. These thoughts were sparked by his brother's death from emphysema, his desire to watch his son grow up, and a recent attempt to become physically fit. He has noticed that he feels extremely winded after running distances he never used to have difficulty with. He has also been experiencing a mild cough in the morning. He has made four major attempts to quit smoking in the past 2 years. While in another state, he was involved in a rapid-smoking/aversive-smoking program, which he did not find helpful. He also involved himself in a program with nine other individuals, during which videotapes were used and he was told to drink lots of water. His most successful attempt lasted 3 weeks, when he used Nicorette gum. He liked the gum but feels he was not really prepared to quit smoking, and this was the cause for his relapse.

FAMILY SMOKING ANALYSIS

The following example illustrates the information that this evaluation component yields:

Mr. H. comes from a family of smokers. Both of his parents smoked while he was growing up, as well as his three brothers and two sisters. One brother was able to stop smoking by going cold turkey but relapsed after a short while off of cigarettes. All of his siblings are experiencing terrible coughs, particularly in the early morning. His father has been diagnosed with emphysema, although he continues to smoke. Mr. H. is currently living with someone who does not smoke. His two children are very distressed by his smoking and are very verbal with their objections. Mr. H. was not aware of his smoking's effects on his daughter's asthma. A family session has been scheduled to discuss his current attempt to stop smoking.

EVALUATION SUMMARY

We have found that this tripart form of evaluation is critical to the entire treatment effort. It represents the most advanced method for evaluation that has come to our attention. This methodology forms the core of our diagnostic evaluative process. We supplemented this core evaluation, additionally, with other widely used instruments. These include the Fagerstrom Tolerance Questionnaire, an eight-item questionnaire introduced by Fagerstrom in 1978, which allows for the assessment of probable physiological addiction to nicotine,[8] and the Addiction Research Unit's (ARU) Smoking Motivation Questionnaire, developed by Michael Russell in 1974.[9] This 24-item questionnaire helps identify primary motivators for an individual person's smoking. The motivators identified are psychological image, hand–mouth activity, pleasure, stimulation, sedation, relief of craving, and automatic behavior.

We have also found it useful to use the Hamilton scales for the assessment of anxiety and depression[10] because the emergence of anxiety and depressive syndromes are, in our experience, quite frequent during the cessation of smoking in individuals with serious nicotine-addiction problems. In addition, we score a 10-item nicotine withdrawal scale, in which each item is scored from 1, (not at all) to 10 (extremely), to assess the presence and severity of the following items: tension, anxiety, irritability, craving, restlessness, impaired concentration, sadness or tearfulness, drowsiness, dizziness, and overall withdrawal symptoms. These two scales (Hamilton and nicotine-withdrawal) are used as repeated measures during the course of the residential treatment period.

Treatment Component

PSYCHOEDUCATIONAL GROUP TREATMENT

This series of groups constitutes a core for the program, in which the patient is provided with a basic foundation of knowledge about the complex interplay of physiological, behavioral, psychological, emotional, and interpersonal factors that contribute to the initiation and maintenance of smoking, as well as the complex factors that lead to frequent relapse when smoking cessation is attempted. In addition, the patient learns about the nature of nicotine addiction and about the health and other consequences of smoking and is assisted in initiating abstinence. The patient is assisted, through this modality, in making changes in attitudes, behaviors, and life-styles that support continued abstinence through learning alternative coping methods.

Each session entails a period of group discussion. In addition, there is an audiovisual session schedule, which provides a source of focus for the group experience. Homework assignments are also used, to reinforce the major learnings of the group session.

The following is a description of the primary theme or themes for each therapy session. In the process of actually leading the group session, a critical task is to maintain the delicate balance between a more psychoeducational approach and a more psychotherapeutic approach. It is crucial that the patients be allowed ample opportunity for expression of the intense emotional reactions they experience during the process of withdrawal and recovery from nicotine addiction. However, acquiring a base of knowledge is also essential if the individual is to have the best opportunity for success in his or her recovery. Finally, actual attitude and behavior change through a process of problem solving and rehearsal of alternative coping skills is also an essential element of the group program.

Session 1: "Reasons for Smoking: Source of Habit/Addiction" primarily focuses on factors involved in the initiation of smoking, reasons for the maintenance of cigarette smoking, and the nature and severity of nicotine addiction.

Session 2: "Reasons for Quitting: Change and Resistance to Change" focuses on each individual's motivations and reasons for smoking cessation. Conscious and unconscious motivations for continuing smoking behavior, including fears regarding cessation, are also explored.

Session 3: "Cigarette Smoke and Nicotine: Effects in the Mind and Body" focuses on the physiological effects of nicotine and cigarette smoke and on the negative biomedical consequences of smoking.

Session 4: "Nicotine Addiction: The Nature of the Beast" introduces the concept of nicotine addiction as a disease. The characteristics of drug dependence in general and of nicotine addiction specifically are presented and discussed.

Session 5: "Nicotine Withdrawal: The Heebee Jeebies and How to Prevent Them" consists of discussions regarding group members' experiences with withdrawal symptoms at times they have attempted to discontinue cigarettes. The risks and benefits of pharmacotherapeutic treatments for nicotine withdrawal are also explored in this session.

Session 6: "Abstinence: The Initial Phase or 'Getting Over the Hump'" encourages patients to assist each other in developing positive methods of coping with their withdrawal symptoms. The video "The Ordeal of Arnold Hertz" is viewed and is used to stimulate a discussion of craving and the ways in which people, places, and things that have been intimately associated with smoking can create pressures toward, or actually precipitate relapse to, smoking. In addition, the videos "Gambling," which deals with the need for changes in life-style necessary to facilitate recovery, and "How to Sabotage your Treatment" are viewed.

Session 7: "Long-Term Abstinence: Holding Steady" comprises further discussion of common causes of relapse. The concept of relapse prevention as developed by Marlatt and Gordon[11] is presented. Patients begin to anticipate and prepare for difficult situations in which they might be prone to relapse and are assisted in planning specific strategies for dealing with these situations. Patients also learn to reframe incidents of relapse as temporary slips that may be turned into important learning experiences in which they can review and consider the need for changes in their coping mechanisms.

Session 8: "Interpersonal, Social, and Family Aspects of Long-Term Abstinence" focuses on interpersonal aspects of smoking and nonsmoking. The need for social support is emphasized, and the group discusses important individuals in the patient's life and the influence their attitudes and behaviors about the patient's smoking and nonsmoking can have on their own recovery.

PSYCHOTHERAPY GROUP

The psychotherapy group does not have a specific educational focus. Rather, it aims at facilitating the expression of strong feelings associated with smoking and the relinquishment of smoking. It focuses principally on the intrapsychic and interpersonal aspects of smoking behavior and nicotine use. Issues discussed in such a group involve the symbolic value of cigarettes, the nature of grieving in relation to quitting smoking, and the transition of identity from a smoker to a nonsmoker. Feelings of rage and failure in familial relationships and issues of autonomy and independence in relationships with authority figures are frequent topics of discussion. The group is run with a here-and-now focus for the main body of the meeting, shifting prior to termination of the session to a future relapse-prevention focus with regard to the issues raised.

INDIVIDUAL BEHAVIORAL MODULES

There are four major tasks that are scheduled for accomplishment with each patient in an individual setting. They are the following:

1. Behavioral assessment and goal setting
2. Relaxation training and learning to cope with withdrawal
3. Relapse-prevention planning
4. Planning for generalization of learned skills

Behavioral Assessment/Goal Setting

After a smoker decides that he or she wants individualized attention, it is important to evaluate the environmental, cognitive, and behavioral contingencies that support the smoking behavior. In this session, patients are interviewed about factors in their homes, work settings, and recreational involvements that need to be changed. Thought patterns that distort perceptions and alter self-esteem are evaluated. Reinforcements and secondary gains of smoking are determined. Patients then develop mutually agreed-on goals with the therapist and make a commitment to change these contingencies.

Relaxation Training/Coping with Withdrawal

At the early stages of recovery, patients need to tolerate the extreme physical effects of nicotine withdrawal. Diversion techniques, relaxation training, and educational materials are utilized, to help patients reach a more manageable state in their recoveries. Postacute withdrawal signs are also discussed.

Relapse-Prevention Planning

Each individually treated patient receives a relapse-prevention workbook, which is aimed at self-exploration of factors related to failed attempts at smoking cessation. Patients are encouraged to develop a list of warning signs that have had predictive validity in the past. Workbooks address cognitive, behavioral, biological, and social factors.

Planning for Generalization of Learned Skills

The preceding techniques are useless without application to the patient's natural environment. This session addresses ways in which patients can recognize warning signs and can respond readily without picking up a cigarette. Environmental changes are emphasized (e.g., changing cues at home which have been associated with smoking, avoiding smoking environments, coping with momentary urges caused by contact with cigarette smoke, and recognition of dangerous situations). Application of relaxation techniques is discussed. Role-playing techniques are utilized, in order to combat potential peer pressure. Finally, responses to slips are delineated.

FAMILY MODULE

Typically, two to four family sessions are held. In a program such as this, the number of family sessions is usually determined by the availability of family members, their willingness to participate, and the relevance for the patient of issues in the family. The goals of the family sessions are

1. To educate the entire family regarding the nature of nicotine addiction and the issues involved in the cessation of smoking
2. To elicit appropriate and effective family support
3. To counteract any negative processes present in the family situation
4. To involve the family in an effective aftercare plan

SELF-HELP MODULE

The core component of the self-help module is the Nicotine Anonymous meeting. These meetings are conducted in something of a *rap-group format*, in which a successful nonsmoker "tells her or his story." Through the Nicotine Anonymous group, the patients are educated in the 12-step model for the maintenance of abstinence. Additionally, patients are encouraged to attend an aftercare group, which provides a continuing base for support of the abstinence effort.

BIOMEDICAL MODULE

The biomedical module refers to the decision to treat the patient with a variety of medications that are available to assist in nicotine withdrawal and relapse prevention. These include Nicorette gum, a nicotine-replacement treatment; clonidine, an alpha-2 agonist used to decrease the symptoms of withdrawal due to its effect on the locus coeruleus; and an antidepressant, such as Sinequan doxepin, acting through an unknown mechanism, perhaps for the relief of the associated depression, to avoid subsequent nicotine use. These treatments are used depending on the severity of the person's nicotine dependence, physical condition, and psychological state.

HEALTH AND NUTRITION MODULE

The health and nutrition module consists of a series of exercise and fitness sessions, as well as nutritional education, to help rectify and stabilize the person's eating habits and to introduce a health-oriented life-style.

Program Implementation Issues

The Importance of Staff Education

It cannot be assumed that staff who are well-trained in general psychiatric or in chemical dependency care are adequately prepared to deal with nicotine addiction. This is a specialized form of biobehavioral disturbance, which requires specialized training. It is critical that the staff receive a thorough education themselves in the nature of nicotine addiction, the health consequences and effects of smoking, and, particularly, the phenomenology of nicotine withdrawal. They must be thoroughly familiar with the program philosophy, its treatment goals, and its treatment methodologies.

Lack of Familiarity with Psychiatric and Medical Disorders

The major indications and reasons for residential care will involve patients with some significant comorbidity. As a result, the staff must be both familiar with and comfortable with serious medical and psychiatric problems. Clearly, the nature and location of the residential treatment facility will dictate which staff will be selected and the nature of the patient population. For example, severely ill pulmonary patients will probably be treated in a general hospital program. Nonetheless, the main point to be made here is that staff must be able to understand and manage the nature of the associated illness of a particular patient population using their program.

The Presence of Countertherapeutic Forces

Despite extensive training and particular dedication, the treatment staff remains a microsociety of our larger society. As a result, it will harbor and reflect the same prejudices and values of that society. In particular, the tendency to minimize both the problem of nicotine addiction as a health consequence of smoking and the severity of the difficulty of managing successful withdrawal and abstinence from nicotine will be present. The patients will, further, be apt to generate this sentiment in the staff via regression, complaining, derogatory behavior, and lack of adherence to the treatment regimen. A forum for staff discussion, continuing staff education, and appropriate managerial intervention must be present in order to manage these countertherapeutic situations.

Coordinating and Integrated Multimodal Treatments

This is a problem of all intensive and comprehensive treatment programs. An effort to accomplish this integration is present both in program design, where each therapeutic intervention has its own particular purpose, and through the mechanisms of the treatment team and the treatment planning process. For each patient, the assessment yields a concrete and specific set of goals to be accomplished within each of the treatment modules. Treatment efficacy is assessed based on the degree to which each of these goals is accomplished.

Discharge Planning and the Importance of Aftercare

Despite the intensive effort that is made in the residential program, it constitutes only the beginning of treatment. It is critically important that the patient understand how essential it is that aftercare treatment continue, following discharge. The patient must be provided with a detailed discharge and aftercare plan, specifying the nature of the interventions and the patient's participation with them. In this regard, it is also important that the patient be introduced to the 12-step program and that interface with this program in the format that appears most appropriate for the individual patient be accomplished prior to discharge or plans for its continuation following discharge.

Summary

Based on the grim statistics regarding the prevalence of cigarette smoking, the dangers of cigarette smoking, and cessation-success rates, it is apparent that we need to strengthen our treatment efforts to contend with the seriousness of nicotine addiction.

Residential treatment for nicotine addiction is an intrinsic part of this effort. Inpatient care offers benefits not available in other forms of treatment; it provides a secure therapeutic environment in which patients have access to supportive staff, intensive treatment, and an atmosphere condusive to smoking cessation.

The program outlined in this chapter, we feel, is comprehensive and complete. It provides the necessary diagnostic and therapeutic interventions, psychoeducation, and a secure and supportive setting to help remediate obdurate addictions. For those individuals who have proven unable to quit smoking in other settings or for whom smoking has become exceedingly dangerous, residential treatment is an invaluable opportunity.

References

1. U.S. Department of Health and Human Services. The health consequences of smoking: Nicotine addiction (a report of the surgeon general). Washington, DC: U.S. Government Printing Office, 1988.

2. Hunt WA, Matorazzo JD. 3 years later: Recent developments in the experimental modifications of smoking behavior. J of Abn Psychol 1973; 81: 107–114.
3. Kottke TE, Battista RN, et al. Attributes of successful smoking cessation interventions in medical practice. A meta-analysis of 39 controlled trials. JAMA 1988; 259: 2882–2889.
4. Hughes JR: Clonidine, depression and smoking cessation. JAMA 1988; 259: 2901–2
5. Flanagen J, Maany I. Smoking and depression. Am J of Psychi 1982; 139: 541.
6. MacLellan AT, Luborsky L, Woody GE. Predicting response to alcohol and drug abuse treatments: Role of psychiatric severity. Arch of Gen Psychi 1983; 40: 620–625.
7. Proprietary material available through Health Enhancement Services. 42 Natka Drive, PO Box 539, Centerville, MA 02632
8. Fagerstrom K. Measuring degree of physical dependence to tobacco smoking with reference to individualization of treatment. Addict Behav 1978; 3: 235–241.
9. Russell MAH. Smoking motivation questionnaire London, England: Addiction Research Unit, 1974.
10. Hamilton MA. A rating scale for depression. J of Neurol Neurosurg Psychi 1960; 23: 56–62.
11. Marlatt GA, Gordon JR, eds. Relapse prevention: Maintenance strategies in addictive behavior change. New York: Guilford, 1985.

22
Smoking Cessation in the Workplace

CHRISTINE S. GLIDDEN and GEORGE LUTZ

A corporate culture that values health and well-being makes people feel good about themselves and improves their productivity. If a corporation approaches its employee population with open respect and sheds past attitudes of paternalism, it empowers all concerned to achieve a win-win balance.

As American business corporations recognize that they can have high impact on their employees in ways other than financial, and as insurance costs continue to skyrocket, smoking-cessation programs conducted in the workplace are a natural choice. In this way, businesses need no longer bear the heavy price of medical repair when a combination of individual employee responsibility and some corporate resources can prevent the most costly consequences of one of the nation's biggest killers.

The Workplace

Over the years, numerous and various workplace attempts have been made to help employees quit smoking.[1] The reasons for these programs are well documented and include lower rates of illness, mortality, absenteeism, and health-insurance-benefits usage. Clearly, smoking-cessation programs make economic sense. However, on a more idealistic level, some forward-looking corporations choose to make societal contributions by offering programs such as these, which have a potential of affecting the employee on the emotional, social, and spiritual levels, above and beyond cost savings. It is true that major corporate cultural shifts occur only when both economic need and popular support coexist; let us not undervalue the willingness of upper management to respect and respond to the needs of the employee popultion.[2]

The workplace is a powerful force in today's society. With both men and women working in such great numbers, this facet of our societal life has grown in impact. People spend a large portion of their lives at work. Before, business was dominated and populated by men while women demonstrated their value at home and with the family, but today, the workplace is shared with women in ever-increasing numbers. As a result, business continues to affect men, and it grows in its influence on women and the family.

People identify themselves a great deal with how they make money. Typically, the question asked after meeting someone for the first time is, "How are you?" The second question is, "What do you do?" To varying degrees, workplace culture often provides identity, defines values, and suggests behavioral norms for its participants. The way we dress, the value we place on rigidly following the rules or being innovative, and, by extension, the degree to which we are health-conscious at home are subtly, sometimes unconsciously, determined by our collective mentality called "culture." Using the power of the corporate culture to minimize smoking behavior is a very useful beginning to a successful smoking-cessation program.[3]

Changing the Culture

Changing the culture occurs in several ways at several levels. The motivation to change is in place; smoking cessation makes economic sense, and on some level and for some personal reason, virtually all smokers know that they want to quit.

Structurally, the work organization begins by limiting and ultimately eliminating the number of locations where smoking can occur.[4] Insurance-benefits contributions by the employee are lowered for nonsmokers. Funds and resources are released for wellness programs and facilitates and, specifically, for smoking-cessation programs.

As with all culture shifts, gaining the support of upper management is immeasurably useful. Releasing funds is one thing; getting management smokers to participate in the program and to enforce smoking regulations in the boardroom and with their important customers, is often another.

Probably, the single most significant factor in successful culture change is a thorough, constant, relentless, but varied bombardment of messages repeated to employees, signaling that a healthy lifestyle is in their own best interest. This positively based message probably begins as a general encouragement toward health and is backed up by specialized programs in areas including physical fitness, nutrition, stress management, meditation, cardiac stress testing, weight management, cholesterol testing, parenting, avoidance of alcohol and other drug abuse, and many, many others. Complements to these programs are cancer-detection methods, caretaking of elderly parents, and, of course, smoking cessation.

This wellness culture may take years to accomplish, but recent public media have given us some help. The key here is to get employees talking about and thinking about health in its various forms. Even employees who are suspicious, resentful, or resistant on these issues are at least thinking about them. The level of initial resistance to these programs is directly related to their ultimate success. Posters, educational presentations, newsletter promotions, contests, and the modeling of healthy behavior are mediums for the bombardment of the message. Coordinating events with the date that the organization goes smoke-free is useful. A sense of deadline and time urgency is created. Or perhaps smoking can be hooked into an existing corporate program. Other than wellness, perhaps smoking cessation can be marketed as a safety program mentioned at safety meetings or at first-aid trainings.

As the culture assimilates the wellness message, peer pressure opposing smoking will develop. When nonsmokers complain about smoking permitted in bathrooms, when smokers feel uncomfortable restricted to only a small area in the lunchroom, or when an off-site meeting occurs and only one person smokes and everyone collectively acknowledges that fact, peer pressure is working.

The Holistic Partnership

Many approaches to smoke cessation have been attempted, typically in the form of a single-focused effort. A hypnotherapist might be hired by the *Employee Assistance Program* (EAP—a free mental health counseling service available to all employee); or the wellness department might offer smoking-education training and exercise and nutritional guidance as a support for interested parties. The medical department might prescribe nicotine gum for those who fear quitting "cold turkey" (i.e., abruptly stopping, without any medical assistance or nicotine replacement). All of these worthwhile programs accomplish several things: (1) a continuation of the "smoking is unacceptable" message bombardment; (2) a forum for people who—even if they do not participate—can learn more; (3) an informative experience for participants who fail; and (4) a method for people to successfully give up smoking. Each of these treatment programs can be effective, but just not for everyone every time. Relapse should not be interpreted as failure because the more times a smoker tries to quit, the more likely it is that the smoker will eventually quit.

The piece that is missing in these singularly focused programs, however, is professional teamwork and cross-expertise. What really works best once the health consciousness of the employee population is raised, is an intensive coordinated effort by medical,[5] EAP, and wellness personnel. As corporate health departments grow in expertise and sophistication, all programs will be delivered by this combined partnership.

The members of this partnership need to expect several things from themselves and from each other. First, each individual needs to be nicotine free. Second, each individual must have a working knowledge of addiction and must have personally experienced the difficulty of terminating a compulsive behavior, be it eating, shopping, drug taking, worrying, working, exercising, caregiving, or whatever. The EAP counselor can be helpful to those who are unclear on these issues. Third, the partnership members need to value and support each other's efforts. A certain amount of emotional investment goes into a program such as this, and burnout can easily occur. Partnership support meetings should be scheduled, to enhance a well-orchestrated and unified treatment team. Finally, the partnership needs to understand that it is in this for the duration. Short-term quick fixes are ineffective and disorderly. Failure should be seen as temporary, an interlude between successes. This positivism will permeate the program and will relieve the pressure on the participants.

A Sample Smoke-Free Program

ETHICON, a major manufacturer of wound-closure products, including surgical sutures and stapling devices, has approximately 6000 employees at seven locations in the United States and Puerto Rico. The program described here originated at the headquarters location in Somerville, New Jersey, where there are approximately 2400 employees. This sample program is being gradually disseminated to the company's other locations. A sophisticated Live for Life Partnership has evolved over the past 10 years, with active communication and cross-referral among the core modalities of medical, EAP, and wellness personnel. This partnership is proactively involved in a holistic and preventive approach to occupational health management, including addictions, stress management, and ergonomics.

Early in 1989, the company announced that it will have become totally smoke-free on October 1, 1990. This was a catalyst to an innovative and intensive smoke-free process for the employees, which started in January, 1989. Several key elements combined at this time to facilitate the smoke-free process: (1) the Live for Life Partnership approach to tobacco smoking behavior as an addiction, similar to addiction to alcohol or other drugs included the use of a pharmacological treatment to block nicotine withdrawal craving; we chose to use scopolamine skin patches[6] (any pharmacological treatment with which the physician is familiar can be used). (2) The combined peer pressure of society, management, and fellow employees was used to minimize and ultimately eliminate the cigarette smoking in the workplace. (3) The approaching smoke-free workplace deadline served as an incentive to smoking cessation.

Previous smoking-cessation programs of this Live for Life® Partnership had included the use of clinical hypnosis and nicotine gum. The use of the scopolamine skin patch or disc is discussed in chapter 18 of this book, but briefly, this patch is placed behind the ear, usually for a period of 6 days, as a chemical blockade to nicotine craving. One of the advantages of this method is that the smoker is almost immediately able to abstain from nicotine without suffering withdrawal. However the bad news is that slight side effects may be present; if a side effect occurs, it usually sends the smoker back to medical, wellness, or EAP professionals, where the smoker is monitored, supported, and counseled. The more contact the smoker has with a professional resource, the more help he or she will absorb.

After the partners are clear on their roles and everyone is prepared to start, the program is advertised, and informational sessions are announced, including dates and locations. A few visible, self-disclosure-prone smokers are encouraged to attend. At the first session, the chemical basis for nicotine addiction is explained. Use of the scopolamine patch and clinical hypnosis is detailed. Attendance at *all* sessions and groups is emphasized.

After the first session, smokers are invited to sign up. Group size ranges from 10 to 25 participants. Some smokers report that after signing up, their enthusiasm is so high that they stop smoking in anticipation. That is fine. It does not matter when they quit or how they quit or whether they succeed, it is only important that they quit.

Those who sign up are scheduled for short medical and psychological readiness evaluations. Each smoker is checked by a nurse for blood pressure, medications, alcohol usage, preexisting conditions, and any other complicating issues. The EAP counselor interview examines for signs of depression, alcohol or other drug abuse, psychosis, previous treatment, and existing crises. At this point, some smokers will be advised to wait or to drop out entirely. Those who are accepted need to be convinced to attend all sessions, to commit to regular self-hypnosis, and to ask for help if they need it.

Within 48 hours, the day to quit arrives, and a second group session occurs. At this session, questions are answered, the scopolamine patches are distributed, a group hypnosis with a three-part message is introduced, and tapes of the hypnosis are given out for individual use. The group at this session creates a dynamic of its own. Participants talk and share in the groups and in the workplace. The partnership members have all been introduced and their roles identified. Smokers are sizing up who they will go to if they encounter a problem. A hotline number is announced for after-hours concerns. Everyone feels a connection to this group effort. Smokers go home, have their last dose of nicotine, and put on the patch.

During the next 48 hours, each smoker (now ex-smoker) is contacted at least once by the EAP counselor. Anyone suffering a reaction of any kind is encouraged to schedule a visit. Those experiencing physical side effects are directed to the medical personnel. The ex-smoker feels supported and special.

Approximately 2 days later, a third group session is held. By this time, the group has really coalesced. People are sharing experiences before the session is called to order. Stress-management techniques are introduced; diet and exercise regimens are described as being especially important at this time. Losing one's best friend, the cigarette, often leads to bereavement. Another group hypnosis is performed. Ex-smokers begin deeper forms of self-disclosure on such issues as family support, grief and loss, and fear of failure or success. Ex-smokers are encouraged to connect with one another between sessions. Peer pressure becomes peer support.

At this point, nearly everyone is smoke-free and doing well. Those who are not need undivided, individual attention. Again, losing one's cigarette friend can result in anxiety, depression, or increased abuse of alcohol or other drugs. Many ex-smokers are exercising and eating well and may have undergone individual fitness screenings and exercise evaluations.

One week later, a fifth session is held, to discuss triggers, the red flags of relapse, and general progress. Many people will drop out after this session, as subsequent sessions are voluntary, so effort is made to encourage everyone to continue attending. The topic of smoking, though still popular, takes second place in aftercare groups to discussion of relationships, compulsive behaviors other than smoking, and stress. This is where the power of the group is most evident. People share their feelings and are supported. This, in turn, encourages others to take similar risks.

The question of confidentiality may arise, and if it does not, the partnership facilitator should bring it up. Sharing may expose the group members' vulnerabilities, and these feelings need to be honored and handled with respect. Virtually all employees in any given workplace keep a side of themselves very secret to coworkers. Employees feel that upon disclosure in group, these secrets will be spread beyond the boundaries of the group. Others who are otherwise willing to self-disclose may resist because they fear breach of confidentiality. Facilitation of a workplace group requires clarifying the issue of confidentiality. Scheduling individual sessions or group sessions at the end of the day may be helpful. Otherwise, referring an ex-smoker to an external resource is also an alternative.

Subsequent sessions are held weekly, and as more programs are conducted, additional ex-smokers are fed into ongoing weekly groups, or a group may request to be closed to newcomers because of size or to cultivate a sense of continuity and group intimacy. The topics of discussion in aftercare groups gradually dwell more and more on nonsmoking issues. However, depending on the expertise of the facilitator, the group can resemble a therapy/support group or can adhere strictly to the 12-step model of Nicotine Anonymous. Membership is fixed in the case of a therapy group.

Special Problems

For those organizations that offer shift work, special strategies need to be considered. Effort should be given to include second- and third-shift employees. Depending on the number of shift employees and the number of smokers within the shift, the extent of the resources is determined. The other consideration is partnership availability. One smoking-cessation program should be made available to these smokers, with the understanding that a second convenient program is questionable. Programs offered in the evening are probably ideal because spouses and children of day-shift employees may attend. Family members are regular users of benefits and also may make or break the effort of the smoking employee to kick his or her own habit. A list of local Nicotine Anonymous meetings should also be distributed.

Another problem encountered in such programs is the sense of entitlement some employees have when improved health is perceived to be the responsibility of the company and not of the individual. The investment of the employee's precious time and payment of a fee create a sense of owenrship and responsibility vital to success. The fact that the partnership members (medical, EAP, and wellness) are free, accessible, and so encouraging of emploees often allows the employee to undervalue their roles. For this reason, the members of the partnership need to maintain a professional stance with employees. Individual sessions are scheduled; drop-ins are not allowed except in emergencies. To a point, encouargement is helpful, but when encouragement becomes enabling behavior (doing the smoker's emotional work for him or her), partnership members consciously need to keep each other honest. After all, smoking is an addiction, and addicts seek out enablers. Be careful not to allow an individual or the whole partnership effort to be seduced into that role.

Determination of the quit rate is based on self-reported data. Naturally, all participants want to succeed and to be seen as successful. Some participants may feel enough pressure from family, friends, coparticipants, and themselves to be less than completely honest. There is no best way to deal with this problem other than to emphasize directly that relapse is expected from a certain percentage of people and that trying again is always a feasible option.

A Perspective on Success

Let us evaluate the success of this holistic approach. The fact that a certain percentage of smokers are nicotine abstinent is not the only form of success. We are certainly satisfied that after 1 year, 60% of the first group[6] remains smoke free, but let us consider other forms of success even for those who relapsed.

Participants had the opportunity to learn more about the effects of smoking and the value of proper nutrition and regular exercise, and though they may still be smoking, perhaps a positive change in diet has occurred. Participants now know their current blood pressure. Participants learned what the addictive process is and are now able to apply that model to their drinking, eating, spending, or work addiction. The model is universal and applicable to all compulsive behaviors. For example, a so-called failed smoker may visit the EAP office next time for help with his or her gambling. In fact, because we know that addiction does not exist in a vacuum, terminating one addiction typically exacerbates another. In other words, squeezing the balloon at one end only forces the air to the other end. Historically, we have considered smoking to be an emotionally innocent habit. This is untrue. Many, many of these smokers are satiation addicts. If you take away their cigarettes, they will seek out satiety in other forms—eating, alcohol, sex, TV, and so on. Many of these people eventually present with dissatisfying relationships of some kind. Fortunately, at the workplace, group and individual counseling can be made available to those people. Of course, upper management, which needs to fund these services, needs to understand the direct correlation between personal health and productivity.

In addition, if persons are experiencing low-to-medium dissatisfaction with their lives, there is only a moderate chance they will seek professional help until the progression develops to the point of crisis. With any smoke-cessation program, particularly if it includes scopolamine, dissatisfaction is usually exacerbated by loss of the tobacco friend and/or the cessation's side effects. This quickly forces the person into more intense sad or angry feelings, without a lot of resultant behavioral changes, which typically incur consequences. This, in effect, raises the so-called bottom that most people need to hit to desire change. Without a raising of that bottom, most people would continue to slowly self-destruct and experience further deterioration of self-esteem and relationships. So, as some of these smokers feel these feelings, they fall into the ready and capable safety net of medical, EAP, and wellness.

Participant are very much aware that a caring, professional, helpful resource is available to them for any personal problem encountered in the future. They have names, faces, and some history with a resources person who can see to it that help will be provided. If handouts are included as part of the educational process and participants take them home, family members at least have a resource with a name and phone number attached.

Another form of success concerns itself with information the partnership has been able to gather on individual participants and on the employee population as a whole. The next time the employee visits medical, EAP, or wellness personnel, a personal profile of some kind will exist, which gives the staff member a head start on understanding who this employee is. Also, in talking to the individual participants and observing interactions in the groups, the partnership can better understand through extrapolation the values and needs of the entire employee population. Program development should then reflect those needs.

On a systems level in which organizational mental health is monitored, programs such as these are invaluable because they provide for the monitors, the luxury of putting a fleeting but accurate finger on the pulse of the organization. People talk if you listen, and they tell you what is happening in their departments. Listening with a trained and experienced ear allows the monitor to evaluate the system for stressful changes; for burned-out departments; for high-impact, anxiety-provoking managers; for work overload areas; for stress-causing policies; and for general morale. Intervention strategies can be developed where possible. For example, if competition is particularly fierce within a department, team-building exercises could be introduced; or on a large scale, if work overload is substantiated across the board, training in work prioritizing and a cultural shift in the way the organization views the performance of work could be very beneficial.

Brief Mention of Schools

There is little difference between the workplace and the schoolroom. School is simply the early workplace. A school is an organization with its own culture, set of rules and policies, values, rewards, punishments, and versions of power—who has it, who does not, how it is used, and how much of it is synonymous with control. One would hope that a medical department, a student assistance program, and some form of wellness program exist. The components and the process are the same.[7,8] In general, medications should be avoided when treating addescents who use nicotine. Bibliotherapy is very useful with this predominantly nondependent population.[9] Fading and minimal-intervention self-help aids are also useful.

The one difference that does exist between work and school is the age of the participants. The younger the person, the less likely that he or she has begun to smoke. For this reason, greater effort should be placed on prevention. Cigarette smoking is considered a gateway to other drugs, including alcohol and marijuana. Successful prevention of cigarette smoking, therefore, is especially important. The concept of "just say no" is helpful for those children who are not smoking or who are contemplating cigarette smoking, but past these two stages, this simplistic approach then begins to feed the denial mechanism present in all addictions.

Summary

Traditional, one-dimensional smoking-cessation programs administered at the workplace can provide a useful beginning for a smoke-free employee population. However, a broader, more logistic approach will foster much greater results.

Creating a corporate culture that regards total health as desirable and smoking as unacceptable will go a long way in motivating people to stop smoking and in turning peer pressure into group support. Upper-management commitment and policy changes can help initiate this culture change.

A holistic approach that includes the physical, psychological, social, and spiritual aspects can be achieved by combining the expertise of wellness, medical, and EAP personnel. Benefits gained by this are innumerable and exceed smoking cessation alone. Making a contact such as this with an employee often touches the employee intimately and assures him or her that an effective resource is available for the resolution of any type of problem. Supported, functioning, and aware people make productive employees, responsible parents, and contributing societal members.

References

1. Bibeau DL, Mullen KD, McLeroy KR, et al. Evaluations of workplace smoking cessation programs: A critique. Am J of Prev Med 1988; 4(2): 87–95.
2. Blyth-Bristow B. Implementing a smoking policy at work—A case study. Occup Health 1989; 6: 163–165.
3. Sorensen G, Pechacek TF. Implementing nonsmoking policies in the private sector and assessing their effects. New York State J of Med 1989; 1: 11–15.
4. Biener L, Abrams DB, Emmons K, Follick MJ. Evaluating worksite smoking policies. New York J of Med 1989; 1: 5–10.
5. Fisher EB, Bishop DB, Mayer J, et al. The physician's contribution to smoking cessation in the workplace. Chest 1988; 2: 56s–65s.
6. Cocores JA, Goias PR, Gold MS. Treatment of nicotine dependence in the workplace. Ann of Clin Psychi 1989; 1: 237–240.
7. Olds RS. Promoting child health in a smoke-free school: Suggestions for school health personnel. J of School Health 1988; 58(7): 269–271.
8. Glynn TJ. Essential elements of school-based smoking prevention programs. J of School Health 1989; 59(5): 181–187.
9. Cocores JA. The clinical management of nicotine addiction. In: Miller NS, ed. A handbook of drug and alcohol addiction. New York: Marcel-Dekker, 1990.

23
Treatment of Nicotine Dependence in Chemically Dependent Inpatients

ARYEH L. KLAHR

"Primum non nocere"—First, do no harm—has been the credo of physicians for centuries. As substance-abuse specialists, we are violating this dictum by not aggressively addressing nicotine dependence in rehabilitation programs. Omission of nicotine treatment during rehabilitation or aftercare promotes further dependence and "enables" patients to continue smoking. Nicotine is the single most preventable cause of morbidity and mortality and is, by far, the most widespread manifestation of drug dependence in our society today.[1,2]

Smoking kills more people annually than twice the number of combined deaths from other addictions. Nicotine is now considered to be as addictive as heroin. Proportionately, there are fewer social smokers than drinkers or other drug users. Significant numbers of alcoholics and other addicts state that it is more difficult to give up smoking than to discontinue their other drug of choice.[3–7]

Smokers, like other addicts, continue to compulsively use nicotine regardless of the consequences, yet we continue to treat smoking as a bad habit rather than as an addiction. We help our patients to recover from alcoholism and other drug dependencies and largely ignore the hazards of nicotine dependence.[8–11] Ninety percent of recovering alcoholics are nicotine dependent.[12–16] Dr. Bob and Bill W., the founders of Alcoholics Anonymous, both died from smoking-related illnesses. Why do we neglect to address the problem of dependence on nicotine? There is increasing evidence that the ill effects of smoking may be worse in alcoholics and addicts, due to the synergism of alcohol, nicotine, and other drugs in promoting certain cancers and health problems.[7,9,12,17,18]

The population as a whole is rejecting smoking. The number of adult males who smoke has dropped from 50% in 1965 to 31% in 1987. Unfortunately, there has not been a proportionate decrease in smoking among recovering alcoholics or other drug addicts.[4,6–12,14,17,19,20]

Nicotine dependence has not been forcefully treated in chemical dependency units, mainly due to the myth that such treatment would affect one's maintenance of sobriety and our denial of nicotine as a devastating addiction. The long-held belief that a recovering addict should not stop smoking until the primary addiction is stabilized is not supported by scientific evidence.[4,8,18,21-23]

Conversely, there is evidence that smoking cessation enhances one's ability to maintain abstinence, serves as a model for cognitive confrontation of all drug craving, and aids in acquiring skills for relapse prevention applicable to treating other drug dependencies. A strong phenomenological link between nicotine addiction and alcoholism is being recognized. Smokers are more likely to drink than nonsmokers. Drinkers are more likely to smoke than nondrinkers.[6,7,9,17,20-22] Most people smoke more when they drink, and some only smoke when they consume alcoholic beverages. Heavy drinkers smoke more than light drinkers, and heavy smokers drink more than light or nonsmokers.[15,16,19] Cigarette smoking is being studied as a predictive marker for alcohol-abuse severity. Alcohol and nicotine have both depressant and stimulant actions and may act on the same pathways in the brain. One may serve as a trigger for the use of the other. Nicotine's psychoactive or mood-altering effects, as well as withdrawal symptoms, are well known to every smoker and are documented in the literature. We continue to deny these problems when directing our patients to abstain from all mood-altering substances, explicitly omitting nicotine.[18,20,24-27]

It is time to "walk the walk" and not just "talk the talk." Patients are now requesting treatment for nicotine addiction. Our society is less tolerant of smoking—not only in what it can do to harm the smoker, but in the passive sidestream smoke that poses a danger to the nonsmoker.[28]

Alcoholics Anonymous and the recovering community have led the world in helping millions of people lead happier and healthier lives by recognizing and vigorously promoting treatment and education of alcoholism and other addictions. We have lagged behind in the treatment of nicotine dependence and in preventing its devastating progression and fatal consequences, especially among the ranks of recovering people.[6,9,12,17,18,20]

This chapter examines the extent of the problem, attempts to understand how the problem arose, and proposes methods for change. It explores how addiction professionals and chemical-dependency units have properly educated their patients and have integrated the treatment of nicotine dependence into their programs.

Extent of the Problem

In 1987, 29% of all adults were smokers. This represents a significant decline from the 40% of all adults who smoked in 1965. Unfortunately, the numbers of alcoholics and other addicts who smoke has remained fairly constant at 90%, according to multiple studies conducted over the past 20 years.[9,14,15,19,21]

Alcohol consumption increases tobacco consumption, and the reverse appears to be true. In rats treated with nicotine, ethanol consumption increased. It is hypothesized that nicotine induced a state of hyperactivity (which the rats counteracted by alcohol use) and that cross-tolerance exists between alcohol and nicotine, which may cause use of one to lead to increased use of the other. As mentioned previously, both alcohol and tobacco have stimulant and depressant properties; both act on common pathways in the brain and may increase the metabolism of the other.[18,25–27]

The implications of these findings are that contrary to long-held beliefs, abstaining from one while using the other may be more difficult than abstaining from both and that the continued use of either can act as a stimulus for the other.[9,12,18,20,29–31]

In a survey of 311 alcoholism-treatment professionals, 23% indicated they would never support encouraging a recovering alcoholic to attempt cessation of nicotine use, and 46% stated that they individually did not do so. This was particularly true among 57% of respondents who indicated that they were recovering alcoholics who still smoked, as opposed to 30% of nonalcoholic smokers.[9,11] In a survey conducted at the Veterans Administration (VA) Medical Center in Minnesota, 63% of 410 admissions stated that they had attempted to quit smoking, and 36% indicated the desire to do so.[20,32,33]

Seventy-two percent of chemical-dependency program directors believe that nicotine addiction deserves the same attention as other addictions, yet only 11% include its treatment in their programs. Another 23% felt that smoking cessation would interfere with recovery from other dependencies. Eighty-three percent felt it would be more difficult for patients to stop smoking than to stop their drug of choice.[20,32,33]

The concept of cross-addiction and the need to treat polysubstance abusers by abstaining from all mood-altering chemicals is readily accepted in relation to alcohol, cocaine, marijuana, and other drugs, but it continues to be denied in relation to nicotine. However, this is changing. It is now accepted that those who attempt to stop smoking while continuing to drink report that relapse to nicotine was often preceded by drinking.[29–31]

Health Consequences of Combined Drug Dependence

The risks for oral, pharyngeal, esophageal, pulmonary, and other cancers are greatly increased by combined alcohol and tobacco consumption. Men who drink are 6 times more likely to develop oral cancer. Smoking increases the risk 7 times, and the combination of smoking and drinking increases it to 38 times. Clearly, alcohol and tobacco act synergistically in increasing the risk of cancer and other health problems, such as hypertension, heart disease, and diabetes.[6,9,11,12,19]

It is known that marijuana is cancer-promoting. It is known that pulmonary damage follows the use of marijuana and crack cocaine.[34] Although studies are lacking, it is suspected that the addition of cigarette smoking to the use of other smokeable drugs such as "ice" (amphetamine) results in an additive influence on pulmonary dysfunction.

Barriers to Treatment

Historically, the treatment of alcohol and other drug dependencies were separated. In some programs, opiate abusers were told that they could drink. Today, treatment has merged, and polysubstance use is the norm. Treatment goals include abstention from all mood-altering chemicals, with the noted exception of nicotine. This situation exists because of the myth that nicotine is less harmful than other drugs. This myth persists because of the following reasons: cigarettes are legal and more socially acceptable, and the damage is less immediate, apparent, and chaotic when compared to alcohol and other drugs.[7,9,12,17,18,20,21,32,33,35] Cultural factors play a role as well. Advertisers have portrayed smoking as sexy, macho, sophisticated, and in the past, even healthy. One of the reasons is public denial. Many of the people who make the rules and set policy are active nicotine addicts.[17]

Contradictory reasons for not addressing nicotine dependence on chemical-dependency units exist. Nicotine is minimized as an addiction. It is believed that the patient can be left to deal with this addiction at a later date. Yet, it is also believed to be too stressful to attempt smoking cessation simultaneously with abstention from alcohol and other drugs because it may precipitate return to other drug use. Another fear is that the recovering drug addict will focus on nicotine and will make nicotine recovery a priority over recovery from other drugs.[9,12,17,21,32,33,35]

Data indicate that substance abusers crave nicotine as much as or more than their other drug of choice. Data also suggest that addicts are not very successful in stopping on their own. Drug addicts who smoke are more likely to score higher on nicotine-dependence rating scales and therefore to be more nicotine dependent than non–drug addicts. Data are emerging, suggesting that smoking cessation does not precipitate drug relapse; on the contrary, it may enhance the ability to maintain abstinence from all drugs, including alcohol. In a sample of recovering alcoholics who attempted to abstain from nicotine, not one reported relapse to alcohol because of smoking cessation.[7,9,12,14,17,18,20,21,32,33]

On chemical-dependency units, the most notable barrier to instituting a smoking-cessation program is the resistance from nicotine-dependent staff members. They are threatened by the notion that they are actively chemically dependent. Their attitude conveys denial, rationalization, and minimization to patients. Staff members are also uncomfortable with the individual willpower model, which 95% of people who stopped smoking have used to succeed.[17,24]

Administrators fear patient loss, marketing difficulties, and difficulties in enforcing a smoke-free policy. To date, no hospital that has gone smoke-free has experienced a significant change in admissions or occupancy as a result of a smoke-free policy.[9,17,20,21,32,33]

Methods for Change

Administrative commitment is the first step in implementing a smoke-free unit. As societal opposition to smoking increases, with its ban from airlines, subways, buses, and other facilities, it will become increasingly difficult for hospitals, dedicated to promoting health, to permit smoking. In 1988, only 8% of hospitals were smoke-free. By the year 2000, former Surgeon General C. Everett Koop has called for all hospitals to become smoke-free.[32,33]

In some states, chemical-dependency and psychiatric units have been exempted from legislation aimed at requiring hospitals to become smoke-free. In preparation for implementing a smoke-free policy, a survey of attitudes regarding smoking can help focus attention on nicotine dependence. Staff denial and resistance to accepting nicotine as a true addiction and as a gateway drug can be dealt with by education. Lectures, seminars, workshops, and the dissemination of written material will aid in confronting denial and will assist in acceptance of the need to treat nicotine dependence. Staff commitment and cohesion is essential for success; otherwise, they will sabotage the program.[17,32,33]

Recovering staff members make a lasting impression on patients. Smokers are less effective in promoting smoking cessation than nonsmokers. Therefore, counselors who are recovering from nicotine dependence will greatly enhance the implementation of a smoke-free unit and should be sought for employment.[17,21]

Many alcoholics and other addicts who wish to stop smoking are easily discouraged by their fear of failure and require a lot of support and encouragement. Recovering staff members who have been successful in abstaining not only from alcohol and other drugs, but from nicotine as well, serve as a powerful example. Staff members who undermine or discourage smoking cessation are the greatest barrier to implementing a smoke-free chemical-dependency unit. All efforts to hire nonsmoking staff members and to encourage those smoking staff members to stop should be undertaken. Having smoking staff members on a smoke-free unit and attempting to counsel patients in smoking cessation is similar to employing an active marijuana smoker as a drug counselor.[17]

The process of change requires approximately 1 year if an aggressive stance is taken. Smoking-cessation programs and education seminars should be made available to employees, with the support of administration.[17,32,33]

Smoking cessation is more effective when techniques and strategies are tailored to the needs of alcoholics and other addicts. The advent of Nicotine Anonymous World Services—(415) 922-8575—and their promotion of meetings and adoption of the 12 steps of Alcoholics Anonymous as a cornerstone of recovery from nicotine dependence will aid the recovering community with nicotine dependence.[9,10,17]

Chemical-dependency units should begin to include assessment of nicotine use and consequences during the initial intake process. Diagnosis of nicotine dependence should be included in the patient's chart. A comprehensive nicotine policy statement setting guidelines and outlining parameters for implementation of a smoke-free unit should be formulated. It should include informing patients of the smoke-free nature of the unit and should outline staff responses to violations of policy.

Detoxification from nicotine can be accomplished simultaneously with detoxification from alcohol and other drugs. The specific method—clonidine, antidepressant, hypnosis, acupuncture, nicorette gum, or fading—is best left to individual preference until it is ascertained whether there is a preferred method of detoxification from nicotine in alcoholics and other addicts.

Bibliotherapy and audiovisual materials, as well as didactic lectures addressing the pharmacology, psychoactive properties of nicotine, and its shared features with other addictions, should be incorporated into the treatment program. Nicotine should be addressed in group and individual counseling sessions as well.

Relapse-prevention strategies, including stress management and behavioral and cognitive techniques for dealing with cravings, urges, and environmental cues, should be offered. Recovery-oriented principles learned from treating alcohol and other drug addiction should be applied to nicotine recovery.[17,36]

Aftercare plans should include encouraging attendance at smoke-free Alcoholics Anonymous and Narcotics Anonymous meetings. Recovering addicts in need of additional support should also attend Nicotine Anonymous, to deal with the chronic relapsing nature of nicotine dependence and to be part of a supportive peer group.

Early Results

Reports from chemical-dependency units treating nicotine addiction along with other chemical dependencies are encouraging and indicate the feasibility of treating nicotine dependence simultaneously with alcohol and other drugs without threatening total recovery, although long-term results are not fully known. At the very least, such treatment has increased the awareness of nicotine dependence and the potential to be nicotine free. Fears regarding loss of patients or staff have not been realized, and resistance to implementing the smoke-free units is less than was anticipated.[7,9,17,20,21,32,33]

Conclusion

It is clear that smoking/nicotine dependence among alcoholics and other addicts represents a greater threat to their long-term health than their identified drug of choice. Treatment centers and the recovering community have long ignored this, partly because of myth and partly because of denial.

To promote health among our patients, this link between nicotine, alcohol, and other drug dependencies must be appreciated and addressed. Methods for overcoming resistance to treating nicotine dependence need to be identified and pursued.

The acceptance that the use of one substance may trigger relapse to the use of the other[36] should help motivate us to include nicotine in this message. Simultaneous abstention from alcohol, nicotine, and other drugs does not threaten sobriety, and by eliminating cues, triggers, urges, and cravings, induced by one substance for the other, actually reinforces it.

The health consequences of this association between alcohol, tobacco, and other drugs justifies further research clarifying their interrelationship. Specific areas to be examined include how best to integrate and tailor smoking-cessation programs to the needs and treatment of alcoholics and other addicts and to establish and test long-term relapse-prevention techniques and strategies.

References

1. Mann LS, Johnson RW, Levine DJ. Tobacco dependence: Psychology, biology, and treatment strategies. Psychosomatics 1986; 27: 713–718.
2. U.S. Department of Health and Human Services. Reducing the health consequences of smoking: 25 Years of progress (a report of the Surgeon General). Washington DC: U.S. Government Printing Office, 1989.
3. U.S. Department of Health and Human Services. The health consequences of smoking: Nicotine addiction (a report of the Surgeon General). Washington DC: U.S. Government Printing Office, 1988.
4. Kozlowski LT: Comparing tobacco cigarette dependence with other drug dependencies. JAMA 1989; 261: 898–901.
5. Sees KL, Clark HW: Use of clonidine in nicotine withdrawal. J of Psychoactive Drugs 1988; 20: 263–268.
6. Kozlowski LT, Jelinek LC, Pope MA. Cigarette smoking among alcohol abusers: A continuing and neglected problem. Can J of Public Health 1986; 77: 205–207.

7. Kozlowski LT, Skinner W, Kent C, Pope MA: Prospects for smoking treatment in individuals seeking treatment for alcohol and other drug problems. Addict Behav 1989; 14: 273–278.

8. Bobo JK, Gilchrist LD, Schilling RF, et al. Cigarette smoking cessation attempts by recovering alcoholics. Addict Behav 1987; 12: 209–215.

9. Bobo JK. Nicotine dependence and alcoholism epidemiology and treatment. J of Psychoactive Drugs 1989; 21(3): 323–329.

10. Bobo JK, Schilling RF, Gilchrist LD, Schinke SP. The double triumph: Sustained sobriety and successful cigarette smoking cessation. J of Psychoactive Drugs 1986; 3: 21–25.

11. Bobo JK, Gilchrist LD. Urging the alcoholic client to quit smoking cigarettes. Addict Behav 1983; 8: 297–305.

12. Battjes RJ. Smoking as an issue in alcohol and drug abuse treatment. Addict Behav 1988; 13: 225–230.

13. Maletzky BM, Klotter J. Smoking and alcoholism. Am J of Psychi 1974; 131: 445–447.

14. Burling TA, Ziff DC. Tobacco smoking: A comparison between alcohol and drug abuse inpatients. Addict Behav 1988; 13: 185–190.

15. Dreher KF, Fraser JG. Smoking habits of alcoholic out-patients. Int J of Addict 1967; 2: 259–270.

16. Istvan J, Matarazzo JD. Tobacco, alcohol, and caffeine use: A review of their interrelationships. Psychol Bull 1984; 95: 301–326.

17. Cocores JA. The clinical management of nicotine addiction. In: Miller NS, ed. Handbook of drug and alcohol addiction. New York: Marcel Dekker, 1990.

18. Zachny JP. Behavioral aspects of alcohol tobacco interactions. In: Galanter M, ed. Recent developments in alcoholism. Vol. 8. New York: Plenum Press, 1989; 205–219.

19. Carmody TP. Affect regulation, nicotine addiction, and smoking cessation. J of Psychoactive Drugs 1989; 21: 331–341.

20. Knapp J. Nicotine dependency: How are we dealing with it? CD Professional 1989; April, May, June: 2–5.

21. Joseph AN, Kristin NL, Willenbring ML, et al. Beneficial effects of treatment of nicotine dependence during an inpatient substance abuse program. JAMA 1990; 263(2): 3043–3046.

22. Miller WR, Hedrick KM, Taylor CA. Addictive behaviors and life problems before and after behavioral treatment of problem drinkers. Addict Behav 1983; 8: 403–412.

23. Hedlund JL, Vieweg BW. The Michigan Alcoholism Screening Test (MAST): A comprehensive review. J of Operational Psychi 1984; 15: 55–65.

24. Jones RT. Tobacco Dependence Chapter 171. In: Meltzer HY, ed. Psychopharmacology the third generation of progress. New York: Raven Press, 1987.

25. Collins AC, Burch JB, deFiebre CM, et al. Tolerance to and cross-tolerance between ethanol and nicotine. Pharmacol Biochem Behav 1988; 29: 365–373.

26. Schuster CR. Theoretical basis of behavioral tolerance: Implications of the phenomenon for problems of drug abuse. In: Krasneger NA, ed. Behavioral tolerance: Research and treatment implications. NIDA Monograph Series 18, USDHHS Publication No. (ADM) 78-511. Washington DC: U.S. Government Printing Office, 1978: 1–17.

27. Burch JB, deFiebre CM, Marks MJ, et al. Chronic ethanol or nicotine treatment results in partial cross-tolerance between these agents. Psychopharmacology 1988; 95: 452–458.

28. U.S. Department of Health and Human Services. The health consequences of involuntary smoking (a report of the Surgeon General). USDHHS Publication No. 87-8398. Rockville, MD: Author, 1987.

29. Wise RA. The neurobiology of craving: Implications for the understanding and treatment of addiction. J of Abn Psychol 1988; 97: 118–132.

30. Shiffman S, Read L, Jarvik ME. Smoking relapse situations: A preliminary typology. Intl J of Addiction 1985; 20: 311–318.

31. Burling TA, Stitzer ML, Bigelow GF, Russ NW. Techniques used by smokers during contingency motivated smoking reduction. Addict Behav 1982; 7: 397–401.

32. Knapp JM, Kottke TE, Heitzig C. A controlled trial to implement smoke free hospitals. Minnesota Med 1989; 72: 713–716.

33. Knapp J. Smoking in Minnesota's chemical dependency facilities: Survey results. CD Professional 1989; April, May, June: 4–5.

34. Klahr AL, Miller NS, Roehrich HG Chapter 6 Marijuana. In: Giannini, JA, Slaby, AE, eds. Drugs of abuse. Oradel, NJ.: Medical Economics, 1989.

35. Carroll JF, Malloy TE. Combined treatment of alcohol and drug dependent persons: A literature review and evaluation. Am J of Drug Alcohol Abuse 1977; 4: 343–364.

36. Cocores JA. The 800-COCAINE book of drug and alcohol recovery. New York: Villard Books, 1990.

24
Nicotine-Dependent Psychiatric Patients

WANDA TAYLOR, JAMES A. COCORES, and MARK S. GOLD

The treatment of psychiatric disorders requires a constant awareness of the various factors that affect outcomes in both a negative and a positive manner. For example, we know that the social support derived from friends, spouse, or other family members is an unquestionable positive factor in not only improving but also in maintaining optimal mental health. However, schizophrenic patients do better in a low-emotional-expression setting in which family members minimize the amount of feelings expressed toward the schizophrenic member.[1]

Another factor that requires careful consideration and that can have a positive effect on treatment outcome of psychiatric disorders is the choice of psychotropic medication. On this path, one needs to be aware of the biochemical and psychosocial variables associated with the particular disorder, as well as the targeted neurochemical pathway of the medicine selected. An adequate trial of the medicine selected at an appropriate dosage and duration is essential.

The importance of the effect of several substances, such as alcohol, illicit drugs, and nicotine, on mental health has been investigated extensively.[2–5] Studies clearly indicate that alcohol is a central nervous system depressant, and after a few hours, alcohol contributes to central nervous system irritability, expressed as tension and anxiety. It has been established that as many as 50–60% of psychiatric patients abuse alcohol. The treating practitioners do not hesitate in advising depressed as well as other psychiatric patients to refrain from the use of alcoholic beverages. The alcohol deters improvement of the depression, and the depression deters progress with alcohol and other drug recovery.[6] Similarly, the symptoms of anxiety disorders temporarily improve with alcohol and then worsen because of the alcohol withdrawal phase. Anxiety fuels alcohol abuse, and alcohol use fuels anxiety disorders. The goal of dual-diagnosis treatment is to disrupt this morbid synergism by managing each illness separately but concurrently.

What is not as clear are the effects of nicotine on mental disorders. It is estimated that 50–84% of psychiatric patients smoke cigarettes[7] and that the majority of these patients are schizophrenic or bipolar. O'Farrell and associates studied addictive behavior among a group of hospitalized psychiatric patients.[8] They surveyed 309 veterans on 10 psychiatric wards. Alcohol and other drug abuse treatment units were excluded. Their findings revealed that 83% of patients were smokers.

Another study examined the prevalence of smoking in a group of psychiatric outpatients.[7] There were 277 patients surveyed in the Minnesota general psychiatric clinic. Controls included two groups: 1,440 Minnesota residents and 17,000 U.S. citizens collected by the National Health Interview Survey. Socioeconomic variables, alcohol abuse, and marital status were controlled for; the psychiatric patients had a 1.6-fold higher rate for smoking, compared to the general population. The smokers tended to be younger and showed a higher prevalence of schizophrenia, mania, depression, and anxiety. There was also a higher incidence of being prescribed psychotropic medications in smokers.

While there is a recognition that the majority of psychiatric patients smoke, there is a reluctance to advise these patients to abstain from smoking as we would with those who drink alcohol or use illicit drugs.[9] This reluctance may be based on several prevailing facts and questions: (1) Nicotine appears to calm some psychiatric patients and to alleviate stress. (2) Very little is known about the effects of nicotine on behavior, the brain, and prescribed psychoactive medicines. (3) Concern has been expressed that nicotine abstinence will lead to exacerbation of psychiatric symptoms. (4) It is not known which nicotine-dependence-management methods will be most beneficial in a particular psychiatric population. (5) Once the method of nicotine-dependence management is mutually agreed upon, clinicians must determine when it is to be initiated and by whom.

Regulation of Affect and Pain

Nicotine is rapidly absorbed from tobacco smoke across alveolar membranes into the bloodstream. A very small amount is absorbed across the buccal mucosa. Buccal absorption is described more extensively in Cocores's chapter on smokeless tobacco. Nicotine from cigarettes reaches the brain within 10 seconds, with blood levels that are elevated in minutes.[10] Hence the physical and psychological effects of nicotine are experienced almost immediately. Nicotine is known to have a biphasic response on cholinergic receptors. At low doses, there is a stimulatory effect, but at higher doses there is blockade. The chronic effect is one of initial stimulation, followed by the depressant effect of blockade.[11]

Nicotine affects the release of acetylcholine, norepinephrine, dopamine, and serotonin. Nicotine also acts on neuroendocrine transmitters such as beta-endorphin, adrenocorticotropic hormone, vasopressin, prolactin, and growth hormone.[12]

A few of the physical effects include increased heart rate, increased blood pressure, increased stroke volume, and decreased peripheral blood flow. These and other physical effects of nicotine mimic anxiety and sedative withdrawal.

There are many reports in the literature on the effects of smoking on anxiety and pain reduction.[13-20] Pomerleau and associates investigated the pain response in subjects by using a cold pressor test and induced anxiety by using unsolvable six-letter anagrams. Results showed both pain and anxiety reduction following cigarette smoking. This response may be due, in part, to beta-endorphin release. Seeking relief from emotional discomfort, pain, and anxiety are all common explanations given by smokers for their smoking behavior.

Nicotine and Medication

Results of the Boston Collaborative Drug Surveillance Program showed the reaction of nicotine and commonly used medicines.[21] Smoking offsets the pain-relieving effects of propoxyphene and reduces the sedative effects of benzodiazepines and neuroleptics.[22] It is hypothesized that the liver microsomal enzymes are stimulated, which increase the metabolism of these and other medicines. Nicotine also effects tricyclic antidepressant metabolism and blood levels. Therefore, the blood level of many medicines tend to be lower in smokers when compared to nonsmokers on comparable doses of medicine. The blood level of many medicines can abruptly increase with nicotine cessation. Propranolol, acetaminophen, amobarbital, cimetidine, furosemide, heparin, and oral contraceptives are also affected by nicotine.[22,23] It is essential to assess the nicotine use status of all psychiatric patients.

Psychiatric Disorders

One thing that must always be kept in mind with the dually diagnosed patient[6] is that both disorders must be treated. Ideally, this is done concomitantly and in a parallel fashion. However, the parallel treatment approach is not always possible with psychiatric smokers, though it is with alcoholic smokers. I remember when I was in training, I discussed with an analyst the treatment of alcohol dependence in a depressed patient. The question was, Which do you treat first, the addiction or the depression? The response surprised me as to its simplicity, as well as its commonsense approach. Her response was, "Which illness is going to harm the patient most immediately? If the patient is outside standing on the window ledge, you first have to bring him inside the room before you can do any other

TABLE 24.1 A partial list of medical mimics of psychiatric disorders.

Category	Medical mimic
Substance abuse	Illicit drugs, over-the counter, prescribed, and alcohol use
Endocrine disorders	Hypothyroidism, diabetes, Cushing's disease, Addison's disease
Central nervous system	Alzheimer's disease, multiple sclerosis, partial seizure disorder, Huntington's chorea
Infectious disease	Syphilis, mononucleosis, pneumonia, tuberculosis, AIDS
Cancer	Lung, pancreatic, carcinoid syndrome
Nutritional and toxic disorders	Lupus
Collagen vascular diseases	
Metabolic	Wilson's disease, porphyria

treatment." In the treatment of nicotine-dependent psychiatric patients, this consideration always needs to be kept in mind.

Another important consideration when dealing with nicotine-dependent psychiatric patients is the possibility of medical mimics.[24,25] Table 24.1 illustrates a partial list of medical mimics of psychiatric disorders. For example, when a patient is being evaluated for depression, one must consider medical mimics of depression, such as thyroid disorders, anemia, diabetes, or occult cancer.

Only after the psychiatric disorder is stabilized is the nicotine dependence treated. This general rule does not apply to all psychiatric patients or to all psychiatric disorders. However, it applies to most.

Affective Disorders

The management of nicotine-dependent bipolar patients and nicotine-dependent depressed patients are essentially identical, although the bipolar nicotine-dependent patient can be more challenging.

If a patient is diagnosed with major depressive disorder and symptoms that include fatigue, appetite disturbances, sleep disturbances, loss of concentration, irritability, hopelessness, and suicidal thoughts, the first step in treating this dual diagnoses scenario would be to stabilize the depression first. Depressed patients must first restore their interest in pleasure, concentration, memory, desire to live, and other cognitive functions in order to extract, accept, and practice the behavioral and cognitive elements needed to recover from nicotine dependence.

Glassman and his associates treated smokers in an outpatient setting for smoking cessation and found that 61% of patients had histories of depression.[26] Patients with current presentation of depression were excluded. Many who were nicotine-dependence treatment failures had a history of depression. There are several suggestions for the correlation between smoking and depression: depressed people self-medicate themselves with nicotine, low self-esteem may predispose people to smoke, the loss of a significant other (nicotine) is followed by bereavement, or nicotine influences neurotransmitters that play a role in depression.

Glassman used clonidine, an alpha-2 noradrenergic receptor agonist, for smoking cessation. The use of clonidine is based on other studies showing beneficial use of this medicine in opiate withdrawal.[27] The overresponsiveness of the locus coeruleus, leading to increased firing, is believed to be responsible for many of the withdrawal symptoms seen. Clonidine acts to decrease the firing rate of the locus coeruleus. This has been shown to be beneficial in aiding smoking cessation by a similar mechanism. However, alternate treatment modalities may be warranted for patients presenting with a past or present history of depression.

Several investigators have used tricyclic antidepressants as treatment for smoking cessation.[28-31] This has been done with the idea that dysphoria experienced from nicotine withdrawal would respond to the use of these agents. Also, these medicines may affect neurotransmitters in ways similar to nicotine's effects. Edwards et al. studied the effects of doxepin versus patients who stopped "cold turkey" (i.e., abruptly and without medication such as nicotine replacement or antidepressant) in a 5-week pilot study.[28] They excluded those patients with clinical depression. Inclusion criteria were women between the ages of 26 and 70 who were highly motivated for treatment, had previous failures with smoking cessation efforts, and had experienced withdrawal symptoms in previous cessation attempts. Eight of 29 patients started doxepin in titrated doses up to 150 mg/day. Self-rated withdrawal symptoms revealed that dropouts were more frequent in the cold-turkey group. There was a positive effect of doxepin in decreasing subjective withdrawal symptoms.

Doxepin is an antidepressant with strong anticholinergic effects. Patients appear to know when they are taking active ingredients because of the common side effects of drowsiness, dry mouth, and blurred vision. In the preceding study, it may be that the patients perceived that a medication was at work, and this may have affected their ability to stop smoking. On the other hand, antidepressants act on neurotransmitters, such as acetylcholine, dopamine, norepinephrine, serotonin, and other substrates that are also acted on and released by nicotine, which are related to depression. Also, the anticholinergic properties of doxepin may have assisted with smoking cessation, as discussed by Climko in chapter 18.

The treatment of nicotine-dependent affective disorder patients begins with a thorough assessment of current and past symptoms of affective illness. In many cases, nicotine dependence can be treated without medication after the affective disorder is stabilized. If behavioral–cognitive techniques and nicotine fading alone are no match for nicotine withdrawal symptoms then the antidepressant being used can be increased. If an antidepressant is not being used to treat the affective disorder, then one can be added for nicotine-withdrawal symptoms and bereavement for about 3 months.

A common scenario is the presentation of a seemingly motivated nicotine-dependent patient with a history of multiple relapses; further investigation of a possible underlying masked affective illness is in order with chronic relapsers. Chronic nicotine relapsers often turn out to be dually diagnosed with either another chemical dependence or a major psychiatric disorder, or both.

Anxiety Disorders

The use of an antidepressant along with a comprehensive treatment plan that includes behavioral–cognitive therapy and wellness (stress management, nutrition counseling, exercise program) components may be adequate for nicotine-dependent anxiety patients, as is the case with depressed smokers. Again, the anxiety disorder will have to be stabilized first in most cases.

Medical mimics of anxiety disorders should be considered prior to making a diagnosis. Too often, insomnia and anxiety disorders are addressed before addressing the underlying caffeine dependence. Caffeinism is an extremely important differential diagnosis. Caffeinism contributes to depression and mimics anxiety disorders. Caffeinism also may limit the recovering nicotine-dependent person in obtaining long-term recovery.

If nonmedicine approaches have been unsuccessful, then the clinician should consider medicating the nicotine-dependent anxiety patient. First, consider manipulating the patient's anxiolytic medicine upward temporarily (for about 3 months or until smoking cessation is facilitated). Naturally, medicine alone is not the answer. The increase in dose should be accompanied by a smoking-cessation program.

If the patient is not on medication or a medication needs to be added, then medical treatment with clonidine may be appropriate, as this decreases the firing rate of the locus coeruleus. In addition, clonidine can be effective treatment for some anxiety disorders.

Benzodiazepines have always been very fashionable treatment of anxiety disorders. In the past, diazepam (Valium) was overprescribed, and today, similar practices hold true for alprazolam (Xanax). Although, the benzodiazepines may be useful in managing anxiety for a few months, most anxiety patients need to take medicine for years. This increases the risk of developing tolerance and benzodiazepine dependence. Benzodiazepines have also been piloted for smoking cessation, with relatively poor results. In fact, benzodiazepines function similarly to alcohol, in that the resulting disinhibition often results in increased smoking behavior. Benzodiazepines should never be prescribed to alcoholics or other drug addicts for smoking cessation.

Clonidine, or the tricyclic antidepressants are probably more appropriate with anxiety-disorder patients. Usually, the medicine is started and a nicotine-fading schedule is started (i.e., gradual reduction of nicotine intake each day for about 3 weeks). Before the zero-nicotine target date, behavioral and cognitive techniques are reviewed, stress management is reviewed, an anxiolytic diet is outlined, and an exercise program is initiated.

If tricyclic antidepressants or clonidine are inappropriate, then other medicines may be useful. Other experimental medicines that have been used to ease nicotine withdrawal symptoms are discussed elsewhere in this text and include beta-blockers, calcium-channel blockers, buspirone (BuSpar), and fluoxetine (Prozac). Nonmedicine approaches such as hypnosis can be especially useful with nicotine-dependent anxiety patients.

Psychotic Disorders

Psychotic patients are a very heterogeneous group. Some schizophrenics decompensate in a group therapy setting. These patients are difficult to treat for schizophrenia, and these patients are the most difficult to treat for nicotine dependence, using traditional methods. In fact, it is close to impossible. These are the patients who many psychiatrists hopelessly recall when faced with the dual diagnosis dilemma. The reality is, however, that many psychotic patients and most psychiatric patients can be helped with smoking cessation.

There is another group of stabilized psychotic patients who can be treated. They are more socialized and higher functioning. Nicotine fading is useful with this group in conjunction with a complete individual-therapy smoking-cessation program.

Some specific medications and smoking-cessation methods can aggravate psychosis. For example, the use of antidepressants in psychotic patients can often exacerbate the illness. Bromocriptine or scopolamine can precipitate psychosis. The use of hypnosis is contraindicated in psychotic patients.

Attention Deficit Disorder [32,33,34]

Nicotine-dependent attention deficit disorder (ADD) patients are difficult to treat for the former (nicotine dependency) without first or parallel treatment of the latter (ADD). Individuals who have difficulty concentrating, extracting information, learning, assimilating, and practicing new ways to think and act about nicotine use are incapable of recovery or at least unlikely to recover[32] from nicotine dependence. Also, drug craving has been viewed in terms of dysfunction in attention to recovery;[33] people who have difficulty focusing on the consequences experienced from drug use tend to glamorize drug use—glamorization of drug use is the forerunner of craving.

It is easy to treat nicotine-dependent ADD patients after the ADD is corrected. If traditional ADD medicines are feared or contraindicated (e.g., for a recovering cocaine addict), then consider safer options, such as bromocriptine,[32,33] imipramine, pemoline, and Bupropion (Wellbutrin).[34]

Neuropsychiatric Disorders

Nicotine affects many neurotransmitters. There is evidence of changes within the acetylcholine (cholinergic–nicotinic) receptor sites. Barclay and Kheyfets studied a group of patients with Alzheimer's disease and observed that most lost their desire to smoke many years before the onset of Alzheimer's disease.[35] They also noted a lack of withdrawal symptoms, such as altered appetite, that also preceded Alzheimer's disease. These investigators suggest that there are changes in central nicotinic receptors that precede Alzheimer's disease, which simultaneously facilitate smoking cessation at a neurochemical level.

Newhouse and associates conducted a pilot study in which they infused probable Alzheimer's patients with nicotine and monitored cognitive and behavioral changes.[36] The cognitive and behavioral changes were monitored before, during, and after nicotine infusion. They found an improvement in long-term recall of objects that occurred during the infusion. Behavioral changes included anxiety and depression. The authors felt that the changes were age related and/or reflected changes in nicotinic–cholinergic function.

The effects of nicotine on the dopaminergic system has been investigated.[37] As already mentioned, there is a high rate of nicotine addiction among schizophrenic patients. This is especially true of schizophrenics taking neuroleptic medication. Other studies suggesting nicotine's role as a dopamine agonist include case reports of the use of nicotine gum in conjunction with haloperidol for the treatment of Tourette's syndrome.[38] There is also evidence that smokers are less likely to develop Parkinson's disease. Parkinson's disease involves impairment of the nigrostriatal dopamine system.

Investigators have also looked at the relationship between nicotine and tardive dyskinesia. In tardive dyskinesia, the striatal dopamine function is enhanced. Yassa and associates looked at the question of whether nicotine increased the development of tardive dyskinesia.[39] Patients with the diagnosis of schizophrenia or affective disorder were evaluated, and patients with an organic mental disorder were excluded. Smoking habits, presence of movement disorders, current medication (neuroleptic doses were converted to chlorpromazine equivalents), and duration of illness were studied. Of those studied, 154 were schizophrenic, and 15 had an affective illness. There were 70 men and 84 women. Results were as follows: There were no differences between smokers and nonsmokers in terms of age, gender, or duration of illness. The number of patients on anticholinergic medications were similar between smokers and nonsmokers. The smokers with tardive dyskinesia were on higher neuroleptic doses than nonsmokers with the disorder. The enhancement of dopamine may account for the increased prevalence of tardive dyskinesia. However, the authors did not suggest a direct cause-and-effect relationship between nicotine and tardive dyskinesia and suggest further studies.

Conclusion

There are reports of positive effects of nicotine on stabilization of some schizophrenic patients, on memory in Alzheimer's disease, and in the potentiation of haloperidol in correcting Tourette's syndrome. However, even if these benefits prove to be true, they do not overshadow the benefits of managing nicotine dependence in patients with other stabilized psychiatric disorders. In addition, the possible increased risk of tardive dyskinesia in smokers needing higher doses of neuroleptic medication is another good reason to encourage recovery from nicotine dependence.

Nicotine dependence affects both the physical and mental condition of our patients. There is no single treatment that will fit all psychiatric patients. The clinical management of nicotine-dependent psychiatric patients requires the selection and application of an appropriate smoking-cessation treatment plan carefully matched to the stabilized psychiatric disorder and the individual psychosocial profile. Outpatient psychiatrists are probably the physicians best trained to manage nicotine-dependent psychiatric patients. Psychiatrists should no longer ignore their responsibility for managing nicotine-dependent psychiatric patients. Further research is a necessity in this particular aspect of dual diagnosis.

References

1. Vaughn CE, Leff JP. The influence of family and social factors on the course of psychiatric illness. Brit J of Psychi 1976; 129: 125–137.
2. Dackis CA, Gold MS. Depression in drug abusers. Washington DC: American Psychiatric Press, 1984: 20–39.
3. Kosten TR. Pharmacotherapeutic interventions for cocaine abuse. J of Nerv and Mental Disease 1980; 177(7): 379–389.
4. Kosten TR, Schumann B, Wright D, et al. A preliminary study of desipramine in the treatment of cocaine abuse in methadone maintenance patients. J of Clin Psychi 1987; 48(1): 442–444.
5. Kleber HD, Weissman MM, Roundsaville BJ, et al. Imipramine as treatment for depression in addicts. Arch of Gen Psychi 1983; 40: 649–653.
6. Cocores, JA. Treatment of the dually diagnosed adult drug user. In: Gold MS. Slaby AE, eds, Dual diagnosis patients. New York: Marcel Dekker, 1990.
7. Hughes JR, Hatsukami DK, Mitchell JE, et al. Prevalence of smoking among psychiatric outpatients. Am J of Psychi 1986; 143: 993–997.

8. O'Farrell TJ, Connors GJ, Upper D. Addictive behaviors among hospitalized psychiatric patients. Addict Behav 1983; 8: 329–333.
9. Cocores, JA. The 800-COCAINE book of drug and alcohol recovery. New York: Villard Books, 1990.
10. U.S. Department of Health and Human Services. Nicotine: Pharmacokinetics, metabolism, and pharmacodynamics. In: Nicotine addiction—a report of the Surgeon General. Washington, DC: U.S. Government Printing Office, 1988.
11. Benowitz NL. Pharmacologic agents of cigarette smoking and nicotine addiction. New Engl J of Med 1988; 319(20): 1318–1330.
12. Fuxe K, Andersson K, Eneroth P, et al. Neuroendocrine actions of nicotine and of exposure to cigarette smoke: Medical implications. Psychoneuroendocrinology 1989; 13(192): 19–41.
13. Pomerleau OF, Rosecrans J. Neuroregulatory effects of nicotine. Psychoneuroendocrinology 1989; 14(6): 407–423.
14. Pomerleau O. The effects of nicotine on brain neurotransmitter systems. In Balfour DJK, ed. Nicotine and the tobacco smoking habit. Oxford: Pregamon Press, 1984.
15. Wesnes K, Warborten DM. Smoking, nicotine and human performance. Pharmacol Therapeutics 1983; 21: 189–208.
16. Pomerleau O. Nicotine as a psychoactive drug: Anxiety and pain reduction. Psychopharmacol Bull 1979; 22(3): 865–869.
17. Gilbert D. Paradoxical tranquilizing and emotion—Reducing effects of nicotine. Psychol Bull 1979; 86(4): 643–661.
18. Keenan RM, Hatsukami DK, Anton DJ. The effects of short term smokeless tobacco deprivation on performance. Psychopharmacology 1989; 98: 126–130.
19. Ague C. Nicotine and smoking: Effects upon subjective changes in mood. Psychopharmacologia 1973; 30: 323–328.
20. Pomerleau OF, Turk DC, Fertig JB. The effects of cigarette smoking on pain and anxiety. Addict Behav 1984; 9: 265–271.
21. Miller RR. Effects of smoking on drug action. Clin Pharmacol and Therapeutics 1987; 22(5): 749–756.
22. Swett C. Drowsiness due to chlorpromazine in relation to cigarette smoking. Arch of Gen Psychi 1974; 31: 211–213.
23. Dawson GW, Jusko WJ. Smoking and drug metabolism. In: Balfour DJK, ed. Nicotine and the Tobacco smoking habit Oxford: Pregamon Press. 1984.
24. Gold MS. The good news about depression. New York: Villard Books, 1987.
25. Gold MS. The good news about panic, anxiety and phobias. New York: Villard Books, 1989.
26. Glassman AH, Stetner F, Walsh T, et al. Heavy smokers, smoking cessation, and clonidine. JAMA 1988; 259: 2863–2866.
27. Gold MS, Redmond DE, Kleber HD. Clonidine in opiate withdrawal. Lancet 1978; 1: 929.
28. Edwards NB, Simmons RC, Rosenthal TL, et al. Doxepin in the treatment of nicotine withdrawal. Psychosomatics 1988; 29(2): 203–206.
29. Dilsaver SC, Majchrzak MJ, Alessi NE. Chronic treatment with amitriptyline produces supersensitivity to nicotine. Biol Psychi 1988; 23: 169–175.
30. Hughes JR. Clonidine, depression, and smoking cessation. JAMA 1988; 259(19); 2901–2902.
31. Churchill CM, Pariser SF, Larson CN, et al. Antidepressants and cessation of smoking. Am J of Psychi 1989; 146(9): 1238.

32. Cocores JA, Patel MD, Gold MS, Pottash AC. Cocaine abuse, attention deficit disorder, and bipolar disorder. J of Nerv Mental Disease 1987; 175(7): 431–432.
33. Cocores JA, Davies RK, Mueller PS, Gold MS. Cocaine abuse and adult attention deficit disorder, J of Clin Psychi 1987; 48(9): 376–377.
34. Wender PH, Reimherr FW. Bupropion treatment of attention-deficit hyperactivity in adults. Am J of Psychi, 1990; 147(8): 1018–1020.
35. Barclay L, Kheyfets S. Tobacco use in Alzheimer's disease. Clin Psychi News 1988; 16(12): 9.
36. Newhouse PA, Sunderland T, Tariot PN, et al. Intravenous nicotine in Alzheimer's disease: A pilot study. Psychopharmacology 1988; 95: 171–175.
37. Hall GH. The pharmacology of tobacco smoking in relation to schizophrenia. In: Hemmings G, ed. Biochemistry of schizophrenia and addiction. Baltimore: University Park Press, 1980.
38. Sanberg PR, Fogelson HM, Manderscheid PZ, et al. Nicotine gum and haloperidol in Tourette's syndrome. Lancet 1988; 95: 592.
39. Yassa R, Samarthji L, Korpassy A, et al. Nicotine exposure and tardive dyskinesia. Biol Psychi 1987; 22: 67–72.

25
Relapse Prevention

PEGGY O'HARA

The most difficult aspect of working with smokers is handling relapse. Most smokers do want to quit smoking. Once they build up their courage to finally attempt the very difficult task of quitting smoking, it is very discouraging to relapse back to cigarettes. Yet, three fourths of smokers who quit even for a short period of time do relapse within 1 year.[1] An important question for clinicians is how to prevent relapse for those who do want to become nonsmokers but do not want to repeat the same discouraging relapse cycle again.

Definition of Relapse

In cigarette smoking, the problems with relapse begin with definition. How is the occasional cigarette or puff of a cigarette defined? What about the ex–cigarette smoker who has now begun use of pipes, cigars, or smokeless tobacco? When is an ex-smoker considered to have a full-blown relapse? The National Institutes of Health and the National Heart, Lung & Blood Institute Workshop Conference on Relapse[2] worked to define *slips*, *lapses*, and *relapses* so that researchers and clinicians can achieve some consistency in identifying smoking abstinence and relapse.

In order to define *relapse*, it is necessary to determine that a smoker has successfully quit smoking. A period of 24 or 48 hours of total abstinence from cigarettes or other tobacco products is accepted as an attempt to quit.[3] If an expired carbon monoxide level is used to validate abstinence, the level of 8 parts per million (ppm) is generally accepted as the cutoff level between smokers and nonsmokers.[4] Considering the short half-life of carbon monoxide (3 to 5 hours) the 8-ppm level can be achieved by many smokers after 48 hours of abstinence.

For the smoker who *quits* (that is, remains abstinent for a 24- to 48-hour period), and then has even one puff from a cigarette, a "slip" is said to have occurred. The recommended definition of *slip* is that it is an isolated smoking episode that does not occur over a period of more than 6 consecutive days. Once the quitter smokes for 7 consecutive days or more, then the definition changes from a *slip* to a *relapse*. A *relapse* is said to occur when smoking any amount (even one puff of a cigarette) has occurred for a period of 7 consecutive days. The one problem with this definition of *slip* is that it does not pick up the pattern of slipping that sometimes occurs with the social smoker, one who smokes regularly on weekends but not during the weekdays. The definition also misses the smoker who smokes regularly at work, but not at home on weekends.

Validation by carbon monoxide may be difficult if the relapsed smoker is having only occasional puffs throughout the day, even though they occur on the 7 consecutive days, as stated in the definition.

In the earliest relapse studies, Hunt, Barnett, and Branch[5] showed that of smokers who quit, only 35% will maintain abstinence the first 3 months. By 12 months, 75 to 80% will have relapsed. Most of the relapse that occurs tends to happen very early in the quitting process. Smokers who are able to sustain abstinence at 1 year after quitting are usually those who have not experienced slips and relapses throughout the process. Patterns of slipping and relapsing that occur after initial quitting usually precipitate what is described as the "full-blown relapse." When quitting patterns of abstainers versus relapsers have been compared, the relapsers are more likely to appear as slippers within the first 14 days after a quit attempt.[6] The smokers who sustain abstinence for 1 year are more likely to show no slips within that initial 14-day period. Glasgow and Lichtenstein's[7] work on smoking relapse shows that while most relapse does occur relatively soon after quitting smoking, some relapse does continue beyond 6 months and can even continue as long as 2 years after quitting smoking.

Some smokers slip and resume baseline levels of smoking (this is called a "full-blown relapse"), while other smokers appear to have occasional slips over a period of time. Curry, Marlatt, and Gordon[8] showed that the inital reaction to a slip is important in determining whether the outcome will be a full-blown relapse. This reaction is called the "abstinence violation effect" (AVE). Two factors were observed in the AVE: One is that there is a causal attribution of responsibility for the slip, and second, that an affective reaction takes place along with the attribution. When ex-smokers resumed smoking in an actual smoking situation, those who slipped gradually over time were compared with those who smoked a single cigarette and then experienced a full-blown relapse. The relapsers gave more internal attributions (such as a lack of willpower, which is perceived to be uncontrollable) and global attributions than those slipped and remained *occasional* slippers.

The Process of Relapse

Quitting can be viewed as a process of change with distinct and separate stages rather than a pass–fail attempt in which a smoker makes a decision, tries to find a foolproof method of quitting, and then either succeeds or fails at becoming a nonsmoker.[9] In this change process, as many as five stages have been defined[9] for self-changing smokers. These stages are (1) *precontemplation*, which occurs prior to quitting; (2) *contemplation*, when the smoker is thinking about giving up smoking; (3) *action*, the stage where the smoker is motivated to quit smoking; (4) *maintenance*, where long-term abstinence from smoking now becomes a reality and the initial enthusiasm and motivation begin to wear off; (5) *relapse*, a stage where slips occur and the ex-smoker comes to grips with abstinence violation and either proceeds to recover from a slip or proceeds to a full-blown relapse. Smokers tend to move in and out of these five stages and not necessarily in a sequential order. Sudden events, such as illness, pregnancy, a new child or grandchild, or changes in smoking policy at work, can motivate the precontemplator into an action phase. In working with smokers, the assessment of their stage of change is crucial to the type of intervention that will have beneficial effects for them and one they will accept. Most smokers go through the quitting process an average of three times before a quit attempt finally results in nonsmoking behavior.[10]

Predictors of Relapse

Numerous studies have attempted to determine which ex-smokers are likely to resume smoking after a quit attempt.[11-14] In a study of 5,500 ex-smokers hospitalized for tobacco-related cancers, variables of gender, age, education, occupational level, religion, and the number of years of smoking were evaluated in an attempt to determine those most likely to remain abstinent. For those smokers able to achieve at least 1 year of abstinence, the male obstinence rates increased across age and time periods more than did the female abstinence rates. Among males, absti-nence rates increased along with higher education levels. The same was true for occupational levels, with men experiencing higher abstinence rates in higher occupational levels, but those rates did not hold for women. The women who quit smoking had smoked fewer years than the men, and they had smoked fewer cigarettes. In both genders, there were lower abstinence rates for divorced and separated than for married persons, higher abstinence rates among Jewish smokers than other religious groups, and in both female and males, the abstinence rates increased as the interval between waking and smoking the first cigarette of the day increased. Additional work in smoking relapse shows that life stress is a significant factor in predicting smoking relapse. With a smoking-cessation clinic population, Gunn[13] showed that high life stress scores were strong pre-dictors for men not to stop smoking and to drop out of a clinic smoking-cessation program. The women's number of life stressors (which happened to be the same number as the men's) did not predict their lack of success. In the Multiple Risk Factor Intervention Trial (MRFIT), when participants were evaluated, both the number of life stressors and the number of cigarettes they smoked predicted who would maintain abstinence.[14]

Specific situations appear to be factors in predicting relapse among ex-smokers. Shiffman's[15] work has shown that relapse is more likely to occur in social situations where alcohol is present. Another high-risk situation for the ex-smoker is when negative mood states are experienced and the smoker is alone. In a study examining gender differences and relapse events, Borland[16] has demonstrated that men were more likely than women to relapse in the context of alcohol, and when women were sad and depressed they tended to relapse more frequently than men.

Influence of Household Smokers and Spouse Support on Relapse

The number of smokers existing in a household where a person is attempting to quit smoking is a significant factor in achieving nonsmoking status.[17] While it is generally accepted that the smoking habits of spouses are important in achieving nonsmoking, there is some question about the importance of social support in the quitting process. It is important to look at the different stages of the process of smoking cessation in order to determine the impact of support on each one.[18] In initial quitting, success is associated with a smaller proportion of friends who smoke and who have spousal support for quitting. Achieving and maintaining short-term abstinence appears to be positively related both to such spousal support and to stress-reducing support. However, in long-term abstinence, those smokers who have been shown to perceive an availability of support do not show greater success in quitting. In summary, it does appear that social support is one of many influences on smoking behavior and preventing relapse. However, social support is not a variable that is easily manipulated to produce greater results in overall abstinence.

Relapse-Prevention Programs

Considering the high prevalence of relapse in smoking and other forms of substance abuse, investigators have attempted to identify common relapse situations and to develop relapse-prevention programs. There is sound evidence that the use of coping skills is important in maintaining non-smoking status.[19-21] Shiffman's[20] study of smokers who responded to a relapse hotline has shown that successful ex-smokers report.

1. Using a greater number of coping responses than relapsers
2. more frequently using problem-solving techniques than relapsers
3. using both behavioral and cognitive coping strategies more than relapsers

Some effective behavioral coping strategies are food or drink substitutes for smoking, physical activity as a substitute for smoking, relaxation, delay techniques, and escape from a tempting situation. The cognitive coping strategies include distraction, thinking about the positive health benefits of not smoking, thinking about negative consequences of smoking, will-power, punitive thoughts, and self-talk. In an evaluation of subjects on the smoking hotline,[20] a combination of behavioral and cognitive coping was shown to be effective in preventing relapse, but the quantity of coping skills used in a crisis was no more effective than the use of one coping skill. In this study,[20] the most frequent behavioral skill used was the consumption of food or drink, and the most frequently used cognitive skill was distraction. Those subjects who attended smoking-cessation clinic programs used relaxation techniques and exercise as coping strategies, while those who did not attend clinics rarely did.

Hall, Rugg, et al.[21] evaluated common relapse situations that are seen in alcohol and heroin dependence, as well as nicotine dependence. Most of the common situations involve negative affect, and direct and indirect social influences to use the drug (in smoking, these include the presence and use of alcohol). The relapse-prevention program developed was based on a model that emphasized the interacting role of coping strategies and commitment in maintaining change in the addictive process. The model combined training in both behavioral and cognitive skill components. When the trained groups were compared with a discussion-only group; the ones that received the behavioral skills training reported greater use of coping skills and achieved greater abstinence rates than the discussion-only groups.

In a study of women smokers comparing exercise-maintenance programs with behavioral-maintenance strategies for achieving abstinence over a 1-year period,[22] the women abstainers showed significantly lower tension reduction levels than those women who relapsed. In the Hall et al. study[21] abstinent subjects showed less mood disturbance than smoking subjects. So, while the ex-smoker may relapse back to smoking as a means of coping with stress, it does appear that resuming smoking actually enhances tension or disturbance of mood states.

Program Components

Assessment

In a program to prevent relapse, the initial assessment includes a history of prior quit attempts; the withdrawal symptoms experienced, as well as their duration; and the length of abstinence the smoker was able to maintain. Other factors included in the assessment are the number of household smokers present, the support system that is available, and the difficulties that may be present in the smoker's social and work environment.

One of the most important components of the assessment is questions to evaluate the smoker's stage of readiness in the quitting process. There are three basic questions that indicate whether the smoker is in precontemplation, contemplation, or the action stage:

Question 1. Have you been thinking about your smoking habit? (If no, the smoker is likely to be in the precontemplation stage).

Question 2. Have you considered quitting smoking? (If yes to Question 1 and 2, the smoker is probably in the contemplation stage).

Question 3. Are you ready to set a date for quitting smoking in the near future? (If yes to Questions 1, 2, and 3, the smoker is probably in the action stage and ready to quit smoking).

In this early assessment, there should be a question to determine the smoker's self-efficacy in achieving and maintaining abstinence. Questions such as, "How confident are you that you can quit smoking?" and "If you do quit smoking, how confident are you that you will remain a nonsmoker 1 year from now?" will alert the clinician as to how confident the smoker is going to be in specific high-risk situations without cigarettes available as a coping strategy. Condiotte and Lichtenstein[23] were able to match self-efficacy scores in smokers who experienced slips in specific situations along with their actual relapses in later quit attempts and found remarkable agreement. These specific situations that have caused problems for smokers in prior quit attempts can be a basis for instruction in skills training for future attempts.

EDUCATION

An education component needs to be a part of relapse prevention. Smokers need to have realistic expectations of the quitting process, the difference between initial quitting and long-term quitting, and the changes in behavior that will need to be made. For some smokers, it may require total avoidance of alcohol or specific social situations that will be initially high risk for relapse. Other smokers may need to plan eating and work breaks in nonsmoking areas. At this point, it is useful for the smoker to have an understanding of nicotine dependence and the withdrawal process. Many smokers will have heard others talk about cravings that seem to last for years beyond quitting. In the initial prequitting stage, the smoker needs to understand the difference between initial, frequent cravings and those that will occasionally occur months or perhaps years after quitting smoking. Smokers should be educated about the fragile period of the first month after quitting, when most relapse occurs. Smokers need to understand that an occasional puff or slip during that period can reduce the probability for long-term abstinence.

BEHAVIORAL AND COGNITIVE SKILLS TRAINING

The smoker can be given smoking-cessation materials with lists of coping skills that can be practiced in high-risk or tempting situations. There are four basic first-line strategies that work for smokers in most tempting situations.[24] The four basic coping strategies are avoidance, escape, distraction, and delay. The smoker needs to know that it is important to focus on using many different strategies so that if a high-risk situation is encountered, there will be choices that have been previously tried and practiced.

RECOVERY FROM A SLIP

When a slip does occur, the smoker needs to go through a debriefing period in order to understand the events that occurred prior to the slip, as well as during and after the crisis period. A series of questions is asked, which are to focus specifically on events following the first cigarette that was smoked. The questions are, Where were you? What were you doing at the time of the slip? Were others present? If so, were they smoking? Where did you get the cigarette? Was there food or alcohol present? Did you use coping strategies in an attempt to prevent the slip? How did you feel after the slip occurred? Did you continue to smoke after the first cigarette was smoked? How motivated are you to go back to total abstinence?

Once the data is collected, the clinician can determine the smoker's vulnerabilities in specific situations and use of coping responses. Discussion of how this situation could be different if it does reoccur will lead to some problem solving and the development of an action plan for future high-risk situations. The debriefing assessment that takes place after a slip should be nonjudgmental and should encourage the smoker to take an objective view of any smoking behavior rather than become subject to the AVE.

Physician's Role in Preventing Relapse

The physician has a unique role in smoking cessation and relapse prevention. Through physical examination and tests for smoking-related symptoms and diseases and family history, the physician can determine the individualized risk factors unique to the smoker. Once the physician has determined whether the smoker is in a precontemplative or contemplative stage of change, work then is focused on moving the smoker through the process of quitting toward the action stage.

Discuss with Patients the Risks of Smoking and the Benefits of Quitting

When symptoms are present that relate to smoking, such as cough, sputum production, or shortness of breath, the physician can offer direct advice on the benefits of quitting smoking. Russell, Wilson, Taylor, and Baker[25] showed that by giving direct physician advice for quitting, a leaflet, and a plan for a follow-up visit, 5% of patients in a general office practice were motivated to give up the smoking habit. Additional opportunities for talking about smoking occur when test results or diagnosis of disease and risk factors are given to patients. When risk factors for coronary heart disease such as high blood pressure, elevated cholesterol, and diabetes, exist, the physician can discuss the combined risk caused by smoking. For women patients, specific situations such as pregnancy or use of oral contraceptives present an opportunity to deliver a message about quitting smoking. The physician can also educate patients about the effects of smoking on clinical tests and the effects of smoking on drug therapies. While scare tactics are not effective with patients, discussion of the health benefits of quitting smoking can help a long-term smoker decide that becoming a nonsmoker is worth the effort.

Provide Intervention Materials and Referrals to Community Programs

Smokers who have had numerous quit attempts on their own and have not been able to maintain abstinence can benefit from the ongoing contact with support groups in smoking-cessation programs. The physician can provide a list of local resources in hospital and community groups. In most cities, local agencies, such as the American Cancer Society or the American Lung Association, can be of assistance in getting information on local smoking-cessation groups.

Recognize and Treat Tobacco Dependence

According to the American Psychiatric Association's *Diagnostic and Statistical Manual of Mental Disorders* (3rd ed.),[26] individuals who are considered tobacco dependent are those who have used tobacco continually for at least 1 month and have one of the following: (1) They have made serious attempts to stop or to significantly reduce the amount of tobacco used on a permanent basis, but they have been unsuccessful; (2) their attempts to stop smoking have led to the development of physical withdrawal symptoms; (3) they continue to use tobacco despite a serious physical disorder that they know is exacerbated by tobacco use. For those nicotine-dependent individuals, the use of a nicotine-replacement product, such as nicotine chewing gum, can be benefical in the first few weeks or even months of quitting until nonsmoking behavior is firmly established.[27]

The Clinician's Role in Relapse Prevention

1. Assess the stages of change. The goal is to move the smoker from one stage to another. Very few patients are in the action stage.
2. Educate patients about relapse as a process.
3. Refer, if necessary, to a smoking-cessation program.
4. Follow up. Continue for as long as 1–2 years to monitor the health benefits of quitting smoking and any side effects of quitting smoking (such as weight gain), as well as to encourage changes in other life-style behaviors.

References

1. U.S. Department of Health, Education and Welfare. Smoking and health (a report of the Surgeon General). Washington, DC: U.S. Government Printing Office, 1979.
2. Bigelow G, Ossip-Klein DJ. Task Force I: Classification and assessment of smoking behavior. In: Shumaker S, Grunberg N, eds. Proceedings of the National Working Conference on Smoking Relapse. Health Psychol 1986; 5: 5–6.
3. U.S. Department of Health and Human Services. The health consequences of smoking: Cardiovascular disease (a report of the Surgeon General). Washington, DC: U.S. Government Printing Office, 1983.
4. Kozlowski LT, Herling S. Objective measures. In: Donovan DM, Marlatt GA, eds. Assessment of addictive behaviors. New York: Guilford Press, 1988: 214–235.
5. Hunt W, Barnett L, Branch L. Relapse rates in addiction programs. J of Consult Clin Psychol 1971; 27: 455–456.
6. Marlatt GA, Gordon JR. A longitudinal analysis of unaided smoking cessation. J of Consult Clin Psychol 1988; 56: 715–720.
7. Glasgow RE, Lichtenstein E. Long-term effects of behavioral smoking cessation interventions. Behav Ther 1987; 18: 297–324.
8. Curry S, Marlatt A, Gordon JR. Abstinence violation effect: Validation of an attributional construct with smoking cessation. J of Consult Clin Psychol 1987; 55: 145–149.
9. Prochaska JO, DiClemente CC. Stages and processes of self-change of smoking: Toward an integrative model of change. J of Consult Clin Psychol 1983; 51: 390–395.
10. U.S. Department of Health and Human Services. The health consequences of smoking (a report of the Surgeon General). Washington, DC: U.S. Government Printing Office, 1988.
11. Kabat GC, Wynder EL. Determinants of quitting smoking. Am J of Public Health 1987; 77: 1301–1305.

12. Shiffman S. Relapse following smoking cessation: A situational analysis. J of Consult Clin Psychol 1982; 50: 71–86.

13. Gunn RC. Smoking clinic failures and recent life stress. Addict Behav 1983; 8: 83–87.

14. Ockene JK, Hymowitz N, Sexton M, Broste SK. Comparison of patterns of smoking behavior change among smokers in the Multiple Risk Factor Intervention Trial (MRFIT). Prev Med 1982; 11: 621–638.

15. Shiffman S. Maintenance and relapse: Coping with temptation. In: Nirenberg TD, ed. Advances in the treatment of addictive behaviors. Norwood, NJ: Ablex, 1987: 353–385.

16. Borland R. Slip-ups and relapse in attempts to quit smoking. Addict Behav 1990; 15: 235–245.

17. Hanson BS, Isacsson S, Janzon L, Lindell S. Social support and quitting smoking for good. Is there an association? Results from the population study, "Men born in 1914," Malmo, Sweden. Addict Behav 1990; 15: 221–233.

18. Mermelstein R, Cohen S, Lichtenstein E, Baer JS, Kamarck T. Social support and smoking cessation and maintenance. J of Consult Clin Psychol 1986; 54: 447–453.

19. Marlatt G, Gordon J. Determinants of relapse: Implications for the maintenance of behavior change. In: Davidson P, Davidson S, eds. Behavioral medicine: Changing health lifestyles. New York: Brunner/Mazel, 1980: 438–445.

20. Shiffman S. Trans-situational consistency in smoking relapse. Health Psychol 1989; 8: 471–481.

21. Hall SM, Rugg D, Tunstall C, Jones RT. Preventing relapse to cigarette smoking by behavioral skill training. J of Consult Clin Psychol 1984; 52: 372–382.

22. Russell PO, Epstein LH, Johnston J, Block D. Smoking cessation: Aerobic exercise vs. a behavioral maintenance strategy. Addict Behav 1988; 13: 215–218.

23. Condiotte MM, Lichtenstein E. Self-efficacy and relapse in smoking cessation programs. J Consult Clin Psychol 1981; 49: 648–658.

24. Shiffman S, Read L, Maltese J, Rapkin D, Jarvik ME. Preventing relapse in ex-smokers: A self-management approach. In: Marlatt GA, Gordon JR, eds. Relapse prevention: Maintenance strategies in the treatment of addictive behaviors. New York: Guilford Press, 1985: 472–520.

25. Russell MAH, Wilson C, Taylor C, Baker CD. Effect of general practitioners' advice against smoking. Brit Med J 1979; 2: 231–235.

26. American Psychiatric Association. Diagnostic and statistical manual of mental disorders. 3rd ed. Washington, DC: American Psychiatric Association, 1981.

27. Schneider NG. Use of 2 mg and 4 mg nicotine gum in an individual treatment trial. In: Ockene JK, ed. The pharmacologic treatment of tobacco dependence: Proceedings of the World Congress, November 4–5, 1985. Cambridge, MA: Institute for the Study of Smoking Behavior and Policy, 1986: 233–248.

26
Wellness Component of a Long-Term Maintenance Strategy

Patricia R. Flynn

Any number of methods (or combination of them) can help smokers to achieve abstinence. Whatever method is used, however, should help the client actively in treatment to enhance self-attribution.

Leading causes of relapse are anxiety, stress, anger, weight gain, and lack of inner resources. Eating excessive and drinking coffee or alcohol also contribute to relapse. Those smoking programs, then, with a good maintenance component will show the best long-term success.[1]

Social support, training in coping strategies, and the use of exercise as an intervention bolster maintenance. Adopting a healthy life-style and taking responsibility for one's health are all part of the long-term maintenance strategy for the new nonsmoker.

Balanced Nutrition and Weight Management

Most sucessful ex-smokers find substitutes both during and after quitting. Gum-chewing, deep breathing, relaxation exercises, eating more, and physical exercise are common. Deep breathing, exercise, and relaxation are valuable interventions. Overeating, however, leads to frustration and often to relapse.

Many ex-smokers find themselves eating too much, and some fear quitting smoking because of weight gain. There is some foundation for this fear. Some evidence links cigarette smoking with a faster body metabolism. This suggests that an ex-smoker who eats the same amount of food and does not increase physical activity will store the extra calories as body fat. A smoker who has a small weight gain after quitting can get back to normal weight by combining a balanced diet with increased activity.[2]

Although managing weight is a popular media subject, aspects of this problem are unique to new nonsmokers. Because smoking has functioned to depress appetite and to increase metabolism, the smoker has often not had to cope with a weight problem. Most know little about nutrition and how to make appropriate food choices.[3]

A new nonsmoker is then faced with an array of potential solutions. Emphasize a moderate approach for long-term success.

Eat a Balanced Diet

Surgary and starchy snacks add extra calories and can make blood sugar rise steeply and then drop, causing fatigue. Cigarettes have a similar effect on blood sugar levels—causing cravings. Choosing low-calorie snacks and eating three regular, balanced meals lead to good nutrition, as well as a way to fight cigarette cravings.

The following guidelines outline a program for optimal nutrition.[4]

Introducing even a few of these into daily eating patterns will make a big difference in helping to prevent relapse for the new nonsmoker.

1. Balance calorie intake with exercise to attain and maintain desired body weight.
2. Eat fresh, wholesome foods.
3. Establish consistent eating patterns (do not skip meals).
4. Eat more complex carbohydrates. Good choices are fruits, vegetables, whole-grained and enriched cereals, rice, pasta, and beans.
5. Eat more dietary fiber. Good choices are bran, whole grains, fresh fruits, and vegetables.
6. Eat less fat. Avoid fried foods, butter, oils, nuts, commercial pastries, high-fat dairy products, fast foods, and high-fat meats.
7. Eat less sugar. Substitute fresh fruit for desserts, candy, and soft drinks.
8. Eat less cholesterol. Limit intake of egg yolks, organ meats, and dairy products.
9. Limit sodium. Avoid processed meat, canned foods, and frozen dinners.
10. Limit caffeine to 0–2 cups of caffeinated beverages daily.
11. Limit alcohol.
12. Drink at least 8 glasses of fluid daily, 4 of which are water.

Daily Guidelines

Follow these guidelines, which provide 1200–1500 calories from a variety of foods.

Protein	2 Servings (3 oz.)	Poultry, fish, lean red meat, tuna
Dairy	2–3 Servings (1 cup or 1 oz.)	Lowfat or nonfat dairy products
Complex carbohydrates	4 Servings (½ or 1 slice)	Dried beans, cereals, rice, bread, pasta

Fruits and vegetables	4 Servings (1 med. or ½ cup)	Oranges, grapefruits, tomatoes, leafy greens, spinach
Fat	3 Servings (1 tsp.)	Polyunsaturated: corn, safflower oil
Water	6–8 Servings (8 ozs.)	Water

Sample Balanced Menu (1500 Calories)

Breakfast: ½ Cup orange juice
½ Cup nonfat milk
1 Cup branflakes
1 Small banana
2 Glasses water

Lunch: Turkey sandwich:
3 oz. turkey
2 Slices whole wheat bread
Lettuce, tomato
1 tsp. Mayonnaise (or no-cholesterol mayonnaise)
Carrot sticks
1 Small orange
1 Cup nonfat milk

Dinner: 4 oz. Broiled fish with lemon
1 Baked potato with 1 tsp. margarine
½ Cup broccoli
Tossed dinner salad with 1 tbsp. dressing
1 Small dinner roll
½ Cup mixed fruit
2 Glasses water

Coping with Stress

Many ex-smokers used smoking as a primary way of coping with stress. After quitting, they need new ways to deal with day-to-day stresses.

Many feel depressed or anxious after quitting. Nicotine withdrawal can cause tension, irritability, low energy, depression, and low concentration. Deep breathing, relaxation training, and physical exercise can be helpful.

Other methods include

1. A brisk walk or any enjoyable outdoor activity
2. A hot shower or bath
3. Pleasant daydreams
4. Talking with a friend

5. Enjoying art, music, or a good book
6. Playing with a child or a pet
7. Prayer

Physical Activity

Benefits

There are many reasons to include exercise in a relapse-prevention strategy for new nonsmokers:

1. It provides the client with a replacement or substitute activity
2. It helps offset the feeling of deprivation that many clients experience
3. It increases self-efficacy as the client gradually masters an improved life-style[5]
4. It counteracts lowered metabolism and helps with weight maintenance[6]
5. It is incompatible with a smoking life-style

Type of Exercise

Most people know that exercise is important for their health but will argue that they lack the time to participate. Another obstacle to beginning a regular program is lack of information on how much and what kind of exercise someone needs. Clients need to understand that exercise does not have to hurt and that they do not have to become athletes or runners to enjoy its rewards.

The type of exercise to include in a maintenance program is aerobic. Aerobic exercise is not just aerobic dance classes. *Aerobic* means "with air," and it refers to activities that are of moderate intensity, can be kept up for long periods of time, and use large muscle groups, such as the legs and arms. Examples are walking, cycling, swimming, and jogging.[7]

Getting Started

Beginning exercisers need to start slowly and gradually increase the frequency, intensity, and duration. Some may experience some mild muscular discomfort, but this goes away after the first 2 or 3 weeks.

Brisk walking on a daily basis is an excellent choice for many individuals because it is pleasant and relatively easy to perform.

Whichever activity the client chooses, the exercise should start with a 5–10 minute warm-up and muscle-conditioning period and should end with a 5–10 minute cool-down. For clients who have rarely exercised in the past or for whom exercise may represent an increased health risk, a complete physical examination by a physician is recommended.

Although most people will have no problems with exercise when they follow the guidelines, problems occasionally arise that may need medical attention. Warning signs include

1. Chest pain or pain in the arms, neck, jaw, or upper back
2. Nausea
3. Dizziness or light-headedness
4. Unusual or severe fatigue
5. Severe leg pain or cramps
6. Severe shortness of breath

STARTING A WALKING PROGRAM

1. Gradually increase the length of the walk.
2. Speed is not crucial in the first few weeks of adjusting to exercise. More important is just getting out and doing it and building up the ability to sustain longer periods of exercise.
3. Wear comfortable shoes.

WALKING GUIDELINES

Week	Exercise sessions per week	Minutes per session
1	3	20
2	3	20
3	3	25
4	4	25
5	4	30
6	4	30
7	5	35
8	5	35

Summary of Exercise Recommendations[8]

Frequency	3–5 Times per week
Intensity	60–80% Of maximum heart rate *or* moderate intensity that still allows you to talk while exercising
Time	20–60 Minutes of aerobic activity per session
Type	Continuous activities such as walking, stationary cycling, swimming, or jogging

Staying Motivated

Some suggestions to help clients stay motivated to exercise:

1. Choose an activity they enjoy
2. Include exercise as part of a healthy lifestyle (e.g., walking to do errands, gardening, nature hikes)

3. Exercise with friends or family members
4. Keep it simple
5. Progress at their own pace

References

1. Marlatt G, Gordon J. Relapse prevention. New York: Guilford Press, 1985.
2. Farquhar J. The American way of life need not be hazardous to your health. Stanford, CA: Stanford Alumni Association 1978.
3. Nash, J. Taking charge of your smoking. Palo Alto, CA: Bull Publishing, 1981.
4. Select Committee on Nutrition and Human Needs. U.S. Senate dieting goals for the U.S. Washington DC: U.S. Government Printing Office, 1988.
5. Condiotte M, Lichenstein E. Self-efficacy and relapse in smoking cessation. J of Consult Clin Psychi 1981; 49: 648.
6. Cooper K. Controlling cholesterol. New York: Bantam, 1988: 216.
7. Cooper K. Running without fear. New York: M. Evans and Co., 1985: 100.
8. American College of Sports Medicine. Guidelines for graded exercise testing & exercise prescription. 2nd ed. Philadelphia: Lea and Bebiger, 1980.

27
Nicotine Anonymous

JAY L.

The organization now known as Nicotine Anonymous was founded in California in 1983, based on the "Twelve Steps" and other principles and traditions of Alcoholics Anonymous. Originally known as "California Smokers Anonymous" or "Smokers Anonymous,"[1] it originated virtually simultaneously in Los Angeles and San Francisco, with one meeting group in each location, each unaware of the other's existence. As of 1990, Nicotine Anonymous has over 400 weekly meetings in 43 states, as well as dozens more in Canada, Europe, Central and South America, Australia, and elsewhere in the world.[2]

The the surprise of many, Nicotine Anonymous is not a smoking-cessation program per se. To be sure, its primary purpose is to help nicotine addicts obtain and maintain freedom from nicotine. However, it does not offer any magic formula or easy treatment for "quitting smoking." The program focuses rather on a gradual process of spiritual growth as a means of combating the nicotine addiction. Attention is not directed specifically at tobacco or smoking or cigarettes because they all involve just packaging and delivery systems and methodology for getting nicotine into the body. The focus, rather, is on the cunning, treacherous, and deadly drug, nicotine.[3]

---

[1] The name change was required because a private, for-profit smoking-cessation program operator in New York state, unaffiliated with any Twelve-step organization, had registered the name "Smokers Anonymous." Rather than litigate the issue or pay a licensing fee, it was decided in April 1990 to adopt the new name, "Nicotine Anonymous."

[2] Literature, meeting locations, and other information may be obtained from Nicotine Anonymous World Services, 2118 Greenwich Street, San Francisco, California 94123.

[3] "Cunning," "baffling," and "deadly" are adjectives that are used in Nicotine Anonymous to describe the drug nicotine. That the terminology is not exaggerated has been given recognition in the Surgeon General's 1989 report, in which, under the daring leadership of Dr. C. Everett Koop, nicotine's addictive powers officially have been classified on a par with heroin. Recidivism rates—that is, failures to maintain abstinence—are among the highest in the entire drug world. Also the

Without delving into the childhood traumas or other psychological underpinnings to nicotine dependency, suffice it to say that nearly all members of Nicotine Anonymous will give compelling witness to the fact that they became nicotine addicts inadvertently. Nearly all started using nicotine (and for most, this involved smoking cigarettes) deliberately. The motivations are widely varying, and at least at the conscious level, range from "wanting to be one of the guys" to "trying to be a defiant bad girl." In a small survey taken within Nicotine Anonymous in 1988, the average age was 16 years when people now in the group began using nicotine; nearly all thought at the time that they were making a decision that would help them become more "grown up"—irrespective of what was perceived as appropriate for attaining that goal.[4] Nearly all became addicted as soon as they started; for those who tried to quit, they found an inability to do so right from the start.[5] The choice to use nicotine (e.g., to smoke) was deliberate and conscious; inadvertently, addiction to nicotine also came along as part of the deal.

Once the user found that nicotine could provide the change of mood that was perceived to be needed—wherever on the broad spectrum of needs a particular one might fall—it was not long before the drug came to be used for almost every and any perceived need or emotion. One "fix" (i.e., dose of the drug) led to another—just as with other, more widely recognized addictive substances—except that with nicotine, the need for a fix recurs generally every 20 minutes, and the substance is not only legal, its production is subsidized with taxpayer dollars, and its use is promoted with millions of dollars in imagery that ranges from macho cowboys to sylvan springs and flowing skirts in flowering meadows. Take your pick. Its insidiousness is perhaps unique in the drug marketplace.

Given the early age at which most nicotine addicts became hooked, and given the broad panoply of emotions concerning which addicts have used the drug as a crutch, nearly all members of Nicotine Anonymous find that as the years of using have rolled by, they have become older and more

---

official death rate *in just the United States* is approaching 400,000 annually as of the beginning of the 1990s.

[4] This may seem peculiar to those who never have experienced nicotine dependency, but the stated reasons for starting to use the drug—mostly by smoking cigarettes—include a broad range of diametric opposites. Responses to the 1988 sampling within Nicotine Anonymous included that people smoked to feel "in" and to belong, or to be defiant and to be "out." They smoked to "party," as well as to be "sad and lonely," and because of both exhaustion and exhilaration. Nicotine provided a cover for "fear," while it also was bound up with "bravado."

[5] Clearly, not all persons who smoke a cigarette, or use nicotine in some other form, end up being addicted to the drug. However, by definition, for persons in Nicotine Anonymous, we are talking about those who did become hooked—and for them, the addiction took control with great speed, right from the beginning of their careers as nicotine users.

mature, chronologically, but their emotions and emotional growth were left back at the starting block. Members in (chronological) age categories 30 to 40 to 50 to 60 find themselves with grossly stunted emotional growth, as it were, with an average emotional maturity that matches the point in the mid-teens when the addiction took control—grownups with the emotional maturity of 16-year-olds.

Coupled with the stunted emotional maturity, most people also come to Nicotine Anonymous in some stage of terror. There is a gripping fear that comes from traumatic experiences of failure. Failure to quit smoking—to get free of the nicotine monster. Nearly all who have been addicted for any period of time have tried to quit; most have tried to quit innumerable times, and some have been trying to quit ever since starting, sometimes 30 or more years earlier. Yet all attempts have been in vain![6] Failure after failure, with one failure feeding the next, and each failure taking the addict's self-esteem and self-confidence one step lower.

The fear is exacerbated by overwhelming doubt on the part of the addict that he or she can live without nicotine. This facet of the fear syndrome arises out of the fact that virtually every waking act and emotion has become bound up in daily rituals related to nicotine. The first cup of coffee in the morning, talking on the telephone, driving a car, sexual acts, reading a book, writing an essay, having an argument—or a laugh. All of that was accompanied by nicotine. The thought of "the rest of one's life without one's friend" is nearly overwhelming.[7]

Last, but certainly not least, for most nicotine addicts today, there has developed a deep, pervasive denial system as part of the ongoing insanity of the addiction. For decades now, the health warnings have been increasingly ominous, ever clearer and more pervasive and persistent.[8] Virtually no one who smokes today is unaware of the grave health risks connected with the practice. From conversations within Nicotine Anonymous, it

---

[6] Again, to be sure, there are many, many people who have succeeded in quitting smoking. Some quit and "stay quit" (remain abstinent) for the rest of their lives. However, from the perspective of Nicotine Anonymous, by definition, we are talking in most instances about the "hopeless addict" who has tried everything by way of cessation programs and remedies, with all attempts ending in failure sooner or later.

[7] Many members of Nicotine Anonymous relate experiences of the "fear of the rest of life without nicotine" as being a major factor in previous failures to "stay quit." It was simply unimaginable that one could go forever without using the drug again. This provided the opening wedge for the addict to rationalize resumed usage today, knowing that there were a limited number of tomorrows one can survive being abstinent: a classic "junkie game."

[8] The small print that is the "Surgeon General's Warning" confronts the user 10, 20, 40, 60, 80 times a day. Those who were surveyed in 1988 responded to Nicotine Anonymous, in essence, that they saw the warning every time, but did not see it. To continue that type of madness over any period of time requires some sort of sophisticated denial system!

appears that the same also is true of those who chew or sniff tobacco as their way of getting nicotine into their system; they too know of the increased risks of such things as cancer and respiratory and circulatory diseases. Many nicotine addicts, in more candid moments, acknowledge an awareness that they likely are committing suicide, albeit perhaps on an installment basis.

Thus, the portrait of an addict from the perspective of Nicotine Anonymous is of one who inadvertently became hooked on a readily available drug—one of the most pernicious available on the marketplace, yet widely viewed as just a "stupid, smelly, dirty habit"—frightened, loaded with denial, and more or less severely emotionally retarded or stunted. Also, many of them are sick—or as we say in Nicotine Anonymous, "sick and tired of being sick and tired."

Unlike smoking-cessation programs, Nicotine Anonymous recognizes straightforwardly that the addict who is hooked on nicotine has a serious and life-threatening disease, with deep-seated origins and symptoms that pervade every aspect of the addict's waking and sleeping life. Furthermore, given the very nature of drug addiction, we do not believe that there is either an easy or a quick solution, or indeed, even a cure at all. From the viewpoint of Nicotine Anonymous, one who is addicted to nicotine does not simply quit smoking. There is no quitting the addiction. It will be there for the duration of the addict's life. Nonetheless, there is an opportunity for freedom from the drug. Nicotine Anonymous offers the hopeless nicotine addict a program for recovering from the addiction, and a means for staying free of the drug, "one day at a time."

Nicotine Anonymous's program for recovery from nicotine addiction is adapted directly from the "Twelve Step" program of recovery used so successfully against alcoholism by Alcoholics Anonymous. The twelve steps provide a tried and tested gradual process of getting and staying free of the demonic control previously exerted by the nicotine drug. At its core, the program involves a step-process of self-analysis and growth, directed toward enabling each addict to find his or her own personalized source of spiritual guidance and energy and motivation, which enables that individual, with the help of fellow sufferers, to enjoy life in continued freedom from the deadly drug.

These, then, are the "Twelve Steps of Nicotine Anonymous":

Step One: Admitted we were powerless over nicotine—that our lives had become unmanageable.

Step Two: Came to believe that a power greater than ourselves could restore us to sanity.

Step Three: Made a decision to turn our will and our lives over to the care of God *as we understood Him.*

Step Four: Made a searching and fearless moral inventory of ourselves.

Step Five: Admitted to God, to ourselves, and to another human being, the exact nature of our wrongs.

Step Six: Were entirely ready to have God remove all these defects of character.

Step Seven: Humbly asked Him to remove our shortcomings.

Step Eight: Made a list of all persons we had harmed, and became willing to make amends to them all.

Step Nine: Made direct amends to such people wherever possible, except when to do so would injure them or others.

Step Ten: Continued to take personal investory and when we were wrong promptly admitted it.

Step Eleven: Sought through prayer and meditation to improve our conscious contact with God as we understood Him, praying only for knowledge of His will for us and the power to carry that out.

Step Twelve: Having had a spiritual awakening as the result of these steps, we tried to carry this message to nicotine users and to practice these principles in all our affairs.[9]

It should be emphasized that this is a program of spiritual awakening and growth, not religious dogma. The god to whom we refer depends on each individual's definition and understanding and is simply a shorthand for a "higher power" or a " power greater than oneself"—a source of strength,

---

[9] The "Twelve Steps of Nicotine Anonymous" are reprinted with permission of Nicotine Anonymous World Services. However, because the text of the "Twelve Steps," as applied to nicotine are adapted directly from Alcoholic Anonymous, consent from the latter organization to Nicotine Anonymous to use the "Twelve Steps" is conditioned upon the original "Twelve Steps of Alcoholics Anonymous" being set forth in full and acknowledged as such. The original text, as applied to alcohol, is as follows:

Step One: Admitted we were powerless over alcohol—that our lives had become unmanageable.

Step Two: Came to believe that a power greater than ourselves could restore us to sanity.

Step Three: Made a decision to turn our will and our lives over to the care of God *as we understood Him.*

Step Four: Made a searching and fearless moral inventory of ourselves.

Step Five: Admitted to God, to ourselves, and to another human being, the exact nature of our wrongs.

Step Six: Were entirely ready to have God remove all these defects of character.

Step Seven: Humbly asked Him to remove our shortcomings.

Step Eight: Made a list of all persons we had harmed, and became willing to make amends to them all.

Step Nine: Made direct amends to such people wherever possible, except when to do so would injure them or others.

Step Ten: Continued to take personal inventory and when we were wrong promptly admitted it.

Step Eleven: Sought through prayer and meditation to improve our conscious contact with God as we understood Him, praying only for knowledge of His will for us and the power to carry that out.

Step Twelve: Having had a spiritual awakening as the result of these steps, we tried to carry this message to alcoholics and to practice these principles in all our affairs.

a moral beacon, a ray of hope—however and wherever a given individual can find or conceive of such things for him- or herself.[10]

A basic understanding of the Twelve Steps in operation may be facilitated by dividing them into four main groupings, with Group I composed of the first three steps, Group II consisting of Steps Four through Seven, followed by Steps Eight and Nine as Group III, and concluding with the last three steps in Group IV.

Group I

The first three steps are generally concerned with the addict confronting his or her own powerlessness over nicotine, confronting the situation as it really is—rather than continuing to live by using various denials as a means of being able to rationalize slow suicide—and recognizing the need for help and forming the basic desire to be willing to be helped with regard to nicotine addiction.

The concept of powerlessness contained in Step One requires a revolutionary change of thinking for the addict. All previous attempts as quitting smoking had been focused on winning the upper hand as the means for stopping. Powerlessness, in contrast, connotes defeat and surrender and requires admitting that the drug has won the war—and that it will continue to win the war for as long as we choose to fight. Powerlessness has nothing to do with stopping smoking, or stopping anything else for that matter, other than stopping fighting the drug and the denial of addiction. It has to do with admitting defeat, of losing, and of giving up. In our goal- and success-oriented society, these are all concepts that are at diametric odds with our basic value systems. Step One is not easy.[11]

---

[10] To be sure, many of the spiritual themes found in the Twelve Steps echo ideas of Christianity and Judaism, as well as other major religions of the world. However, Nicotine Anonymous is not affiliated with any religious organization or sect. Its only teachings are that the Twelve Steps are the guides to obtaining and maintaining freedom from nicotine, and its only purpose is to give assistance to those seeking to obtain those ends. It has no dues or fees but is fully self-supporting through members' contributions. No outide support is sought or accepted. The only requirement for membership is a *desire* to be free of nicotine; one need not already have quit using nicotine to attend meetings. Anonymity and confidentiality are guiding principles and are designed to further rigorous honesty as an antidote to the denial associated with nicotine use. No member can tell another member how to find or maintain freedom from nicotine *other than* through sharing his or her own personal experience, strength, and hope.

[11] Because we view nicotine addiction as incurable, accepting one's own powerlessness is not something one does just as part of taking the first step toward recovery. It is a continued crucial ingredient in continuing abstinence. Just as the addiction continues, so does the need for the addict to remember that he or she is powerless over the drug. We help to remind ourselves of our own powerlessness by introduc-

For most, the true realization of the hopelessness of the battle with nic-otine is a devastating experience. Not only does it require cracking through all of the years of denial, but it also amounts to an acknowledgment of the dishonesty that has pervaded all that has gone before. The surrender and defeat are truly humiliating and leave most newcomers feeling even more terrified and terrible than before.[12] Almost out of necessity, one must look for solace and for help.

If the nicotine addict really believes he or she is powerless, there is almost an instinctive reaction to seek help—somewhere, somehow. That is the lead-in to Step Two and coming to believe that a power greater than ourselves can restore us to sanity. Again, though, the concept of *restora-tion to sanity* carries with it the inherent requisite of admitting *current insanity*, something that few of us are readily willing to believe about our-selves. However, clearly, nicotine addiction is an insanity, and all who have experienced it know that to be true. The trick is to become willing to accept—to come to believe—that somebody, something other than oneself might help to restore sanity.[13]

Taking it one step further, Step Three calls for a willingness to surrender control of our will and our lives[14] to a god of our own creation—to some power greater than ourselves.[15] This step requires, for many, a true leap of

---

ing ourselves at meetings by saying, "My name is _____, and I am power-less over nicotine." Silly and trite it may seem to outsiders, and indeed to many newcomers in the program. However, once an addict understands the significance of the concept of powerlessness, the incantation flows easily and with feeling.

[12] Often, the psychological impact of Step One occurs roughly simultaneously with the physiologic nightmare of initial detoxification and ongoing withdrawal from nicotine poisoning. Most members of Nicotine Anonymous recall the period as one of the darkest of all times. These very difficulties associated with the experience, however, help explain a cliché of Nicotine Anonymous—namely, that "It won't happen before it's time." An addict cannot admit powerlessness before he or she hits bottom. Admitting defeat can occur when one is beaten. Health-care profes-sionals, like members of Nicotine Anonymous, can make information available that Nicotine Anonymous exists. The nicotine addict cannot be forced to attend "before it's time."

[13] Part of the brilliance of the Twelve Steps is that they are one step at a time, each step in order. Step Two does not require that one have a fully defined belief system in respect to a deity. We only need to have stepped as far as recognizing that *some* power *might* restore us to sanity.

[14] The surrender of control of our will and our lives does not call for an abdication of our free will or an irresponsible "cop-out" on responsibility for our own life. The Serenity Prayer of Nicotine Anonymous makes an important distinction in this regard: "God, grant me the serenity to accept the things I cannot change, the courage to change the things I can, and the wisdom to know the difference." Sur-rendering only that over which one has no control, while retaining the courage to change that which one can change, does not equate with abdication of responsi-bility. It calls for wisdom to know when one is, or is not, charging at windmills.

[15] Yet another cliché of Nicotine Anonymous is, "If you have trouble believing in somebody else's God, invent your own." Each member is free to define, under-

faith, a plunge over the abyss. However, by the time one reaches this step, freedom from nicotine probably will have been a reality for some period of time. For the addict, that fact probably exists as evidence of at least the beginning of a miracle. Each day that the miracle of abstinence continues makes the trust in some other higher power easier to fathom, easier to believe in, and the leap becomes less incomprehensible, and smaller.

Group II

The three steps in this group involve taking a hard look in the mirror, and the theme is set in the two adjectives used to describe the Fourth Step inventory—"searching and fearless." The introspection is to be vigorously honest, in contrast to the dishonesty and denial associated with nicotine addiction.

The objective of the Fourth Step's "moral inventory" is to get a clear picture of the chaos and unmanageability of our lives as addicts. According to the dictionary, *inventory* derives from a Latin word meaning "to come upon, discover," and *moral* has to do with separating right from wrong. The inventory thus is a fearless and searching discovery of what is right and wrong about us. By making this discovery, we can see what has been working in our lives, and we can separate that from what has not been working—seeking to get free of the useless patterns of our past that had for so long held us captive to our addiction. We seek freedom from our old selves—seek freedom from yesterday so that we may live today, each day, one day at a time.[16]

Through making the inventory, we dissipate the chaos of the past. Also, from the honesty that we summon, we receive a gift of being able for the first time to distinguish between truth and lies about ourselves, thereby freeing ourselves from our own muck.

Step Five involves going public with our inventory—admitting to ourselves, to our higher power, and to another human being what we have found.[17] There is an act of surrender and humbleness is these self-admis-

---

stand, and relate to his or her own higher power. As a result, the concepts run the gamut from the more traditional deities of organized religious groups, to the flame of a candle, to the power of the group, and beyond.

[16] The "one day at a time" theme is very important in Nicotine Anonymous. It frees us from the incomprehensibility of never being able to use our drug again, because all we need to focus on is staying free of it *today*, each day. It also can be expanded to all aspects of living, providing a focus that is manageable, and enabling us to live life here and now, rather than escaping today's realities via a drug fix.

[17] Steps Five through Seven use terms that many consider denigrating and guilt-ridden: "our wrongs," "defects of character," "shortcomings." The language was inherited from Alcoholics Anonymous and comes from several decades past. In

sions, and the notion of sharing them with others is designed to further our own vigorousness in being honest. By becoming honest, and sharing our honesty, we further free ourselves of the chains of the past and from the sufferings that have held us captive to nicotine addiction. Usually, in the process of sharing with another person, we learn that we are not as hopelessly unique as we had thought. Instead, we discover that we suffer from the human condition.

Step Six then is a meditative step, preparatory to asking our higher power to relieve us of our past ill-suited behavior patterns. All that is required is to *become ready* to be free.[18] Once we are ready, then we ask for help in Step Seven in having removed the roadblocks that have kept us unhappy and afraid to confront life without the drug nicotine.

Group III

While the second group of steps involves primarily internal housecleaning, the third group involves external tidying-up—that is, vis-à-vis others whom we have harmed through our unhealthy behavior. In Step Eight, we make a list of persons we have harmed, and in Step Nine, we make amends to all of them unless doing so clearly would be counterproductive from the perspective of others. While the object is to apologize, it is for purposes of cleaning up one's own life, not taking care of the other person's life. We are continuing to free ourselves of our own past, not fixing anything for anyone else—unless of course, that happens as part of the spillover from cleaning up our own past.

Group IV

By the end of Step Nine, the nicotine addict will have performed a major transformation of his or her life. However, because the addiction to nicotine is a lifelong disease, the program of recovery is ongoing, and Steps Ten through Twelve are the guides for the rest of the process.[19]

Nicotine Anonymous, we have retained the language but prefer to focus on the concepts that these terms represent to us—namely, old behavior patterns that have disserved us.

[18] Like the Second Step, Step Six is a step of preparation, of meditation, and of increased understanding. One does not seek help from a higher power to be freed from the muck of the past until one is really ready, upon reflection, for that to occur.

[19] We talk in Nicotine Anonymous about the recovery process being like peeling another layer off the onion. There's always another layer, and one just keeps peeling to a new level (of awareness). Again though, we keep ourselves from being

Step Ten calls for continued inventory taking and appropriate remedial action, on an ongoing basis. It is the beginning of the rest of our lives. It helps us stay in check with ourselves and our progress on a daily basis. In that manner, we continue to avoid the chaos of the past by continuing to keep our honesty foremost in our lives. Thereby, we stay all right with ourselves, with those around us, and with our higher power. It helps remind us to keep our side of the street clean.

Often, the triviality of each day seems unimportant and insufficient. One day at a time frees us from fear of the future but deprives us of perspective. We have found that the way out of this trap is by trying to increase our contact with our higher power, and through prayer or meditation finding the larger setting for the "mundaneness" of a given day, putting it into the perspective of some greater scheme of things.[20] We seek no specific answers or solutions or material things through prayer, but rather wisdom and guidance on how to continue to live free of nicotine. Also, as always in Nicotine Anonymous, the god with whom we seek to establish an increased level of conscious contact is a god of our own individual creation and understanding.

The theme of the Twelfth Step is the rest of our life with freedom from nicotine. Upon reaching this point, the addict will have experienced an awakening of his or her spirit or soul. The distance traveled will have been great, and the miracle of escaping the deadly drug will have become clear. That freedom will have occurred only as the result of the help of our higher power. The spiritual awakening has been gradual—step by step through these Twelve Steps.

As unquestionable as the awakening has been, we cannot be lulled into a sense of false security because we remain addicted to nicotine. Also, the junkie in us is always ready to come knocking again—in cunning and baffling ways. Recidivism is always an option with this drug—thus, the second part of the last step: carrying the message to others who continue to be addicted to nicotine.

We have learned that the best antidote against our own resumed madness is by helping others—in sharing our own miracle. By sharing our freedom, we help others, and thereby help ourselves.[21] Proselytizing is

---

overwhelmed by the infiniteness of the process by remaining focused on today, each day, one day at a time.

[20] As with the lack of a definition of a god, Nicotine Anonymous prescribes no set manner of prayer or meditation. However one can become introspective and find the tranquility to reflect on a "higher power" qualifies as prayer or meditation. One can be running or sitting, as well as kneeling.

[21] One is reminded of "the golden rule" as it is expressed in various religions. The principle is the same—what goes around, comes around. As applied to nicotine addiction, we do unto others for purposes of saving ourselves from renewed enslavement to our drug.

ineffective because the person still suffering probably will continue to do so until he or she is ready to change. However, for those who are willing to try to get free from nicotine addiction, we can offer our own example, and our own experience, strength, and hope—and that is all that we have to offer. Each addict must find his or her own higher power, his or her own way—with the help and support of, and through sharing within, the group. Remaining true to these principles of the program, we give the greatest gift of all—hope of freedom to someone else, thereby confirming our own miracle.